Good Pharmaceutical Freeze-Drying Practice

Edited by
Peter Cameron

Contributors
L. David Butler
Peter Cameron
Kevin Kinnarney
Peter Monger
Kevin Murgatroyd

informa
healthcare

New York London

Informa Healthcare USA, Inc.
52 Vanderbilt Avenue
New York, NY 10017

International Standard Book Number-10: 1-5749-1031-0 (Hardcover)
International Standard Book Number-13: 978-1-5749-1031-5 (Hardcover)

Library of Congress Cataloging-in-Publication Data

Good pharmaceutical freeze-drying practice / edited by Peter Cameron.
    p. ; cm.
  Includes bibliographical references and index.
  ISBN-13: 978-1-5749-1031-5 (alk. paper)
  ISBN-10: 1-5749-1031-0 (alk. paper)
  1. Freeze-drying. 2. Drugs--Drying.
  I. Cameron, Peter.
  II. Murgatroyd, Kevin.

  RS199.F74G66 1996
  615'.19--dc21   96-39290

Visit the Informa Web site at
www.informa.com

and the Informa Healthcare Web site at
www.informahealthcare.com

CONTENTS

Commissioned in the UK by Sue Horwood of Medi-Tech. Publications Limited, Storrington, West Sussex, on behalf of Interpharm Press, Inc., USA. General Scientific Advisor: Robin N. Stephens, Manager of International Regulatory Affairs and Clinical Research, AVE Inc., UK

PREFACE

Welcome to *Good Pharmaceutical Freeze Drying Practice*, a book that I hope you will find interesting, useful, and a bit different. Why different? Well, for one thing, it is aimed at people who are looking for some help with actually running a freeze dryer—we can't press the buttons for you, but we can help you to improve the management of your facility and understand what is actually happening inside the stainless steel facade and how to control it. In addition, it can help you to understand the requirements associated with operating these plants and what the regulatory bodies are looking for, acting as a comprehensive guideline.

This book is very much about the practical aspects of freeze drying; there has been a great deal written on the theory and biophysics of the process, but it is very difficult to find any "how to" books. So here we are, trying to plug the gap. The primary concern of the text is the freeze drying of parenteral products, as this involves the most rigorous controls and represents the most exacting operations. However, many of the issues covered also relate to the processing of bulk intermediaries, diagnostic reagents, and most other aspects of the discipline.

In starting off this project, it was our intention to deliver something that will assist pharmaceutical production personnel in attaining a good grounding in all aspects of freeze drying operations. However, this is not meant to exclude others; associated departments should all benefit: engineering, quality assurance, research and development, regulatory, training, documentation, and senior management. To this aim, a small group of practitioners, experts in their fields, teamed up and have set out the intricacies of the process relating to their experiences. The contributors come from diverse backgrounds within the pharmaceutical and allied industries, including regulatory authorities, parenteral production, technical services, and freeze dryer manufacture and supply.

The book is set out in a logical and easy-to-reference manner. Although this is primarily a practical text, the first chapter deals with the theory of the process, detailing the concepts involved, and thereby acting as an introduction to the subject for some and a refresher to others. Perhaps in some way it will dispel the black-art myth that often surrounds freeze drying, a process that is commonly understood only in the rudimentaries. Following this description of the process are chapters on hardware and on the all-important control systems.

Subsequent chapters then deal with the operating and regulatory aspects. Although we would hope and recommend that you read the whole book, the chapters are intended to stand alone, facilitating easy referencing for individual needs. There may, therefore, be a small amount of overlap between different sections and between authors, but I am sure you will find this a bonus.

In the pharmaceutical business, it is impossible to operate without running into the bubbling crucible of regulatory matters, whether it is the discipline of product licences or the network of validation requirements. Although these matters are a source of some anxiety, developing an understanding of them is actually an advantage. We are, of course, talking about Good Pharmaceutical Manufacturing Practice—GMP. Guaranteeing that a process consistently produces quality end products means fewer rejects and less reworking and in-process testing, and enhances knowledge and training, which in turn reduces machine downtime. Most of the practices expected by the regulatory authorities do actually benefit the quality of the process and, therefore, give that extra level of customer assurance. So in this book we constantly relate topics to regulatory issues, alerting the reader to the areas where attention needs to be paid. Added to this theme, which runs through every subject, are two chapters that speak exclusively of the current regulatory issues in Europe and North America. Why two separate chapters? Well, although the moves towards harmonisation across the Atlantic are gathering speed, there are certainly differences of approach and are likely to be for some time. As more and more companies are looking to expand their markets, the level of interest in this area is keen. There will always be differences in emphasis, and companies with an eye to the other side of the Atlantic would do well to listen to the experience of those who have already bridged the "pond".

Freeze drying is a specialised area, and the improvements in technology have been particularly marked over the last ten years. Thus, it is important that everyone in the industry with an interest in lyophilisation be aware of the latest requirements and trends within the pharmaceutical and allied world. It is inevitable that certain information within the book will be out of date in due course, as new technologies are always around the next bend, but I am confident that most of the data and the themes developed in the text will be relevant for years to come. It is the intention, of course, to keep updating and refreshing the contents in future editions.

Peter Cameron
December 1996

ACKNOWLEDGEMENTS

The editor and authors of this book would like to thank the following people, groups, and companies for their help and advice in the preparation of this book:

The United Kingdom Parenteral Society, Freeze Drying
   Technical Group

VirTis Company

Usifroid

Mr Edward H. Trappler, Lyophilization Technology, Inc.

Dr John Levchuk, Food and Drug Administration

Sue Horwood, Medi-Tech. Publications Limited

1

THE FREEZE DRYING PROCESS

Kevin Murgatroyd

Biopharma Process Systems Ltd.
Winchester, United Kingdom

The terms *freeze drying* and *lyophilisation* refer to the same process and can be interchanged with impunity. However, the derivations of the two terms differ. Freeze drying is an obvious English language description of the process. Lyophilisation comes from the Greek and means to make easily dispersed or solubilised (*luo*—loosen, *philos*—loving). The latter refers to one of the characteristics of most freeze-dried materials.

Freeze drying may be defined as the drying of a substance by freezing it and removing a proportion of any associated solvent by direct sublimation from the solid phase to the gaseous phase, without passing through the intermediate liquid phase.

In most freeze drying applications, the solvent is usually water. Within the pharmaceutical and related markets, the target substance is often in true solution. With the exception of coffee and tea, most food applications involve the removal of water from a solid structure. The resultant products exhibit an increase in shelf life and a loss in weight, associated with other important considerations such as retention of biological activity, form, or taste combined with ease of reconstitution.

There are many explanations about how the freeze drying phenomenon was first observed or used. There are tales of how a solitary Inca died high in the Andes mountains just below the snow line. The corpse became frozen in the cold dry air and was freeze-dried in the wind. Certainly this is feasible because it is thermodynamically possible; the ambient temperature would ensure that the body would

1

remain frozen and the dry air would carry away sublimed moisture. The process would be slow, taking several years, because of the Inca's mass, which would also consist of many water resistant membranes. The nearby ice and snow would make a significant contribution to the water vapour pressure in the airflow, also slowing the process.

An alternative scenario explains how the Eskimos dry fish by freezing them and hanging them out to dry in the wind. In this case, although the fish is frozen, it would be at a higher temperature (or more specifically would be a smaller heat sink) than the surrounding ice and snow mass and so sublimation could occur.

Fabrics that have been washed and left out to dry in cold weather can freeze and dry in the frozen state.

Maybe these stories were generated by the travel experiences of the originators, although the latter is a personally observed fact. They are largely irrelevant, but add a human interest to the subject.

All of these scenarios depend on the surrounding air having a low relative humidity. In the first two cases, the presence of air, and, hence, oxygen, would result in a form more similar to that of freezer burn exhibited when food is not properly wrapped in a domestic freezer. In this case, the food undergoes a process similar to freeze drying in that water will migrate, by sublimation, from the food to the coldest part of the freezer (where the refrigeration system's evaporator cools the food chest), the food is oxidised by the air with which it is in contact.

The drying of biological materials by sublimation was known by the turn of the century, and Shackell applied vacuum to his experiments, in order to facilitate the process, in 1909. One of the first medicinal uses of the freeze drying process was by Greaves in 1944, who used it to dry serum for use in treating the victims of World War II. It was at this time that the first crude commercial apparatus became available. This starting point expanded rapidly, by the end of the war freeze drying was an accepted method of preserving medicines and biological materials. Today, the greatest diversity and interest are within the pharmaceutical and life science fields, although food freeze drying probably accounts for the greatest volume of freeze-dried products. It is in the former areas that the largest numbers of freeze dryer users are concentrated, and it is for these workers that this book is primarily intended.

ADVANTAGES OF FREEZE DRYING

Freeze drying is a technique offering many unique advantages to the pharmaceutical production process. It is difficult to ascertain how many labile molecules would not be manufactured into a final presentation if the technique was unavailable. The primary advantages centre around the ability of the technique to dry whilst retaining the original structure and activity.

Retention of Activity

Providing that a substance is suitably formulated, then freeze drying is acknowledged as the most gentle of all methods of drying, and, as such, is often used for the preservation of molecules that exhibit biological or other activity. In some cases, for example proteins, not only the chemical structure but also the agglomeration of subunits, or the retention of other molecules complementary to activity, must be and are retained. The viability of freeze-dried bacteria is another example of the mildness of this technique.

There are several reasons, inherent in the freeze drying process, that contribute to this gentleness:

- The process operates at low temperatures, protecting heat labile species. Even when heat is applied to supply the energy to sublime moisture during primary drying, the "wet" portion of the sample remains frozen by evaporative cooling. As a general rule, materials are more heat stable once they have a low moisture content, protection is, therefore, provided during the higher temperatures encountered during secondary drying.

- The immobilisation associated with freezing prevents contact between chemically reactive molecules.

- Degradative enzymes or bacteria cannot operate at such low temperatures.

- Freeze drying is a vacuum process, where the absence of oxygen prevents oxidative reactions.

Retention of Form

The immobilisation that occurs as a consequence of freezing prevents the migration of nonvolatile molecules on the drying boundary, resulting in a retention of form. A sun-dried plum will become a prune: a freeze-dried plum will still look like a plum, although in this case it will not reconstitute to a plum because of water resistant membranes (and the unlikelihood of having frozen all of the sugar content). This characteristic is of primary interest in the food and specimen industries, in a pharmaceutical environment, it will result in an even cake occupying the same volume as the starting solution, which is seen as cosmetically desirable.

Ease of Reconstitution

When an aqueous solution is frozen, under the correct conditions, pure water will freeze in a branched crystal structure that is often called dendritic ice (Greek *dendrites*—tree). The concentrated solution then freezes interstitially within this matrix. The freeze-dried material structurally consists of a lattice formed by the removal of dendritic water ice from around it. This structure has a large surface area and is, therefore, easily dissolved. The relationship between surface area and ease of solubility is easily demonstrated. Finely divided white granulated sugar, even if formed into a sugar cube, will rapidly dissolve in a hot beverage. Large, brown sugar crystals often found in restaurants will not. This solubility phenomenon is of particular interest when the material is of marginal solubility or cannot be warmed to aid reconstitution as in the case of a pharmaceutical presentation.

Long Shelf Life

The low moisture content, typically below 2 percent, results in good storage stability. This long shelf life eases manufacture, distribution, and storage, thereby potentially reducing the cost of the final product. A classic example is the many animal vaccines for the third world. If these can be reconstituted on-site, they do not have to be transported, as a liquid fill, in refrigerated containers, thus significantly reducing the logistics and cost of the eradication program. The advantages of having human medicines "on the shelf" are obvious.

Accurate Dosing

Pharmaceuticals must be accurately and reproducibly dosed. The material to be freeze-dried will be introduced into its final product container as a liquid fill and can, therefore, be dosed more accurately than a powder fill. There are other advantages associated with a liquid fill, namely, the absence of static and the risk of explosion, the need for accurate particle size milling, and homogeneity of mixing.

Sterile Manufacture

Whilst sterility is not inherent in the freeze drying process, the freeze dryer has evolved in such a way that it can be sterilised and the process can be performed under aseptic conditions.

DISADVANTAGES OF FREEZE DRYING

The advantages of the freeze drying technique are partially offset by the disadvantages that centre around cost and throughput. It is often claimed, although not completely seriously, that freeze drying is reluctantly incorporated into a production protocol only when all other techniques have proven unsuitable. This may seem a harsh assessment of the technique, but the obvious advantages do not easily transfer into the reality of a smooth production material flow. The advantages of the technique as defined above will more than compensate for the disadvantages below, providing that the value of the product is high enough.

Batch Process

Freeze drying is a batch process. Continuous freeze dryer prototypes have been built, but have encountered a great number of technical problems. In any case, the vapour pressure generated by the newly introduced product would prevent a low final moisture content being attained in a product ostensibly approaching the end of drying. Unless multiple chambers were used, a continuous technique could only be used for low grade applications not requiring low final moisture content.

Fortunately, the pharmaceutical industry tends toward batch manufacture rather than a continuous process, so this shortcoming is relatively unimportant. The ability to continuously produce coffee and other foods would be preferable to current batch methods, if such a process were technically feasible.

Speed

Freeze drying is not a rapid process: cycle times are rarely less than 24 hours. With the attendant processes of as defrosting, cleaning, and sterilisation it is unusual that a freeze dryer will produce more than 3 batches per week.

Capital Cost

In common with many items of custom-made capital equipment a freeze dryer represents a significant capital investment. In the case of a freeze dryer, there is the additional constraint of a limited throughput. In a production environment, a reasonable amortisation is required, consequently, the technique is usually restricted to low volume, high value products.

Operating Costs

Freeze dryer operating costs are high, mainly because a freeze dyer is extremely inefficient in its use of energy. A mass of several tonnes of stainless steel, silicone oil, and glass will undergo a large temperature cycle in order to remove or apply heat to a few kilograms of wet product to produce a final dry product that may weigh less than a kilogram. To compound this inefficiency, the freeze dryer is not designed to recycle energy. The heat removed during freezing or condenser cooling is dissipated into the refrigeration group cooling system, whilst the heat for drying is generated de novo by electrical resistance. The engineering capability to make a freeze dryer more energy efficient, by recycling, exists, but the capital cost of this additional engineering makes it uneconomical.

Target Product Characteristics

The cost, both in terms of capital and running costs, and the slowness of batch freeze drying dictate, that at least one of the following characteristics be present or required for a product to be considered as a candidate for freeze drying:

- Lability

- Long shelf life

- Retention of form

- Accuracy in dosage

- Sterility

- High value

- Low volume

- Difficulty in reconstitution

With the exception of the latter, a pharmaceutical presentation will fit all of these criteria, and these account for the majority of the diversity and usage. Laboratory applications will usually centre around lability and are, obviously, of high value to the researcher, even if not in the monetary sense.

The freeze drying of commodity food materials operates in a totally different manner, utilising prefreezing outside the freeze dryer, very high radiant temperatures, and automated loading systems. Rapid throughput and economy of scale make the drying of these products viable. A food freeze dryer would be wholly unsuitable for a pharmaceutical presentation.

TARGET PRODUCTS

The vast majority of applications are in the pharmaceutical, biological, fine chemical, and biotechnology fields. They include, but are not restricted to, the following:

- Antibiotics
- Antitoxins
- Bacteria
- Blood coagulants
- Enzymes
- Fine chemicals
- Growth factor
- Hormones
- Media
- Pathological samples
- Plasma
- Reagents
- Standards
- Tissue (for electron microscopy)
- Vaccines
- Viruses
- Vitamins
- Yeast

Food applications include the following:

- Chicken cubes
- Coffee
- Fruit
- Garlic
- Herbs
- Prawns
- Seaweed

- Tea

- Vegetables

Freeze-dried tea and coffee have raised the general awareness of the technique. The use of freeze-dried rations for use by high altitude mountaineers and polar explorers has resulted in them being commercially available for lesser expeditions. NASA astronauts have used freeze-dried foods on the moon.

Other applications cover a variety of materials. The freeze drying of flowers has great popularity in the United States, and there are many cottage freeze drying industries producing elegant displays or preserving wedding bouquets. Many small specimens in natural history museums are now freeze-dried, it is said that freeze drying is the taxidermy of the future. Silage starters are largely freeze-dried. Books and manuscripts can be salvaged after water damage. Artefacts from marine archaeological digs (e.g., King Henry VIII of England's flagship, *The Mary Rose*) have been freeze dried. The author has been approached with such diverse projects as the freeze drying of human corpses for preservation, superconductor intermediates, and lugworms for fishing bait. Applications are limited only by the imagination of the end user.

THE THREE STAGES OF FREEZE DRYING

The freeze drying process is classically split into three separate stages: freezing, primary drying and secondary drying. Freezing is self-explanatory. Primary drying is the removal of the free moisture that has been frozen. Secondary drying is the desorption of bound moisture. It is important to realise that the three stages are not totally independent of each other.

Evaporative cooling, which will occur when vacuum is first drawn and the product begins to sublime, will slightly lower the temperature of the frozen product. This may cause a change in the crystal structure or even initiate eutectic freezing, or a glass transition, if the material has been inadequately frozen. Some materials will only crystallize when the temperature is rising.

The boundary between primary and secondary drying is not clear-cut. The freeze dryer is grossly operating in a similar way during both stages. It is obvious that some desorption will occur from the dried layer during primary drying, and that the last vestiges of free moisture may be removed during secondary drying.

In the development of a freeze drying cycle, primary and secondary drying are two distinct entities, with slightly different sets of operating conditions. It is usual to commence secondary drying by reducing the pressure to a minimum, and increasing shelf, and thus product, temperature to a point just below the denaturation temperature. There is no mechanism for detecting the exact point of the change from primary to secondary drying, although a pressure rise test will give a good indication. The two processes overlap, and the distinction, in terms of machine control, is relatively arbitrary.

The three stages comprise the actual freeze drying cycle, but ancillary activities may require an equivalent length of time as the freeze drying cycle. A full batch-to-batch protocol is likely to involve the activities listed in Figure 1.1.

This chapter will primarily concentrate on the three stages of freeze drying: freezing, primary drying, and secondary drying. Before these are discussed, it is first necessary to investigate some of the

Figure 1.1. The complete freeze drying cycle.

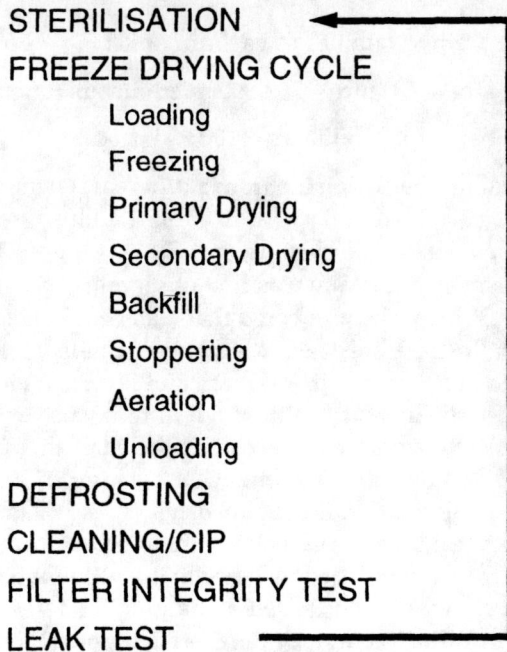

STERILISATION

FREEZE DRYING CYCLE

    Loading

    Freezing

    Primary Drying

    Secondary Drying

    Backfill

    Stoppering

    Aeration

    Unloading

DEFROSTING

CLEANING/CIP

FILTER INTEGRITY TEST

LEAK TEST

physical principles involved in freeze drying—vacuum and vacuum units, matter states, and saturated vapour pressures.

Vacuum Units

Vacuum may be defined as any reduction in atmospheric pressure. Atmospheric pressure is not an absolute and will vary with the height above sea level and with the prevailing meteorological conditions. A standard atmosphere (atm) is defined as that which will support a column of mercury 76 cm high. The units of this standard atmosphere are 760 torr or 1,013 millibars which equate to 14.69 pounds per square inch or 1.033 kilograms per square centimetre.

In the abstract sense, a high vacuum is one that contains fewer gas molecules than a low vacuum. The complete absence of gas molecules—a perfect vacuum—is unattainable.

The torr is the preferred unit of vacuum within North America, whilst Europe tends to use the millibar. The millibar is used within this text but the two units are easily convertible: 1 millibar is 0.75 torr; 1 torr is 1.33 millibars. The inaccuracy of the hot wire vacuum gauges used within freeze dryers result in the two units being, for all intents and purposes, interchangeable at the pressures used during the freeze drying cycle.

There are two families of vacuum units:

1.   1 atm = 760 torr = 760,000 micrometers (often called microns)

2.   1 bar = 1000 millibars = 100,000 pascals

Unfortunately, they originate from a different starting point as 1 atm is 1.013 bars and 1 bar is 0.987 atm. Table 1.1 illustrates the conversion factors between the different units.

Atmospheric pressure was first observed, in a column of water in a well, by Galileo. He discovered that water could not be drawn higher than 10 m. In 1640, Torricelli, a student of Galileo, filled a tube, which was closed at one end, with mercury and inverted it in a mercury bath. The level of the mercury column fell until it was 76 cm high. The column of mercury was 13.6 times smaller than that of water because mercury has a density 13.6 times that of water. The upper end of the tube was sealed and had contained no air, as it had previously been full of mercury so the space above the mercury had to be a vacuum. This was the first recorded instance that a vacuum had been created.

Torricelli was immortalised by naming the torr after him; a torr is equivalent to the vacuum required to support a column of mercury 1 mm high. The micron is based on the same system and corresponds to a column of mercury 1 micrometer high.

Table 1.1. Comparative Values of Vacuum Units

	Atm	Bar	Torr	mbar	Pascal	μm
Atmosphere	1	1.013	760	1,013	101,308	760,000
Bar	0.987	1	750.12	1,000	100,000	750,120
Torr (mm Hg)	0.00132	0.00129	1	1.33	133.3	1,000
Millibar	0.000987	0.001	0.75	1	100	750
Pascal	0.00000987	0.00001	0.0075	0.01	1	7.5
Micrometer (Micron)	0.00000132	0.00000129	0.001	0.00133	0.133	1

Pressure, and a vacuum is still exerting a pressure, is defined as the force per unit area or

$$p = hdg$$

where, for atmospheric pressure, $h = 0.76$ metres; $d = 13{,}600$ kg/m^3, the density of mercury; and $g = 9.8$ m/sec^2, acceleration due to gravity. Therefore,

$$p = 101{,}300 \text{ N/m}^2$$

or, as 1 N = 100,000 dynes

$$p = 1.013 \times 10^6 \text{ dynes/cm}^2$$

A bar is defined as 1,000,000 dynes/cm^2, therefore, the bar can be related to standard atmospheric pressure as 1 standard atmosphere is equivalent to 1.013 bars. The bar was originally defined in the CGS system of measurement but its SI equivalent is 100,000 N/m^2. The SI unit of pressure is the pascal, which is defined as 1 N/m^2 and having a value of 0.01 millibar or 0.00001 bar.

Matter States

Water, and most other solvents, can exist in three states: gas, liquid, or solid. The transition between these states, or phases, is a function of temperature and pressure and is represented by the phase diagram in Figure 1.2. It can be seen that at the critical temperature and pressure (0.0098°C and 6.103 mbar), and in the absence of air, pure water is in equilibrium in all three states. This condition is known as the triple

Figure 1.2. The triple point of water.

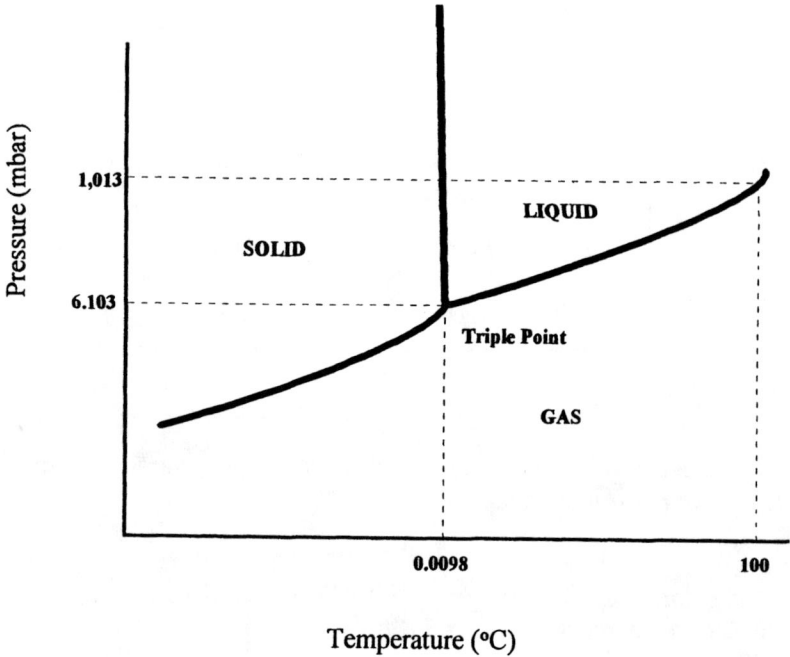

point. In the presence of air, at atmospheric pressure, the pure water equilibrium point is at the more familiar freezing point of 0°C.

Whilst the triple point has little relevance to practical freeze drying, other than that the water vapour pressure must be below it, it is from this point that the phase boundaries radiate. These boundaries are crucial to freeze drying. It can be seen that the transition between phases does not have to proceed through the conventional solid-liquid-gas path, but can occur from solid to gas (sublimation) and gas to solid (condensation). This is exactly what occurs during the freeze drying process. The freezing process is the crossing of the liquid to solid boundary.

Saturated Vapour Pressure

At any given temperature, water, or any volatile substance, will have a vapour pressure above it. The substance will always attempt to evaporate in order to produce a partial pressure of its vapour that is equivalent to its saturated vapour pressure (SVP) at that temperature. As the substance evaporates in order to achieve its SVP, unless a supply of heat is introduced to the substance, this evaporation will cool the substance, and equilibrium will occur at a lower temperature than the starting temperature. The values of saturated vapour pressures for water at different temperatures are given in Table 1.2.

If the SVP is equivalent to the pressure of the system, then the liquid boils. For example, water will boil at 100°C when its SVP is equivalent to atmospheric pressure. The boiling point of water, and any other substance, will vary with atmospheric pressure. This explains why there is a tendency to drink coffee rather than tea on an aircraft.

Table 1.2. Saturated Vapour Pressure/Temperature Chart for Water

°C	mbar	Torr	°C	mbar	Torr
100	1,013.00	760.00	–10	2.60	1.95
50	123.32	92.51	–12	2.17	1.63
40	73.74	55.32	–14	1.81	1.36
30	42.42	31.82	–16	1.51	1.13
20	23.38	17.54	–18	1.25	0.94
18	20.63	15.48	–20	1.04	0.78
16	18.17	13.63	–22	0.85	0.64
14	15.98	11.99	–24	0.71	0.53
12	14.02	10.52	–26	0.57	0.43
10	12.28	9.21	–28	0.47	0.35
8	10.73	8.05	–30	0.39	0.29
6	9.34	7.01	–40	0.13	9.71×10^{-2}
4	8.13	6.10	–50	3.94×10^{-2}	2.96×10^{-2}
2	7.05	5.29	–60	1.07×10^{-2}	8.08×10^{-3}
0	6.11	4.58	–70	2.58×10^{-3}	1.94×10^{-3}
–2	5.17	3.88	–80	5.33×10^{-4}	4.00×10^{-4}
–4	4.37	3.28	–100	1.33×10^{-5}	1.00×10^{-5}
–6	3.68	2.76	–120	1.31×10^{-7}	9.85×10^{-8}
–8	3.11	2.33	–150	7.00×10^{-12}	5.25×10^{-12}

Water boils at a lower temperature because of reduced cabin pressure; this lower temperature does not infuse the whole flavour out of tea and tea tastes insipid.

Ice also has a vapour pressure associated with it, just as if it were liquid water. It is worth noting that as water freezes, there is not a great change in its SVP. Thus, the immobilisation of water as ice does not significantly lower its SVP except by the temperature fall. The same phenomenon occurs with most organic solvents and is of great interest in the freeze drying of solvents that do not freeze at temperatures associated with a freeze dryer.

Freezing

Definition and Purpose

The purpose of freezing within the freeze drying process is merely to immobilise the product being freeze dried. Inclusion of freezing in the process not only defines it but also gives the process its name, if freeze drying were performed in the liquid phase, it would then be vacuum distillation. This is not to say that the freezing stage is unimportant; in actuality, the advantages of the freeze drying technique relate to the fact that the product is immobilised by freezing and that low temperatures are utilised.

Immobility prevents

- Frothing under vacuum and hence the ability to dose accurately. Frothing will cause the loss of a large proportion of the product, as a foam, within the freeze dryer chamber.

- Shrinkage, providing retention of form.

- Solvent, and hence solute, migration, allowing ease of reconstitution and retention of form.

- Degradative reactions by both slowing down the chemical reaction, because of the low temperature, and by separating and immobilising reactive molecules. This would also include enzymatic and microbial degradative or metabolic reactions.

The product structure, size, and shape is fixed after freezing, as are the sublimation and characteristics of the final product. This structure cannot be changed during the freeze drying process without damage, or loss, to the product. Freezing is, therefore, one of the most critical parts of the freeze drying process. Fortunately, most of the mechanisms are hidden and occur without special attention. These are discussed below.

Eutectic Freezing and Glass Transitions

A true solution can freeze in one of two mechanisms, or a mixture of both. Initially, pure ice will supercool, nucleate, and crystallize, and the concentration of the solute will increase to a critical concentration, after which it will concentrate no further. At this critical concentration and at the relevant temperature, the concentrated solution will either undergo a eutectic freezing or a glass transition. Eutectic freezing is a crystallisation. A glass transition is a large increase in viscosity, the material, whilst appearing to be a brittle solid, is in actual fact, a supercooled solution that retains elastic properties.

The classic example of a glass transition, and the origin of the term, is glass itself. Glass is a supercooled liquid and will slowly flow. A glass window will, over a period of many years, become thicker at the bottom than the top. The window is brittle and can be easily broken, but will flex slightly and return to its original shape if gently deformed.

The frozen cake is a lattice of pure, or dendritic, ice within which there are pockets of frozen solute. This may be easily demonstrated by the removal of the concentrated solute from frozen fruit juice. The temperatures in a domestic freezer are insufficient to freeze the sugars in the fruit juice completely, so it is possible to suck out the concentrated juice and leave the ice lattice behind. In ancient times, this freezing of pure water was used as a method of increasing the potency of alcoholic beverages. A jar of cider or wine would be left outside on a cold night and the ice crust would be removed the following morning. After this process had been repeated several times, a more potent beverage was produced.

The eutectic freezing diagram in Figure 1.3 shows the behaviour of a simple two-component system, in this case water and sodium chloride. As heat is removed and the temperature falls, pure water will begin to crystallize at 0°C. The system will then follow the freezing point curve, as the concentration of sodium chloride increases as more pure water crystallizes out as ice. At the point (C_e, T_e), the freezing point curve will meet the solubility curve and eutectic freezing will occur. In the case of a sodium chloride/water system T_e, the eutectic freezing temperature, is -21.4°C and C_e, the composition at eutectic freezing, is 23.6 percent w/w sodium chloride.

It should be noted that T_e and C_e are independent of the initial concentration of the solute, and that the concentration of the solute will always increase. This has important ramifications in multicomponent systems where, for example, a buffer may be used to stabilise a protein. During freezing, the concentration of the buffer will rise, increasing its ionic concentration and possibly altering its pH. This will

Figure 1.3. Eutectic freezing diagram.

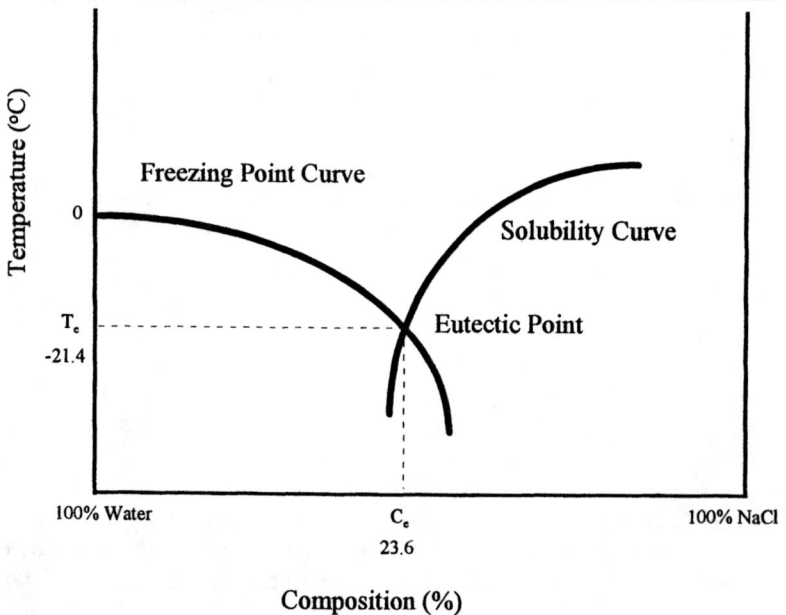

change the environment, and probably the structure and level of activity, of the protein. In order to cryoprotect species that are dependant on other molecules for stability, it is necessary to formulate with molecules that will protect rather than disrupt during the freezing process. As a general rule, these cryoprotective molecules are amorphous on freezing and undergo glass transitions. The rigid crystalline structure imposed by excipients, or buffers, that crystallize on freezing will affect the structure of the molecules of interest with which they are in association.

If the solute will not crystallize and will, therefore, undergo a glass transition the freezing diagram is very similar (Figure 1.4). In this case, the freezing point (melting point) curve will meet a glass transition curve at (C_g, T_g), the glass transition composition and temperature respectively. Most molecules that are freeze dried, or at least a component in the system to be dried, fall into the glass transition category and exhibit amorphous behaviour.

The glass transition temperature is that at which the viscosity of the mixture attains a value where mobility ceases and further solvent crystallisation cannot occur. Prior to reaching the glass transition

Figure 1.4. Glass transition freezing diagram.

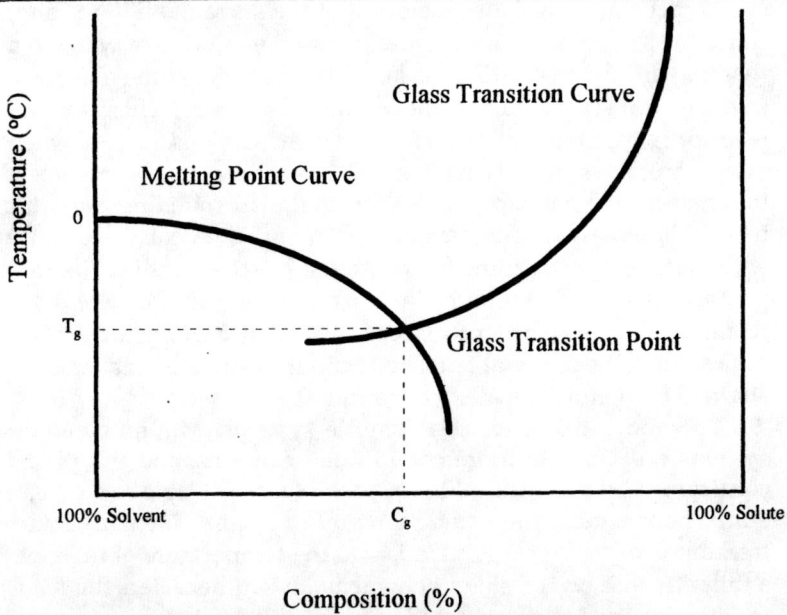

temperature, the freezing mixture passes through a point termed the *collapse temperature,* where the viscosity of the solute/solvent mixture is such that it will retain its structure and form throughout the sublimation process, even when it is not supported by the surrounding dendritic ice. This collapse temperature is of more interest during the freeze drying process.

Multiple component systems are more complicated and may contain mixtures of solutes that will crystallize and undergo eutectic freezing and those that will remain amorphous and undergo a glass transition. It is possible that there is no clearly defined freezing point, or there may be more than the two freezing points expected from the water and the solute mixture. Throughout the freeze drying process, two rules are apparent and irrespective of the type of freezing:

1. The final temperature during the freezing stage must be below the lowest crystallisation or collapse temperature.

2. During drying, the temperature of the frozen material must not rise above the crystallisation or collapse temperature.

If these temperatures are exceeded, then melting or collapse will occur.

Eutectic melting causes solution of the surrounding area and, because the system is under vacuum, a rapid evolution of water vapour that may lift the freeze-dried cake. This will occur at the warmest part of the frozen layer, which is the bottom of the cake, where the sample is in contact with the relatively warm shelf. Collapse occurs when the viscosity of the material drops as the collapse temperature is exceeded; the material cannot support itself once the surrounding dendritic ice has sublimed away. The material puffs and then collapses. Collapse will, therefore, occur at the freeze drying interface. If the collapse temperature is exceeded within the frozen portion of the cake, which it would have to be in order to exceed the collapse temperature at the interface, then the material tends to retain its structure because it is constrained by dendritic water ice around it.

The above refers to ideal, simple systems. Multiple component systems will react in more complicated fashions, and the process is constrained by the physical limitations of the available rate of temperature change, nucleation, and many other factors. The temperature of freezing is not necessarily identical to the temperature of melting. For a fuller treatise on freezing phenomena, the author refers the reader to more specialised texts prepared by acknowledged leaders in the field.

The Frozen Structure and Freezing Rate in True Solutions
For brevity, the remainder of this text will use the term *solidification* to signify either a eutectic crystallisation or a temperature below the collapse temperature, where either case could apply.

The structure of the frozen cake not only defines the final appearance of the freeze-dried product but also how it behaves during sublimation. Ideally, dendritic ice crystals should form a lattice with interstitial pockets of product; if cooling proceeds too rapidly, then the reverse can occur. The overall structure of dendritic ice crystals should also orientate toward the surface of the frozen cake.

The mechanism of freezing with respect to the freezing rate shows that a rapid cooling will nucleate many small crystals of ice within the solution to be frozen. These crystals do not show the hexagonal snowflake structure and are often described as irregular dendrites or having undergone heterogeneous ice formation. They may grow, but in general, remain discrete. During the freezing process the temperature of the solution will fall to 0°C, at which point nucleation will occur, then remain at this temperature until the majority of the water has frozen. At this point, the temperature will fall until solidification takes place, and then fall to the ultimate temperature of the cold source. The ice crystals will be discrete and surrounded by the frozen solute. During sublimation, there are no continuous pathways for the vapour to escape through from the lower layers.

If the solution is cooled more slowly, then the overall mass will fall below 0°C and the solution will be supercooled. Cases of 38 degrees of supercooling have been reported, although 3–8 degrees is more normal. At some point, nucleation occurs, and a freezing front is propagated throughout the solution, forming a matrix of ice with interstitial pockets of solute solution. These ice crystals exhibit hexagonal symmetry and are of the familiar snowflake pattern. They are often referred to as having undergone homogenous ice formation. The temperature of the partially frozen material rises to 0°C, as the negative sensible heat associated with supercooling is negated by the evolution of the latent heat of fusion as the water freezes. As more heat is removed, the ice matrix thickens, usually associated with a steady drop in temperature, until the solidification point is reached, after which the system behaves as before. In this case, the ice matrix is continuous; on sublimation, it will leave channels through which vapour can escape from the lower layers.

The propagation of a freezing front during homogenous ice formation will fix the freezing mass retaining the interstitial pockets of solute solution. If cooling proceeds more rapidly by heterogeneous ice formation, then the growth of ice crystals, which occupy more volume than the liquid form, can squeeze the concentrating solute solution upward. Upon complete freezing, this can leave a nonporous skin on the surface of the frozen cake that will slow the subsequent sublimation. In extreme cases, this can prevent the escape of vapour, resulting in melting as the frozen cake is no longer cooled by evaporative cooling when heat is applied during sublimation. It can be seen that homogenous ice formation is the preferred route, and it is fortunate that the rate of cooling that a freeze dryer is capable of generating will allow this mechanism to prevail.

Material that has undergone rapid freezing and heterogeneous ice formation may often have its sublimation properties improved by warming the frozen mass to above the solidification point but below the ice freezing point. This allows ice crystal growth and coalescence. The material must then be cooled to below the solidification point prior to sublimation.

Whilst the uses of liquid nitrogen or blast freezing are viable methods of freezing externally to the freeze drying chamber, and are necessary for some applications, it is apparent that this method produces heterogeneous ice formation, which does not present the optimal ice crystal structure. Solutions may be frozen, by these methods, as pellets or thin wafers, not unlike the material removed by a paper hole punch, called prills and dried as a layer. The ice crystal structure will not optimise sublimation, but the small product depth within each pellet, and the voids between pellets, will allow a ready escape of vapour and a reasonable rate of drying.

Ice crystal formation tends to be in the direction opposed to heat flow, so a shelf freeze dryer will tend to orientate ice crystals to the surface of the cake. *The desired effect.* However, the site of the initiation of nucleation, the presence of particles, and temperature gradients within the cooling mass will all affect ice crystal orientation. The observation of a frozen cake under a hand lens will verify the diversity of ice crystal orientation. The important criterion is that the pure ice matrix is continuous; the governing factor is, therefore, the rate of removal of heat.

Freezing of Suspensions, Structured Materials, and
Nonfrozen Materials

It is not unusual for suspensions to be freeze-dried. In this case, ice will form around and between particles. Channels for the escape of vapour form between particles as the ice is removed. If particles are suspended in a buffer, then it is necessary to take this into consideration, and the criteria discussed above for true solutions will apply. The inclusion of suspended particles will tend to nucleate ice crystals and it is difficult to obtain a continuous ice structure. Often, the important consideration is to immobilise the suspension quickly in order to prevent settling. Raising the temperature to allow ice crystal growth and coalescence may help.

Structured material, specimens, flowers, foodstuffs, and so on, cannot have their ice structure significantly altered. Freeze drying cycles for these materials tend to be long, and the most efficient method of optimisation of sublimation is by physical means. In the case of specimens, this would be by puncturing the specimen in areas where the puncture would not be visible, to allow vapour to escape along the puncture. Foodstuffs should be diced or minced in order to give a minimum product depth for escaping vapour to cross. Flower heads are removed from the stalks prior to freeze drying. The high concentrations of sugars, especially in vegetable matter, may prevent complete freezing. Fortunately, small unfrozen areas are constrained by the gross structure, and the reconstitution characteristics and fine structure are not as important as in the case of a pharmaceutical presentation.

Some materials will not solidify at the temperatures normally encountered on freeze dryer shelves. Small concentrations of these materials may be locked in place within the ice lattice by higher concentrations of an excipient. Many organic solvents do not freeze within the freeze dryer; these are discussed later in this text.

Eutectic Measurement

A large proportion of freeze drying cycles employ an initial shelf freezing step that freezes down to -50°C or lower. The reason for this is usually that -50°C was the ultimate shelf temperature of the freeze dryer upon which the cycle was developed. As there was no information on the freezing characteristics of the product, then this temperature was incorporated into the cycle. This may appear harsh, but many commercial freeze drying cycles have been developed in this way. In the vast majority of cases, this low temperature is not necessary and only serves to utilise process time and waste energy with no additional benefit.

The criteria for freezing are that the product is completely frozen and that the ice structure is, as far as is possible, homogenous. Providing that the temperature is low enough for solidification to occur, then there is little value in reducing the temperature of the system further.

During freezing a steady temperature may be maintained and the complete product will equilibrate at this temperature. It is at this time that data from the product probes have any real meaning, as the system is not subliming and there are no temperature gradients in operation. Providing that there is little batch-to-batch variation, and if the solidification temperature for the product is known, then the shelf freezing set point is easily defined. This would usually be approximately 5°C below the point where the product is completely frozen. It is necessary to hold the shelf temperature at the freezing set point to ensure equilibrium in order to ensure that complete solidification has been achieved.

It is necessary to know the complete freezing point of the product in order to optimise this freezing temperature. There are two methods in common use: differential thermal analysis (DTA) and resistivity.

Differential Thermal Analysis. DTA makes use of the fact that there is an evolution of heat when freezing occurs. This occurs from the raising of the temperature as a supercooled solution changes state and the evolution of the latent heat of fusion. A thermometer does not have sufficient accuracy to determine this point exactly, so a null method is practised using two opposed thermocouples. One is placed in a sample of pure water, and the other is placed in an identical container containing an identically sized sample of the product. Both containers are placed in a large metal block that can be slowly varied in temperature and has an independent temperature monitor. Heat evolution brought about by the water content of the product is cancelled out by the pure water sample; only peaks generated by solidification are recorded, along with the temperature at which they occur.

Accuracy may be improved by the use of additional opposed thermocouples and integrating the outputs to reduce electronic noise. Thermocouples are used as they have little thermal mass. The rate of change of temperature must be very slow to prevent overshooting the point of interest.

Resistivity. A resistivity measurement is simpler. This technique relies on the fact that as ions are immobilised by freezing, then their ability to pass an electric current is reduced; hence the electrical resistance of the sample increases. This increase may be several orders of magnitude and is easily measured.

A simple resistivity probe consisting of two electrodes is placed in the sample and an alternating current is passed through them. This current is high frequency in order to avoid electrolytic effects. A temperature probe is incorporated into the system. The sample is cooled until fully frozen and then warmed, and data are taken of resistance against temperature.

A logarithmic plot of resistance is made against a linear plot of temperature. The points where there is an abrupt reduction in resistance will mark the temperatures of solidification and give a guideline to the freezing temperature.

DTA and resistivity readings are usually taken in the reverse direction (i.e., when the sample is completely frozen and is being warmed up). The reason for this is that it mimics the freeze drying sublimation process, and that the point of incipient melting (when melting starts to occur) is not necessarily that at which freezing occurs. This will give data on the highest temperature that the sample can be subjected to during the sublimation phase. However, it is necessary to take readings on a falling temperature in order to predict a safe shelf freezing set point.

There are many systems that make use of resistivity in order to attempt to control heat input during sublimation. These systems are suspect in that they are invasive and control the whole batch on the one vial that is known to be atypical, because of the probe. In any case, the position of the probe within the drying cake will determine its temperature, as will be seen in later chapters. The only use for such a control system is as a veto if product temperature is becoming too high, it should never be used to call for additional heat input.

Note should be taken that many complex solutions have more than one glass transition temperature and the determination of the highest does not guarantee complete solidification.

Machine Status

Freezing occurs at atmospheric pressure. All valves to the chamber and condenser, with the exception of the chamber isolation valve, are shut. The vacuum pump is isolated and not running. The control and monitoring systems are on.

If shelves are precooled before they are loaded, then it is possible, and often desirable, to place a dry nitrogen blanket and flow within the chamber. This technique is often used in larger freeze dryers that are loaded one shelf at a time due to the time taken to fill the batch into vials. The nitrogen has two effects:

1. It is inert and will prevent oxidation reactions within the product, or a pH change by adsorption of atmospheric carbon dioxide (although it is probable that the air in the vial may not be displaced).

2. The dryness prevents a build up of frost on the cold surfaces.

Products that are prefrozen prior to placement within the freeze dryer should be loaded onto precooled shelves. The time taken to pull a vacuum and the heat content of the shelves at ambient temperature would otherwise lead to some melting occurring.

Primary Drying

Definition and Purpose

The purpose of primary drying is to remove all of the water that has been frozen, either as pure ice or as ice associated with the solute. The mechanism of this removal of water is by sublimation under vacuum and comprises the crossing of the solid/gas phase boundary. To prevent melting, (i.e., crossing the solid/liquid phase boundary), the partial pressure of water vapour (not necessarily the total pressure) within the freeze dryer must be below that of the triple point (6.103 mbar). In addition, the temperature of the product (not necessarily that of the freeze dryer thermoregulated shelf) must be below that of the solidification point.

In order for the sublimation to occur approximately 680 calories of heat, the heat of sublimation, must be supplied to each gram of water in the product. A calorie, by definition, will raise 1 gram of water by 1 degree Celsius. The heat of sublimation compares to the latent heats of fusion (solid to liquid) and evaporation, which have values of 80 and 540 calories per gram respectively. The heat that must be supplied to sublime 1 gram of ice would be sufficient to raise the temperature of that gram, as water, from an ambient temperature of 20°C to boiling point 8 times. This heat is supplied from thermoregulated shelves but does not effect a comparable increase in product temperature due to evaporative, or more accurately sublimative, cooling. It can be seen how a subliming product can remain frozen when situated on a shelf at +25°C. The relatively high temperature of the shelf is necessary to form a temperature gradient to push heat into the frozen mass. This heat is dissipated as the heat of sublimation and, providing that water vapour can completely escape, and the heating is not excessive, then there is little or no increase in sensible heat within the product.

The structure determined by freezing will become apparent after water is removed. Providing that the material never melts, then the size, shape, and structure remain unaltered.

At the end of primary drying the "dry" cake will have a residual moisture content of around 5–7 percent and will still retain bound moisture. Bound moisture is water associated with the solute molecule, (e.g., water of crystallisation, hydrogen-bonded water cages, etc.).

Primary drying is the stage of freeze drying where the shelf temperature and vacuum level can have the greatest impact on the drying process and, ultimately, the length of the cycle. The understanding of the contribution of both of these parameters to primary drying is essential to cycle optimisation.

The Mechanism of Primary Drying

It is the tendency for ice to attempt to generate its SVP above it that gives the driving force for primary drying. At a temperature of -20°C, such as may be found at the freeze drying interface, ice will have a SVP of 1.04 mbar. The ice on the condenser at -70°C will have a SVP of 0.0026 mbar.

If it is assumed that the transport of water vapour around the freeze dryer is rapid then the partial pressure of water vapour above the material undergoing freeze drying will always be below 1.04 mbar. Providing heat is supplied to replace the heat used in sublimation and the temperature of the drying interface remains constant, then the material will sublime water vapour continuously until either the partial pressure of water vapour in the freeze dryer reaches 1.04 mbar or all of the water in the sample has sublimed.

Meanwhile the condenser is experiencing a partial pressure of water vapour in excess of the SVP associated with its temperature. It will condense this vapour onto its surface. This change of state, and to a lesser degree, drop in temperature will input heat to the condenser surface which would result in a temperature rise. If the temperature were to rise, in this case to –20°C, then freeze drying would stop as the condenser would not condense water vapour being generated by the product, and the product would stop subliming as the vapour above it would become saturated. Accordingly, the condenser must be kept cool, usually by mechanical refrigeration.

The Freeze Drying Interface

Drying proceeds along a front known as the freeze drying interface. This interface initiates on the surface of the solidified material where it meets the vacuum and progresses inwards, leaving a dried layer behind. At normal freeze drying temperatures, it can be assumed that this interface will move at approximately 1 mm/hour, although this is temperature dependant. The rate will be slower for materials that have a low solidification temperature and must be dried at very low shelf temperatures.

A vial or a frozen block in a tray is the simplest system, in that the heat input is from the heated shelf below and the vapour sublimes from the top surface of the solidified mass. The interface then progresses downward until it reaches the bottom of the vial. In actuality, there are edge effects and the interface bows as it descends; the final part of the sample to dry is on the centre line of the vial about 1 mm from the base of the cake.

The input of heat at the bottom of the cake and the initial removal of water from the top result in a temperature gradient being set up within the solidified cake. The warmest part of the sample is at the base of the cake, and the coldest is at the interface. It is this temperature gradient that results in the use of product probes being of dubious value. The use of product probes and probe placement will be dealt with at length elsewhere within this text but it is worth noting that the position of the probe will dictate the temperature that it displays. It is the temperature at the interface that dictates the SVP of the product and the base of the cake where there is the most chance of melting.

Prills, or pellets, will start to dry on the surface, and the front will progress inward until all of the material is dry. The mechanism of heat transport is more complicated and is a combination of convective heat transport by gas molecules and conduction between particles.

In any case, the sublimed water vapour must escape through the dried layer; it is for this reason that the formation of homogenous dendritic ice during freezing is important. The void left by this pure ice after it has sublimed acts as a series of channels for the water vapour subliming from the lower levels to escape through.

If the layer to be dried is deep then there is an increased resistance to flow when the drying interface reaches lower levels. This is where many users miss an opportunity in the development of a freeze drying cycle. If the physical problems associated with changing the temperatures of large thermal masses, (i.e., silicone oil, stainless steel shelves, the fluid circulation system, and the product trays and containers) are temporarily discounted, then the time when the solidified mass will accept the most heat is at the start of primary drying. When primary drying commences, there is little resistance to vapour flow and evaporative cooling is maximal. At the end of primary drying, when the interface is near the bottom of the cake then there is more resistance to the flow of vapour; thus sublimation and, therefore, evaporative cooling, slows. At a constant heat input, generated by a constant shelf temperature, this will result in a rise in cake temperature with the attendant risk of melting. The optimum shelf temperature profile is, therefore, to quickly raise the temperature and to reduce it as primary drying proceeds. Taking the thermal masses into consideration, the optimum shelf temperature profile is at the least flat, but at a high temperature and probably reducing in temperature toward the end of primary drying.

The temperature profile described above will cause two potential problems. If the heat is applied too quickly, then the ice may not be able to conduct it to the interface, and there will be an attendant increase in temperature and melting. The above shelf heating strategy should, therefore, be predetermined experimentally. The second, and trivial, problem is that the temperature profile will place an increased load on the condenser during the initial stages of primary drying as the vapour flow will be heavier. Condenser temperature should be monitored closely. This profile does result in a shorter cycle time than the usual profiles.

The usual shelf temperature profile is to commence at a low temperature and to gradually ramp up the temperature until it is at a maximum at the end of primary drying. This results in the maximum heat input when evaporative cooling is at a minimum. Often, this results in some melting at the base of the cake, which is usually explained as progressing to secondary drying too early in the process. This is incorrect, although an early progression to secondary drying would give the same effect; the real reason is the "usual" shelf temperature profile puts too much heat into the product when the interface is at the bottom of the vial, and this heat input is not easily dissipated.

Optimisation and Heat Transfer

In order to optimise the speed of primary drying, the control of heat transfer is important. The vapour flow characteristics of the solidified cake were determined during freezing. The task is now to balance the flow of heat into the product, by conduction, convection, and radiation, against the evaporative cooling effect. The heat balance is illustrated in Figure 1.5. There are two mechanisms by which the heat input into the product can be controlled: shelf temperature and vacuum.

Shelf temperature is self-evident—the higher the shelf temperature, the more heat will be applied to the product. Temperature profiling was discussed in the previous section. The efficiency of heat transport is largely determined by the level of vacuum.

Strictly speaking, vacuum is not necessary to the freeze drying process. It is the partial pressure of water vapour above the product that is the important criterion. If a current of dehumidified air was constantly passing over the surface of the material undergoing drying, then this would have the same effect. In the case of a freeze dryer

Figure 1.5. Heat transfer during primary drying.

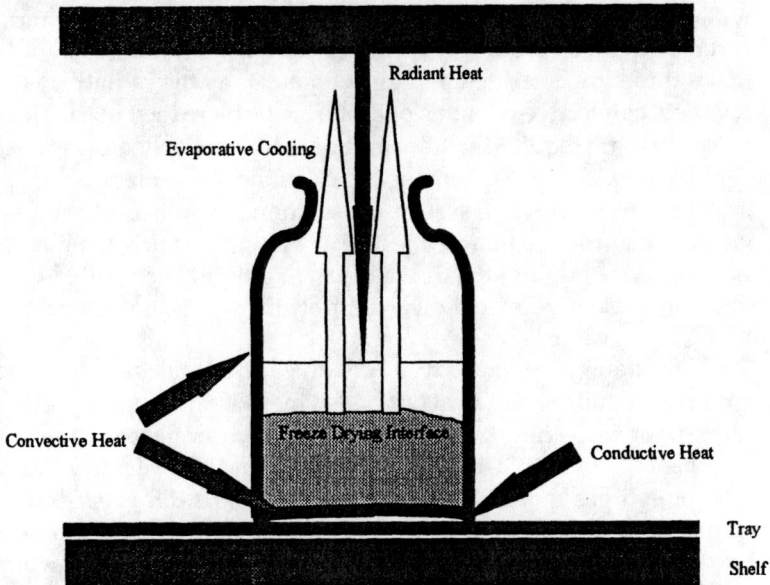

where the water vapour must transport to the condenser, a vacuum is drawn to facilitate this transport. Another way of describing this is that the noncondensable gases—oxygen, nitrogen, etc.—are removed so that water molecules do not collide with them and reduce their mobility. The vacuum also sets up a pressure gradient through the dried layer above the interface that facilitates vapor transport and lowers the local water vapour pressure at the interface.

It is easily seen that the thermal conductivity from the shelf, possibly to a tray, and then to the base of a vial is inefficient because the surfaces are not completely flat. It is apparent that under high vacuum ($<10^{-2}$ mbar), where there are few gas molecules available to perform convective heat transport, the main mechanism of heat transfer is by heat radiation from the shelves. It is for this reason that most freeze dryers have a top, unusable, thermoregulated shelf whose sole purpose is to ensure that the top shelf of product experiences the same conditions as the product on the lower shelves. This requirement is usually of greater importance in secondary drying.

Heat radiation is an accepted method of heat transfer, and is used in the food freeze drying industry; however, it requires very high shelf temperatures to be efficient and is, therefore, wasteful of energy. A food freeze dryer invariably has the product prefrozen outside the freeze dryer, and so the shelves are constantly maintained at elevated temperatures, often by steam, giving energy efficiency to the process.

A biological freeze dryer, where the product is frozen on the shelf, will utilise lower shelf temperatures in order to save energy, and, to a certain extent, to protect the product in a vacuum failure. In order to make these low shelf temperatures efficient, as the radiative effect is reduced, convective methods of heat transport are then used. The molecules that are required to transport heat convectively are supplied by slightly spoiling the vacuum by the use of the air, or nitrogen, injection system. The air injection system is also known by other names, usually vacuum control or calibrated leak. The system comprises a method of passing a dry gas into the freeze dryer, to a tightly controlled vacuum level, by means of a needle valve throttling a solenoid valve or by a modulating valve.

The strategy is to introduce enough gas molecules to give efficient convective transport of heat but not so many that the transport of water vapour molecules to the condenser is compromised. It can be experimentally determined that the optimum heat transfer is when there are enough gas molecules to exhibit viscous, or diffusive flow. Heat transfer is minimal when the vacuum is at a level where the mean free path between molecular collisions is less than the spaces between the shelf and tray, tray and vial, or shelf and vial. Heat transfer rises in the transition vacuum level and maximises when viscous flow is achieved. The likely spaces between the shelves, trays, and vials are usually in the order of 0.5 mm to 1.5 mm and so the minimum vacuum value during primary drying is usually approximately 5×10^{-2} mbar as shown in Figure 1.6.

The mean free path, in cm, between molecular collisions with respect to pressure can be calculated by the following equation:

$$\text{Mean Free Path} = \frac{6.4 \times 10^{-3}}{P}$$

where mean free path is in cm and pressure is in mbar.

For a space between the shelves, trays, and vials of 1 mm the mean free path can be calculated to be 6.4×10^{-2} mbar, which agrees with the experimental data.

The efficiency of the heat transport mechanism can be experimentally assessed by a product temperature probe. If the temperature at a fixed point is measured, at a low vacuum and at a steady shelf temperature, and the air injection system is then stopped, the temperature of the product will fall as the vacuum becomes higher. This can be

Figure 1.6. The absolute lower pressure limit for efficient heat transfer.

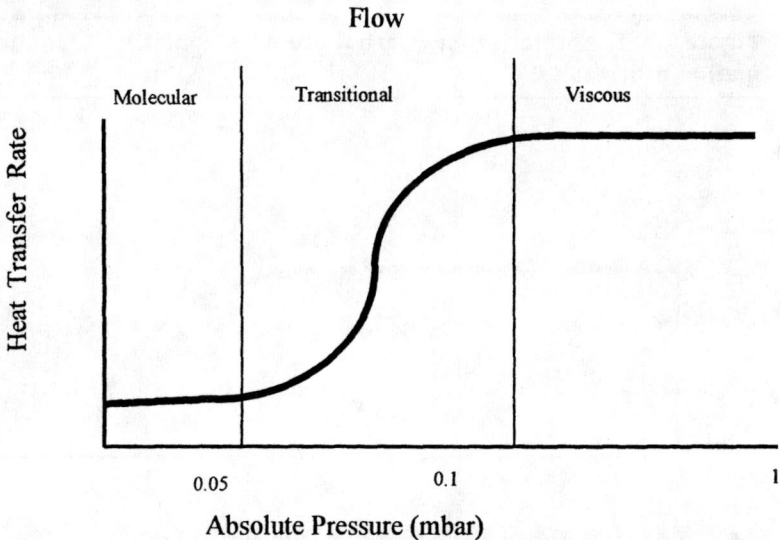

compensated for by increasing the shelf temperature. It is possible that the shelf temperature may have to be raised by up to 100°C in order to achieve the same product temperature.

An upper vacuum level (low vacuum) is theoretically easily determined, but it requires a knowledge of the temperature of the freeze drying interface. Sublimation cannot occur if the partial pressure of water vapour within the system exceeds that of the SVP at the interface temperature. If the water vapour partial pressure exceeds the SVP, then condensation will occur. Providing that a constant interface temperature is maintained, then the rate of sublimation will increase and maximise at a water vapour partial pressure value of approximately half the SVP at that interface temperature. Figure 1.7 shows how the rate of vapour evolution varies with the partial pressure of water vapour.

Unfortunately, the interface temperature is not easily measured except by imperfect or destructive means. The destructive way is to isolate the drying chamber and to let the pressure rise until the SVP is reached, at which point the temperature of the interface can be deduced by reading the pressure and referring to the SVP table. The problems associated with this technique are that the shelf temperature must be that at which you are drying, so it is unlikely to be below the solidification temperature and results in the melting of the sample as evaporative cooling stops. The presence of noncondensable gases will

Figure 1.7. The water vapour partial pressure upper limit for sublimation of ice at –20°C.

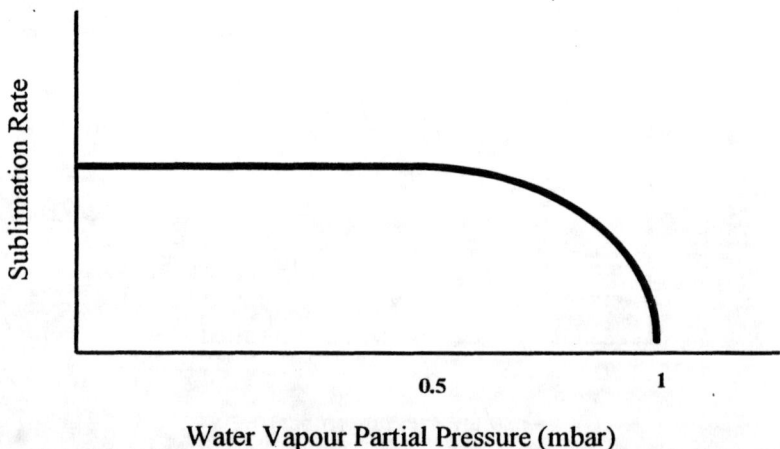

Water Vapour Partial Pressure (mbar)

give an elevated vacuum reading, with subsequent increase in apparent interface temperature. Vacuum gauges are notoriously inaccurate. This method is, therefore, obviously unsuitable.

If a direct measurement is attempted, it is difficult to place a probe on the interface, or to exactly determine when the interface passes a probe on its downward path. An indication can be taken from the temperature when the probe starts to exhibit a steep increase in temperature. As the probe makes the vial that it is placed within atypical, and the probe is invariably wider than the interface, such temperature readings should be taken with some scepticism. They do, however, represent the most accurate method of assessing the interface temperature.

The maximum sublimation rate with respect to low vacuum is measured in water vapour partial pressure; that of the high vacuum is measured in total pressure, so strict upper and lower limits cannot be determined and experimentation is needed to optimise the vacuum level. If the vacuum level is such that heat transfer is maximal, then adjustments of shelf temperature can then be used to vary the heat input level.

The use of an air injection system also destroys the myth that a low condenser temperature is necessary for primary drying. In the absence of an air injection system, and under steady drying conditions, the system pressure would reduce as the temperature of the condenser reduces. A low condenser temperature will reduce the pressure until the convective heat transport effect will no longer operate. In terms of the driving force for freeze drying, the product/condenser temperature differential is not too important. For instance in the previously mentioned case, at a temperature of -20°C, product ice will have a SVP of 1.04 mbar. The ice on the condenser at -70°C will have a SVP of 0.0026 mbar. If the condenser temperature was only -60°C, the SVP would be 0.011 mbar—still a gradient of 100:1, and more than enough to drive freeze drying. The conditions change in secondary drying, where a low condenser temperature is useful.

A low interface temperature, usually necessitated by a low solidification temperature, will have a greater effect on drying time. The low levels of vapour evolved will mean that drying will progress slowly. A cycle for a product with high levels of glucose as an excipient may need a primary drying time 6 times longer than one using mannitol as an excipient. Glucose has a collapse temperature below -40°C, whilst mannitol has a eutectic point of around -3°C.

There is another aspect to the vacuum of the system that is not related to heat transfer but to material being eroded, or ablated, from the surface of the freeze-dried product by the force of the escaping water vapour. The Standard Molar Volume Law states that 1 mole of gas occupies 22.4 L at 0°C and 1 atm. of pressure. One mole of water will weigh 18 g so, to a first approximation, 1 g of water vapour will occupy 1 L at atmospheric pressure. Boyle's Law states that this gas will occupy 5,000 L (5 m³) at 5 × 10⁻¹ mbar and 50,000 L (50 m³) at 5 × 10⁻² mbar.

For a vial with an internal diameter of 30 mm (cross-sectional area, 7×10^{-4} m²), freeze drying 10 mL (product depth 14 mm) in 10 hours at a vacuum of 5×10^{-2} mbar the volume of water vapour subliming per second will be

$$\frac{50 \text{ m}^3 \times 10 \text{ mL}}{10 \text{ hours} \times 3600 \text{ seconds}} = 0.014 \text{ m}^3/\text{second}$$

The speed of the vapour leaving the product will be

$$\frac{0.14 \text{ m}^3/\text{second}}{7 \times 10^{-4}} = 19.84 \text{ m/second}$$

If it can be assumed that the cut-outs in the stopper have 10 percent of the surface area of the cross-sectional area of the vial, then at 5×10^{-2} mbar the speed of the water vapour leaving the vial can be as high as 200 m/second. This speed would almost certainly result in a large quantity of the product ablating from the surface and distributing itself around the freeze dryer and the vacuum pump. This product would be irrecoverable, give inaccurate dosing, could foul the vacuum gauge(s), and would also necessitate a cleaning regimen.

If the drying cycle was performed at 5×10^{-1} mbar then these speeds would be reduced by a factor of 10, which would result in far less, if any, ablation. The mass flow would be identical, but the speed of the vapour flow is reduced. It can be seen that the selection and control of the vacuum level are of great importance in the freeze drying process, affecting both speed and recovery.

The volume of gas at the vacuum levels employed during freeze drying demonstrates the requirement for the condenser. An average bulk drying operation could expect to remove 10 kg of water in 10 hours per square metre of shelf area at 5×10^{-1} mbar. This equates to 5000 m³/hour/m². A large vacuum pump for a 1 m² freeze dryer is capable of pumping 15 m³/hour; 35 of these would be required to pump the vapour, even if the water vapour did not condense into the oil and damage the pump. It is necessary to trap the water vapour for two reasons: the impossibility of pumping such large amounts of vapour and the need to protect the vacuum pump from the water vapour.

Completion of Primary Drying

Once the unbound moisture has been removed, it is usually necessary to perform secondary drying to bring the moisture level down to below 2 percent in order to achieve long storage time stability. Secondary drying conditions will involve higher shelf temperatures; it is essential to ensure that all the unbound moisture has been eliminated to prevent melting. There are five methods of determining the end point of primary drying, but only one good method.

Temperature product probes will show a marked rise in temperature as the evaporative cooling effect ceases and the cake temperature rises to that of the shelf. This method suffers from the usual problems associated with product probes, in that the temperature shown by the probe will be dictated by the position of the probe within the product. The vial containing the probe will also be atypical because of the presence of the probe. Probes are usually, because of the practical aspects of incorporating them, placed in vials on the edge of the shelf. It is well documented that vials on the edge of a shelf dry more quickly than those in the centre that experience higher partial pressures of water vapour.

If vacuum probes are present in both the drying chamber and the condenser, then it will be possible to see the chamber pressure falling until it matches that of the condenser probe at the end of primary drying. This is caused by the cessation of vapour evolution and the subsequent reduction in the contribution to system pressure by the partial pressure of water vapour. Unfortunately, vacuum probes do not have sufficient accuracy to determine the end point with any degree of confidence.

The condenser temperature will minimise at the end of primary drying. The cessation of condensation of water vapour will remove the heat load on the condenser and allow it to reach its ultimate temperature. As the temperature approaches the ultimate, the rate of change slows and an accurate determination is difficult.

If it is possible to see the product, it is possible to see the interface reach the bottom of the vial. Edge effects mean that the interface will reach the bottom of the vial at the edge prior to it reaching the bottom at the centre.

The most effective, and preferred, method is the pressure rise test. It is noninvasive, measures the contribution of all the product, and is easily measured. The test comprises of stopping the air injection system, closing the chamber isolation valve between the drying chamber and the condenser and observing chamber pressure. If primary drying is still progressing, there will be an immediate rise in chamber pressure as water vapour being evolved is physically prevented from being condensed by the condenser. It is important to perform the test rapidly in case primary drying is not completed. Too large a pressure rise could result in the slowing down of vapour evolution with the attendant reduction in evaporative cooling and consequent melting. The expected rises in pressure must be carefully selected. Too high a value could exceed the SVP and would never be achieved; too low a value would mean that the test would never be passed. Most control systems will perform the pressure rise test automatically for the end point determination of either primary or secondary drying, or both. The selection of the correct parameters in automatic systems is critical. It is worth noting, in passing, that the pressure rise test is the only real reason to have a condenser separate from the drying chamber.

Machine Status

As the freeze dryer advances from freezing to primary drying, the shelves are held at the last set point value in freezing whilst the condenser is cooled. Once the condenser reaches a preset temperature, or on older dryers after a predetermined time, the vacuum pump is started. The use of a condenser preset temperature, or time, prevents water vapour passing the condenser and contaminating the vacuum pump. Some systems will start the vacuum pump(s) at the start of condenser cooling, but keep the valve between the pump and the condenser shut. This allows the vacuum pump oil to heat up and further reduces the risk of water vapour condensing in it. The vacuum valve will then open at the preset condenser temperature.

Once the condenser is cold and the vacuum level adequate, the shelf temperature and vacuum profiling starts. The monitoring systems are on.

Secondary Drying

Definition and Purpose

The purpose of secondary drying is to desorb bound moisture from the freeze drying product. At the completion of primary drying, all free moisture, which had existed as either pure ice or ice associated with the product, has been removed. If the sample were allowed to warm up to ambient temperature the material would suffer no immediate adverse degradation with respect to melting and resolution. However, the final water content of 5–7 percent would not be of a sufficiently low value to provide long-term storage stability. In order to achieve the desired stability, the moisture content must be reduced to 0.5–3 percent. This moisture content difference is accounted for by the bound moisture. Although the average weight of bound moisture is approximately 5 percent of that of the dried product, this is product specific and wide variances can be observed.

Although a low moisture content is necessary for stability, the minimum moisture content may not be optimum. Many products can suffer from overdrying. The optimum moisture content must be determined by stability trials. It is possible to measure the final moisture content by means of the Karl Fisher reaction, vacuum drying, chromatographic methods, and physical methods. The disadvantage of these techniques is that the sample absorbs moisture as soon as it is removed from its sealed container. It is usual to determine the moisture content of the sample at different times after breaking the seal and to extrapolate backward to the actual value.

This bound moisture is attached by many different means. Products that crystallize and undergo eutectic freezing generally have waters of crystallisation that can account for a substantial proportion of their weight. Copper sulphate which crystallizes as the pentahydrate, $CuSO_4 \cdot 5H_2O$ will have 45 percent of its weight as water. Materials undergoing glass transitions will have other binding mechanisms, (e.g., the hydrogen-bonded water cage associated with a protein). The removal of a water cage will damage the structure and reduce the activity of the protein. The percentage moisture of substances undergoing glass transitions is generally lower than those undergoing eutectic crystallisations.

The Mechanism of Secondary Drying

As has previously been stated, secondary drying is a desorption process, although the removal of the water of crystallisation to give an anhydrous "crystalline" product is kinetically different. Removing the water of crystallisation is a matter of supplying energy, in the form of heat, to break up the crystal lattice structure and to allow the water molecules to escape.

The desorption process is of more interest. There is a correlation between the relative humidity and the final moisture content of the product. This is illustrated in Figure 1.8. The illustrated curves are isothermal (i.e., they are elements of a family of curves corresponding to the range of possible product temperatures). The higher the product temperature, the lower the final moisture content at a given relative humidity, which may be defined as the pressure of water vapour present as a percentage of the SVP.

The system partial pressure of water vapour is a function of the condenser temperature and will correspond to the SVP of water vapour at the condenser temperature, providing the product is not evolving water vapour. The relative humidity, with respect to the product, will be defined by the partial pressure of water vapour above the condenser as a percentage of the SVP at the product temperature. Ultimately, relative humidity is the ratio of the SVPs at the two temperatures. Pressure gradients cause the desorption of moisture in a

Figure 1.8. Desorbtion isotherms during secondary drying.

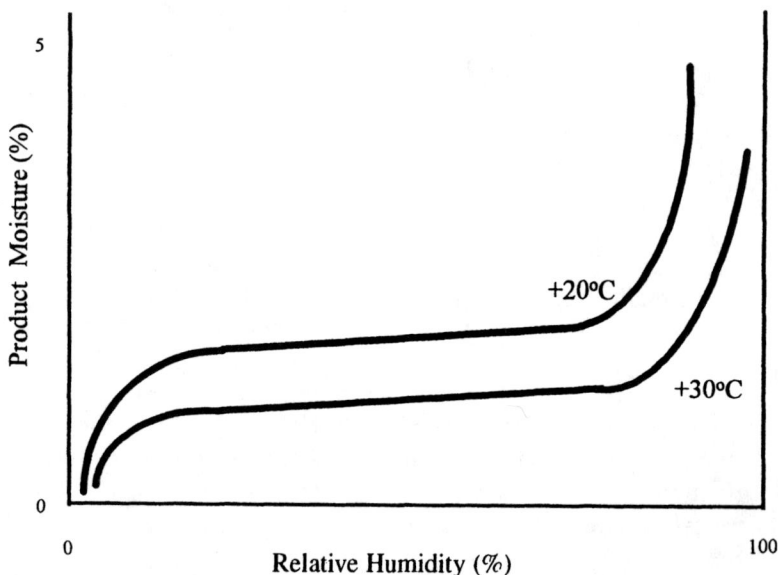

similar method to the evolution of sublimed moisture during primary drying. The final moisture content of the product will be achieved by desorption down the desorption isotherm until the pressure gradient is insufficient to cause more water molecules to desorb.

The higher the product temperature, the higher the SVP and, at a given condenser temperature, the lower the relative humidity. It can, therefore, be seen that the higher the secondary drying product temperature, the lower the final moisture content. It is also apparent that the lower the condenser temperature, the lower the final moisture content. The condenser temperature is usually fixed at its ultimate temperature, so final product temperature can be used to control the final moisture content of the product.

The operating parameters are similar to primary drying. Providing that primary drying is completed there is no advantage in slowly increasing the temperature of the product. In secondary drying a conservative approach to raising the shelf temperature does no harm; it merely prolongs the cycle. The correct shelf temperature profile is usually an immediate rise to the final drying temperature.

The desorption process is not instantaneous and equilibrium must be reached. Secondary drying times are usually 30 percent of the primary drying time.

A common error is to programme the freeze dryer to verify the end of secondary drying with a pressure rise test and then to cool the shelves in order to store the product until it can be processed further. This results in the product moving to a lower temperature desorption isotherm, reabsorbing moisture, and having a moisture content greater than expected. If a storage temperature is set into the freeze drying cycle, it should be preceded by stoppering.

If the product is removed from the freeze dryer without stoppering, (e.g., in a bulk application), then the product will rapidly absorb moisture from the atmosphere. In this case, reabsorption is caused by an increase in the humidity of the air rather than a decrease in product temperature.

During secondary drying small amounts of moisture are evolved and the heat transfer requirement is far lower, despite the product temperature being elevated above that attained during primary drying. Radiant heat becomes more important and can supply sufficient heat for this part of the process. For this reason the air injection system is either shut off or the set point reduced so that a higher vacuum is present. Convective heating, therefore, largely stops, and radiative, and conductive, heating becomes predominant.

The low requirement for heat during secondary drying can be illustrated by considering the freeze drying of 100 g of a 1 percent w/w solution of sodium chloride. In this case, 99 g of water will sublime during primary drying, composed of 94.8 g of pure ice and 4.2 g of eutectic ice. Sodium chloride will crystallize as the dihydrate $NaCl \cdot 2H_2O$. Water accounts for approximately 40 percent of the crystal so only 0.4 g of water would be evolved during secondary drying.

The advantage associated with shutting off the air injection system is that the incoming gas would not be completely dry, and this supplied moisture would increase the system water vapour pressure. It is also true that a higher vacuum will result in fewer noncondensable gas molecules being present to interfere with the process. The vacuum may be slightly spoiled by the use of the air injection system to prevent backstreaming, although backstreaming is rare in freeze drying. Vacuum levels should be far lower than those in primary drying.

Completion of Secondary Drying

The only way to determine the end of secondary drying, during cycle optimisation, is by the pressure rise test. The pressure rise will be smaller than a test that is performed at the end of primary drying. However, a pressure rise test during secondary drying does not have the danger of the product temperature rising and, as there is no ice present, there is no possibility of melting. The test can, therefore, be conducted with a longer time base in order to gain accuracy.

The final moisture content will be a function of product temperature and condenser temperature, providing that equilibrium has been achieved. If drying is complete, and there are no heat losses caused by vapour flow, then the product temperature is identical to the shelf temperature. The optimum method of reproducibly obtaining a desired final moisture content, in production, is by the use of a reproducible, validated cycle operating on a product with little batch-to-batch variation.

Although the final moisture can be determined by the shelf temperature, it will invariably rise to a higher value, often to a value as high as 2 percent by desorption of moisture from the stopper.

Machine Status

The freeze dryer operates in grossly the same way during secondary drying as it does during primary drying. The only difference is that the air injection system is usually shut off. Older machines often had a phosphorus pentoxide trap that was introduced into the vapour flow during secondary drying. The low temperatures achieved with modern condensers negate this requirement.

ANCILLARY FUNCTIONS

It has previously been discussed that the three elements of freezing, primary drying, and secondary drying comprise the nucleus of the freeze drying process. However, in order to translate these elements into a practical cycle, the ancillary functions must be addressed. Freeze drying technology is addressing the time taken to perform these functions. Clean-in-place (CIP), defrost, and sterilisation can now be undertaken at the same time, which will considerably shorten batch turnaround time. Sophisticated loading systems will not only reduce the time spent loading and unloading the freeze dryer, but their use may also reduce the loss of activity if thermolabile molecules are being processed. The in-cycle ancillary functions of backfilling, aeration, and stoppering are briefly discussed. These ancillary functions are shown in Figure 1.1 on page 9.

Sterilisation

The topic of sterilisation is dealt with, in detail, in chapter 6. In general, a new freeze dryer that is intended to freeze dry parenterals must be steam sterilisable. It is unlikely that the regulatory authorities would accept a nonsterilisable plant, and steam sterilisation is usually the method of choice.

It is important to realise that it is the plant that is sterilised, not the product. The product is sterilised by other means. The requirement for the product to remain in the freeze dryer, without closure, in excess of 24 hours demands a great attention to design to assure complete sterilisation of the entire potential product contact area, especially dead legs.

Pure steam, generated from water for injection (WFI, United States Pharmacopeia XXII, or Europharm equivalent) should be used for a steam sterilisable freeze dryer, as filtered boiler steam leaves rust deposits that are a potential source of contamination.

A recent innovation is the use of cooling jackets on the chamber and doors. If these are used in conjunction with mechanical cooling of the shelves, then the time taken to cool after steam sterilisation may be reduced from the region of 6 hours to approximately $1-1^1/_2$ hours. The cooling media is, by necessity, silicone oil. The use of water as a cooling medium is not advised as any retention would result in freezing, with possible damage to the jacket. A complete steam sterilisation cycle will usually take between 7–9 hours or 2–4 hours for a plant fitted with cooling jackets.

Defrosting

Defrosting, or deicing, is the removal of ice that has collected on the condenser. Modern industrial scale plants usually have coil condensers; the techniques employed will also work on plate condensers. There are four main methods of defrosting, these can be used on either separate (external) or in-chamber (internal) condensers:

1. Hot air

2. Flood and flow

3. Spray

4. Steam

The introduction of hot air may be used as a heat source to defrost the condenser. Air, heated by electric resistance, is blown through the condenser by an impeller. The process is neither efficient nor rapid due to the low heat capacity of air. Additionally, the air is generally nonsterile and contamination is bound to occur, although sterility is not an issue if the plant is to be sterilised after defrosting. It is for these reasons that hot air defrosting is rarely encountered. The advantage of this method is that it leaves a dry condenser after defrosting.

The flood and flow method fills the condenser with water and progresses by either spilling the excess water or draining and refilling. The design of the condenser must be such that the top of the condensation coils is below the bottom of the vapour duct to the chamber, or the vapour duct is angled downward toward the condenser, in order to prevent flooding the chamber and clean room. Process efficiency is increased by the use of hot water but this is not essential. If the freeze dryer is not to be sterilised after defrosting then WFI should be used. The disadvantages of the technique are the large volume of WFI used and the increase in weight of the freeze dryer due to the water. This increase can be in the order of several tonnes and floor load bearing becomes important. The advantage is that the technique is quick and performs some cleaning action within the condenser.

Spray was the most common method of defrosting, up to 1991. The technique incorporates either a rotating spray ball or a bar fitted with several static spray heads. Defrost water is constantly drained through the condenser drain valve. The water flow may be in-line filtered, but the use of WFI is preferred, unless sterilisation is to follow defrosting. Water temperature is largely irrelevant although hot water will speed up the process. The cleaning action is maximised, the condenser coils can occupy all of the condenser shell, and floor loading is not significantly increased.

The advent of the almost universal requirement for steam sterilisable freeze dryers and the preference of the regulatory authorities for sterilising before every cycle have resulted in the use of steam for defrosting. Steam is very efficient, searching, quick, and performs an efficient cleaning action. It is normal that defrosting is undertaken as part of the steam sterilising cycle. While ice is defrosting, it is impossible for the condenser drain probe to approach 121.5°C, or for the system pressure to approach the corresponding steam pressure of 2.1 bar$_a$. Consequently, exposure time will not start until all the ice has defrosted and the plant is fully up to temperature. Steam defrosting is the most prevalent method of defrosting in modern plants.

Drum condensers, usually found in laboratory freeze dryers, may be defrosted by other methods. A heater tape can be used to supply heat. Alternatively, a hot gas bypass, where the hot refrigerant gas from the refrigeration compressor passes through the cooling coils outside the drum, can be used. In the case of vertical drum condensers, these may be defrosted by pouring hot water into the condenser. The heater tape is obviously unsuitable for a coil condenser. The use of a hot gas bypass on a coil condenser results in ice falling off the coils. This ice collects at the bottom of the condenser and the ice fragments can freeze together, blocking the drain valve. The use of hot water is similar to the flood and flow method.

Typically, defrosting is not a time-consuming process. Defrosting by hot air may take several hours, but the water or steam methods achieve a total defrost in approximately 20 minutes.

Cleaning/CIP

There can be no doubt that, with the possible exception of validation, CIP systems have caused the most debate within the freeze drying community. Cleaning has always been a necessity, but a manual clean cannot be validated. Unfortunately, CIP has not successfully translated into the freeze dryer, and an automatic, validatable system is not yet available.

The first parameter that must be defined is the nature of the soil. A light dusting of material that has ablated from the lyophilisation of a true solution (i.e., is extremely soluble) is removed far easily than a product that has burnt on or has a hydrophobic component. The question of what the CIP system is attempting to remove is a variable; no guarantee can be given concerning the effectiveness of cleaning.

There are four methods of CIP that have been developed for freeze dryers:

1. Spray bar

2. Spray balls

3. Flood

4. CIP/SIP (steam-in-place)

Spray bars and spray balls work in similar ways. These two methods depend on the spraying of a cleaning fluid(s) through a bar containing nozzles or through revolving spray balls. Steam admission during sterilisation is by the same route, thus ensuring that the inside of the spray bars and the nozzles are sterilised.

CIP was originally developed in the dairy and brewing industries for the cleaning of tanks and pipes that were relatively free from obstructions. The shelf arrangement in the freeze drying chamber, which is a combination of horizontal shelves and vertical shelf supports with diagonal shelf hoses, causes areas that will be in the shadow of other items during the use of a spray. Consequently, they will not be cleaned to the same extent. There is no system that can give a guarantee of 100 percent coverage, never mind a 100 percent clean using a spray system. The question also exists, even in the best-designed system, "Are you pushing the insoluble material into a corner from which it cannot be swept away and where it will reside?" It is also important to ensure that the back of the nozzles and spray bar are effectively cleaned, which is not an insignificant task. The other drawbacks of this system are the vast quantities of cleaning and rinse fluids that are utilised, a final total of 3–4 m^3 would not be unusual for a medium-sized machine.

Various refinements are added; for instance, the drain valve may remain shut and the plant partially filled with the cleaning solution, the shelves may then rise and lower into this liquid using their stoppering mechanism. Floor loading then becomes important as you could have an extra 2 tonnes or more of cleaning fluid residing in the freeze dryer. The various spray bars (usually 4 in the chamber and 1 in the condenser) can be sequenced to avoid a peak load on the supply system and the condenser spray system can double up as a defrosting system. The drain valve must be increased in size, and from a civil side a 100 mm drain, with an air break, becomes obligatory.

If sterilisation is not to follow CIP, then thought must be given to the drying of the chamber as, unless the final rinse is at elevated temperature, the water ring pump is not effective and the only resort is to cool the condenser. The result of this is that the cycle must be started with a layer of ice on the condenser. Additionally, WFI would have to be used as the medium, raising the cost.

The flood system is exactly as it sounds. The drawbacks are the difficulties of cleaning the roof of the chamber, floor loading, and drying. In addition there is a requirement for some form of scouring of the surfaces to effect a clean. Scouring does not occur with a flood system, which should be regarded as a solubility clean.

In SIP/CIP system, the condensate from steam will solubilise, at elevated temperatures, the soil and wash it away. Full coverage is attained, there is a (gentle) scouring effect, and there are no floor loading and drying problems. The process can be enhanced by precooling the shelves to obtain more condensate. It has been reported that shelf cooling can increase the condensate generated by approximately 40 percent. This condensate is formed on the shelves and falls to the floor, the areas that have the greatest probability of contamination. SIP/CIP is probably the most effective method of cleaning, although the scouring action is suspect; however a process guarantee cannot be given.

Probably the most telling point is that only relatively small amounts of liquid are involved. In the case where a toxic substance is involved, then it is possible to collect the spent waste and decontaminate it. This is balanced by the impossibility of putting any form of detergent or solubilising material in the steam.

The most apparent advantage of a SIP/CIP system is that the ancillary functions of defrosting, cleaning, and sterilisation can be combined in one operation.

Validation of a CIP system is difficult, but can be split into two sections:

1. Coverage where you would validate by covering the inside of the chamber with a dye and then visually ensuring that the dye was removed by the CIP process. The dyes used are usually fluorescein or riboflavin.

2. Cleaning where the material to be processed would be used to challenge the clean. Monitoring is by swabbing the inside of the machine; effluent monitoring is not satisfactory. It is important that the actual soil is used for the validation process, as different materials will behave in different ways.

Manual cleaning is still the usual method. Most installed CIP systems are not used routinely. Particular care should be taken, during a manual clean, with the underside of shelves, where there is often a buildup of silicone from stoppers. This sticky layer can lift vials after stoppering, or can remove stoppers from vials. A manual clean can often be facilitated by judicious use of the stoppering system.

Loading/Unloading

Loading increases in complexity as the size of the freeze dryer increases. Small freeze dryers, with shelf areas up to 8 m^2 are usually loaded by hand. Larger freeze dryers often utilise a loading and unloading trolley. The largest freeze dryers often utilise a sophisticated loading and unloading system and may incorporate single height, shelf-by-shelf loading.

The limiting factor in the loading process is usually the speed of the filling line. This will cause the problem that filled material can reside in the vial at ambient temperature for several hours, causing loss of activity in thermolabile species. It is simple to control the temperature of the fill in the holding tank, but it is more difficult once the fill has been dispensed into vials. Thermolabile products will exhibit a lower activity in the first vials filled unless the temperature of the fill is controlled by some method. Unless filling proceeds in a temperature-controlled environment, the most effective method of temperature control is to place the vials on the thermoregulated shelves of the freeze dryer as quickly as possible.

The height of the top shelf and the depth of the shelves can also cause practical problems on manual loading systems. The bottom shelf must be of a sufficient height to still be in the laminar flow region of the clean room HEPA filtering system.

Consideration must be given to the number and type of product trays. It is not unusual to have one set in use, one set being cleaned and autoclaved, and a third set in the engineering department being straightened after they have buckled during autoclaving. Aluminium trays are lighter and may be made of thicker gauge metal than stainless steel, and have excellent conductive properties, but the use of aluminium is not favoured. Stainless steel trays can distort badly unless they are made of heavy gauge sheeting, in which case, they are heavy and difficult to handle.

Manual Systems

Manual systems usually require the operators to place trays of vials on the shelves; unloading is the opposite process. The trays can have bottoms but the use of trays where the bottom can be slid out to leave the vials in a fence is popular. This fence method allows for a better thermal contact between the shelf and the vial and obviates tray bottom distortion problems. The use of fences is mainly restricted to manual systems. Trays, or fences, can be clipped together so that the removal of trays from the rear of the shelf is facilitated.

If necessary, a small freeze dryer may be loaded one shelf at a time. The shelf temperature may be low or even below 0°C, and the door is closed after each shelf is loaded. This will allow some retardation of temperature dependant activity loss, without causing a heavy frosting of the chamber from humid air in the clean area.

Bulk loads that are charged as a liquid fill are usually pumped into a bottomed tray residing on the shelf. Pellets or prills are loaded in the same way as vials into bottomed trays, which are then loaded into the freeze dryer.

Trolley Systems

Trolley systems, often called loading carts, are used for medium- and large-scale freeze dryers. These may be simple, have multiple levels corresponding to the freeze dryer shelf heights, and are manually loaded. When they are securely docked to the freeze dryer, the trays are then manually pushed onto the freeze dryer shelves from static levels. The product trays are clipped together and unloading is achieved by pulling the trays back onto the corresponding level in the trolley. Trolley systems are not usually suitable for bottomless trays.

Additional sophistication may be present in that the trolleys may be electrically powered. This power could drive the trolley, push and pull the product trays on and off the shelves, and supply a HEPA–filtered laminar airflow over the cart contents. The trolley motors must be sealed and are usually battery driven. The sealed for life batteries charge at the docking points at the filling line and the freeze dryer and are only used during transit. Power for loading and unloading is directly through the docking point. The use of systems that require a cable are becoming less popular.

A criticism of these systems is that the trays sliding over the shelves can generate particles. Systems exist that will use lips on the side of the product trays as a means of support. The loading trolley can then raise the trays by a few millimetres, insert them into the freeze dryer on an extending, wheeled rack, and then lower them onto the shelves. This method is wasteful of the freeze dryer shelf area, as an unused space must be left for the frame to enter the freeze dryer.

If the product is thermolabile, then the loading cart may fill the freeze dryer one shelf at a time. This is known as constant height loading and is usually achieved by indexing the shelves to a datum height and sequentially loading at this height. The loading cart only requires one level, and the loading height of the freeze dryer is the same as that of the filling line. It is, therefore, possible to automatically load the cart. If batch turnaround time is quick, a second, multilevel cart may be used to unload the freeze dryer in one operation. This cart, in sophisticated systems, may index down to mate each level sequentially with the capping line. Less sophisticated systems rely on manual unloading of the unloading cart.

In order to avoid frosting of the chamber, a smaller, but shelf width, door is fitted within the main door at the loading height. Loading takes place through this subdoor and unloading takes place through the main door. Alternatively, the freeze dryer may be double ended and be loaded through a small door on an otherwise solid chamber wall, and unloaded through a fully sized door on the other side of the chamber.

If the trolleys are to be used for more than one freeze dryer, then the floor flatness and shelf levels become critical.

Loading Systems

Whilst CIP has possibly caused the greatest debate within the freeze drying community, there can be little doubt that the latest technological advance is in the field of loading systems. The previous technological advance, control systems, is now increasing in sophistication as computing power and software support platforms become more advanced. Loading systems are the new technology and make use of the control technology.

Loading systems are usually fitted to the largest installations because of price considerations, but systems are now installed that can load (and unload) vials directly onto the shelf, without trays or fences,

with no human intervention. The peopleless clean area, or at least total utilisation of isolation technology, is now available.

It is usual that these systems are custom-made for a particular installation. They usually are composed of modules that are connected
by loading carts running on tracks, although automated guided vehi-
cles (AGVs) are possible. The total trayless system will be composed of
some or all of the following modules:

- A collecting area that is attached to the end of the filling line,
  with a buffer zone.

- A transfer system to transfer the vials to a loading cart. This
  may be a push bar, a vibrating table, or a frame mechanism.

- A loading transfer cart that will run on tracks, or is an AGV,
  which will usually load at constant height, although indexing,
  multiple height variants have been manufactured. The cart
  usually employs a frame with a gate that will load the vials
  onto the shelf and then withdraw.

- In the case of constant height loading, or pass-through chambers, a second cart is usually employed for single operation
  unloading. This cart will be multiple level and may index for
  the capping line.

- If an indexing unloading cart is not used, an indexing holding
  area that will feed the vials to the capping line is used.

The systems are computer controlled and interface with the freeze
dryer control system in order to open the freeze dryer door or index
the shelves.

Important considerations in design are floor flatness, shelf flatness, shelf positioning, and, as near as possible, a linear materials flow
with any change in direction being at right angles. Shelf positioning is
critical, usually to within a fraction of a millimetre and hydraulic creep
is a factor in hydraulic stoppering systems. The deflection of a shelf
under load is important, and shelf edges are usually machined to a
square edge rather than being radiused.

Ironically, the use of trays diminishes some of the engineering
problems, but adds the additional complication of putting the gate on
the tray without human intervention or placing the vials within a tray
with four solid sides. This apart, presently there are more installed systems using trays than trayless systems.

Backfilling

Backfilling is also known as preaeration and consists of filling the
vial with a known pressure of inert gas, through the freeze dryer's

sterilising filter, after the completion of secondary drying and prior to stoppering. This operation is usually performed automatically and consists of stopping the vacuum pump and filling the chamber and condenser with the inert gas at the chosen pressure. The normal back-fill specification is between 500 and 900 mbar of dry nitrogen. It is possible to stopper under vacuum by omitting the backfilling step, and many products utilise this method.

There are several advantages in incorporating backfilling into the freeze drying process. The same advantages also apply for a vacuum stoppering regimen. The backfill is inert and prevents oxidation during storage. The pressure is less than atmospheric pressure, which prevents the stoppers from popping out after stoppering and prior to capping; in addition the partial vacuum makes the introduction of the reconstitution medium easier, and reduces frothing during this introduction.

Ideally, backfilling should occur when the shelf temperature is above ambient because of considerations already discussed under secondary drying. A higher temperature will also ensure that the pressure within the vial will fall when the vial is removed from the freeze dryer, as dictated by Charles Law. An extreme combination of a low shelf temperature during backfilling, a high backfill pressure specification, and low atmospheric pressure during storage could result in a positive pressure within the vial.

Stoppering

Stoppering is the closing of the shelves by hydraulic, or other, means that will push the partially inserted stoppers fully into the vials, thus effecting a seal. Some regulatory authorities do not recognise this seal until an aluminium cap has been added to provide a positive locking of the stopper within the vial. This capping takes place outside the freeze dryer.

The same shelf temperature considerations as during backfilling apply. After stoppering the shelf temperature may be reduced to a storage temperature prior to unloading; however this is preferably done after aeration. For this reason stoppering should normally be performed automatically, but a surprising number of standard operating procedures (SOPs) call for manual stoppering. There is no advantage in stoppering manually. Stoppering mechanisms are considered in more detail in chapter 2.

Aeration

Aeration is the release of vacuum at the end of the cycle, which makes it possible to open the freeze dryer door. As most clean areas operate at positive pressure, it is essential that the gas used for aeration is from the clean area or at this pressure, as only a few pascals difference in pressure will result in it being impossible to open the door. The aeration medium is usually air and passes through the sterilising filter, so the supply from the clean area is not essential for sterility. In actuality, a pipework to the clean area causes problems in that it is not sterilised by the freeze dryer sterilisation cycle and is not likely to be penetrated during gassing of the clean area.

PROBLEM AREAS

Product Problems

It is unfortunate, but true, that a freeze-dried product may occasionally come out of the freeze dryer with characteristics that were not desired. This situation is usually more prevalent during cycle development and optimisation than during production.

If the suspect batch was a standard production run, then it is necessary to look for unusual events within the freeze drying cycle; alternatively, a batch variation could be suspected. Whilst these events may be expensive in terms of lost product, the cause is usually easily traceable. More difficult problems are found when a product is in development or is a one-off sample. In this case, the cycle, formulation, and sample concentration must be investigated. Fortunately, it is usually possible to alter these parameters, at this stage, without causing conflict with the regulatory authorities.

Many symptoms of incorrect freeze drying are merely cosmetic and do not affect the efficacy of the product. This is not always the case; gross melting could cause loss of a product from the drying container. Therefore, it is advisable to develop a cycle that will give a homogenous cake, as this will indicate the consistency of quality required within most markets.

Formulation and cycle development are complex subjects that require a great deal of knowledge and a large database to perform correctly. It is not the intention to discuss formulation here. The pitfalls of having an incorrect parameter in the freeze drying cycle are surprisingly few, and the vast majority fall into ten categories:

1. Low product concentration
2. Incomplete solidification
3. Skin formation
4. Poor ice crystal formation
5. Melting

6. Collapse

7. Inadequate primary drying

8. Scorching

9. Opalescence

10. Inadequate secondary drying

These categories relate to the freeze drying of the product. There are other problems that may be caused during stoppering, aeration, or inadequate storage prior to freezing or after freeze drying.

Low Product Concentration

Whilst this is not a freeze drying cycle parameter, it is not an uncommon problem. At very low product concentrations, the structure of the residual cake is very fine and does not possess sufficient strength to survive the handling of the vial. The result is that the cake disintegrates into a powder that distributes itself around the internal surfaces of the vial. This will only occur at very low concentrations, as is illustrated by domestic water, from a hard water area, having a sufficient solids content to form a stable cake of calcium salts when freeze dried. The obvious remedies are to increase the concentration but maintain the dosage by reducing the volume, or, if this is impracticable, to add an excipient to allow a solid, less friable cake.

Incomplete Solidification

Incomplete solidification is caused by not having a sufficiently low temperature during freezing. The cake will appear to be solid, but complete solidification will not have occurred. The usual cause is that the solidification point is below the shelf temperature, but the cause may be insufficient time at the freezing temperature.

Once a vacuum is applied, the semifrozen cake will lift and the free liquid will boil, giving symptoms similar to that of melting. In marginal cases, it is possible that evaporative cooling may induce complete solidification in the remaining mass. If liquid is present, then the end product will not look attractive; the danger of loss of product still exists. Amorphous products may collapse at the product surface, causing an impermeable layer, loss of evaporative cooling, and complete melting.

The simple remedy is to freeze at a lower temperature; if this is not possible then the answer is usually to reformulate so that the formulation has a higher solidification point. It may be possible to prefreeze in liquid nitrogen and to load onto cold shelves. The liquid nitrogen may induce crystallisation, which may persist on warming. Liquid nitrogen freezing and transfer is logistically difficult for large batches and is not a preferred production technique unless the shelves themselves are ultimately cooled by liquid nitrogen.

Skin Formation

Skin formation is often associated with heterogeneous ice formation, small diameter containers, or high solids content. As the ice forms, it expands. This expansion will displace the remaining liquid. As the liquid is contained at the sides and bottom by the vial, it is forced to rise to the surface of the semifrozen mass and will flood this surface. Upon complete solidification, this frozen skin may act as an impermeable layer, preventing the escape of water vapour and reducing or stopping evaporative cooling. The result is that the product melts or collapses. This is a very common problem within freeze drying.

A skin formed on a bulk product often breaks away and skims around the product surface like a hovercraft. The skin is supported on the water vapour evolving from the product below.

If skin formation is apparent, this may be reduced, or eliminated, by altering the freezing rate, thermal treatment, adding a small amount of ethanol to the formulation, or reformulation. If a narrow diameter container is used, then consideration should be given to a larger alternative, although this will reduce the containers per batch within a given freeze dryer.

Poor Ice Crystal Formation

Homogenous and heterogeneous ice formation has previously been discussed. Whilst heterogeneous ice formation itself is not detrimental to the appearance of the dried product, it will slow down the freeze drying process and could cause other problems (e.g., melting). The remedy is to alter the freezing rate or to introduce a thermal treatment step into the freeze drying cycle.

Melting

In the case of a solute that will crystallize, a product temperature above the incipient melting point will cause partial liquefaction. This will normally occur in the base of the vial or tray contents—the warmest part of the frozen cake.

If this melting occurs during sublimation, often due to an excessive shelf temperature, then the likelihood is that the liquid will boil and the vapour will not be able to escape at a sufficient rate. The frozen cake above the liquefied area will therefore lift. In the case, where melting is marginal, it is possible that the vial contents will settle, leaving a ring around the top of the parallel walls of the vial. The uneven base of the cake will slow down heat transfer and freeze drying may go to completion. In this case, the cake at the base of the vial will be pockmarked. The extreme scenario is that the whole cake will eventually melt and boil, totally destroying or losing the product.

The obvious remedy is to reduce the shelf temperature, which will slow down heat transfer and allow a lower product temperature. However shelf temperature is often not the primary cause of melting. The thermal balance that produces a stable product temperature during primary drying is achieved by balancing the heat input from the shelf against the evaporative cooling caused by the ice subliming. If evaporative cooling is impeded, then this balance will not occur and there will be an increase in sensible heat until the product melts. Therefore, it is advantageous to investigate why evaporative cooling may be impeded, rather than reduce shelf temperature and slow down the freeze drying process. Reformulation to give a product that will freeze dry at a higher temperature is beneficial in that freeze drying may proceed more rapidly but it is not an answer to melting. Melting is caused by heating too strongly or by a physical barrier to vapour evolution.

Collapse

The literature on this subject is vast and only a brief explanation is attempted. Collapse is a feature of materials that undergo a glass transition and occurs at the freeze drying interface when the dendritic ice is sublimed at a product temperature above the collapse temperature. The concentrated solution does not have sufficient viscosity to support its own structure without the additional support of the pure ice that had previously locked it into place. When pure ice is sublimed away, the viscous liquid flows into the cavities in the interface and collapses, followed by puffing up due to boiling. This leaves a layer that usually acts as a barrier and reduces evaporative cooling. The product gains sensible heat and the usual chain of events will occur.

Collapse always occurs at the same temperature as solidification. There is no hysteresis effect as is the case with freezing and melting. Although the mechanism of collapse is quite different to that of melting, the causative agents and the remedies are similar.

Inadequate Primary Drying

If a product is removed from the freeze dryer prior to the completion of primary drying, then any ice present will melt as the vial temperature rises and redissolve the dried layers around it. This will leave holes in the freeze-dried cake, which are often described as looking like Swiss cheese. Inadequate primary drying is also characterised by cold vials when removed from the freeze dryer.

If the product is frozen for long periods and heat transfer is initially slow, it is possible for the cake to shrink slightly. If there is any tendency for the product to stick to the glass, this would cause a void at the base of the cake that would reduce heat transfer and slow drying. It is possible that this would only occur in a proportion of the vials in the batch. A tray that has buckled during autoclaving will have the same effect. If the tray is not fully in contact with the shelf, then heat transfer will be reduced in the affected portion. The vials on this section will receive less heat than their companions and dry more slowly.

If, as is usual, secondary drying is to be performed, then the elevated temperatures during secondary drying will cause melting. The melting is usually minimal, except in cases of gross mismanagement, and is usually manifested as a minor scalloping at the cake base. This is probably the most common fault in freeze drying. A pressure rise test to determine the end of primary drying will obviate this problem.

Scorching

Scorching occurs when the secondary drying temperature is above the denaturation temperature of the dry product. The etymology is obvious. The remedy is to reduce the shelf temperature during secondary drying.

Opalescence

Opalescence on reconstitution is often blamed on backstreaming. Backstreaming occurs when vacuum pump oil migrates into the freeze dryer by molecular flow. The high vacuum and low water vapour pressure experienced during secondary drying are the ideal conditions for this to occur. In actuality, backstreaming rarely occurs in freeze drying, and any oil molecules would have to undergo a tortuous path to contaminate the product. If backstreaming does occur, the amount of vacuum pump oil that enters a single vial is scarcely detectable, and certainly not observable. If backstreaming is proven, then the fitting of a Rootes pump upstream of the vacuum pump will prevent the passage of oil by the physical turning of the rotors.

The more normal reason for opalescence on reconstitution is due to the aggregation of molecules to form particles that are large enough to scatter light. This aggregation is caused by too high a secondary drying temperature. The problem is particularly evident for products containing proteins, salts, and sugars, or those containing sodium alginate. A reduction in shelf temperature, at the cost of a lower final moisture content, is the solution.

Inadequate Secondary Drying

The result of inadequate secondary drying, in terms of either time or temperature, is an excessive final moisture content that will reduce shelf life. This problem will only become apparent after analysis and accelerated storage trials. An increase in drying time or shelf temperature will obtain the required result.

Product Probe Placement

It is necessary to control the freeze drying cycle by the three parameters of time, shelf temperature, and vacuum. There have been many attempts to create control systems that use the temperature of the product to control the cycle. These systems do not work well and should only be used as a warning to reduce shelf temperature, not as a method of calling for more heat or to determine end points. The reason for this inadequacy is the paucity of information gathered from the product probes. This information is inadequate for two reasons:

1. The vial that contains the probe is atypical by the fact that it contains the probe.

2. There is a temperature gradient within the frozen cake, so probe position is critical.

The introduction of a temperature probe into a vial has many effects on the freeze drying characteristics of that vial. The product depth will increase by displacement, which will alter the slope of the temperature gradient within the vial, giving it different heat transfer characteristics to the average vial. If the probe is resting on the base of the vial, then it could act as an insulator that would also alter heat transfer rates.

The probe wire will act as a conductor of heat, allowing additional heat into the cake in the same way that a skewer placed through a potato will reduce its baking time. The probe wire will also disturb the ice structure by acting as a nucleation centre, inducing early nucleation during freezing, and also by acting as a fracture plane that will allow enhanced vapour flow. The probe carries an electric current that will add heat to the product.

Because of the difficulty associated with placing a vial containing a probe into a freeze dryer, the vial is almost always on the edge of a shelf. It is well known that vials on the edge of a shelf dry more quickly than those in the centre. The reasons for this are radiative heat input from the chamber walls, easier vapour flow paths, and a lower partial pressure of water vapour on the edge of the shelf.

The freeze drying process will be slowed down by the increased product depth and insulating properties of the probe, and speeded up by all the other points, the nett effect is to speed up the process. If the probe is being used for end point determination, then it is apparent that the process is being controlled by the fastest drying vials. This is a sure recipe for melting or incomplete drying, unless a large enough temperature margin is built into the algorithm to render the system of limited value.

Temperature information is also inexact, as a temperature gradient is present in the cake. The temperature recorded is a function of the position of the probe. This can be illustrated by the way that some temperature probes always lead or lag behind the majority if multiple probes are used. An averaging system assists in obtaining accuracy, but does not negate the shortcomings of the product probe. The temperature gradients in the cake are shown in Figure 1.9.

In any case, what should be measured? If the necessary product characteristics are known, the freeze drying interface temperature is useful to determine if collapse is about to occur. However, the interface is constantly moving downwards, and the probe is immobile. The temperature at the base of the vial would indicate incipient melting, but a probe touching the bottom of the vial would give an erroneous reading and affect heat transfer.

Figure 1.9. Product temperature gradient during sublimation.

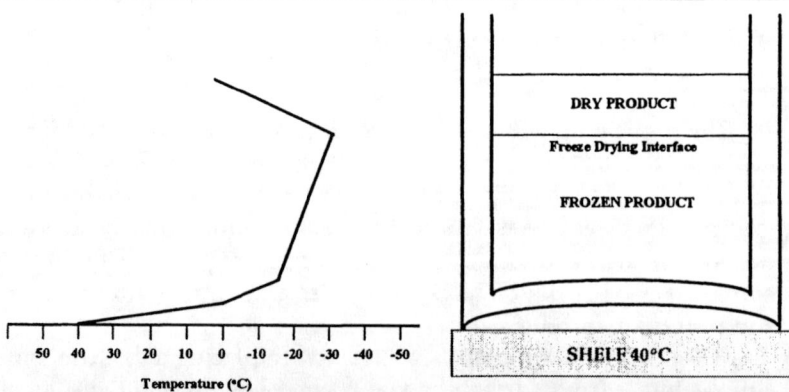

The only time that a product temperature probe can be trusted is at a steady state condition during the hold period of freezing, when there are no temperature gradients or evaporative cooling effects. In the production cycle, there is no substitute for a reproducible, validated cycle. During sublimation, a probe could be used to indicate that there was little or no change in product temperature during a transient power failure, but it has little other value.

Solvents

The use of organic solvents within a freeze-dried formulation is not a new concept; however, particularly in development, it appears to be on the increase. The use of solvents is usually an attempt to increase the solubility of the molecule of interest, but many formulations contain small percentages of solvents as a carryover from previous processing steps.

The incorporation of small quantities of solvents are not usually detrimental, even though the appearance of the freeze-dried cake may be adversely affected. A general rule is that an organic solvent content of up to 5 percent may be tolerated; at higher percentages problems become apparent. This is not to say that concentrations above this are not possible, but the higher the solvent concentration, the more exacerbated the problems become.

Freeze drying may be defined as the drying of a material by passing the volatile component directly from the solid phase to the gaseous phase, without passing through the liquid phase. This definition implies two things:

1.   That the volatile phase must be frozen.

2.   That liquid phase should not be present.

Solvents that freeze, (e.g., acetic acid, formic acid, or t-butyl alcohol with freezing points of 17°C, 8°C, and 25°C, respectively) are not too problematical for the freeze drying process, but may be for the freeze dryer and the environment. High concentrations of solvents that will not freeze at the temperatures normally encountered in freeze dryers (e.g., ethanol and methanol with freezing points of –114°C and –97°C) are almost impossible to freeze dry.

Industrial freeze dryers usually have a lower shelf temperature capability of between –50°C and –60°C. Ethanol has a freezing point at –114°C and will not freeze. Low concentrations of ethanol may result in a finely dispersed mixture that will appear to be frozen, but at the end of freezing will contain droplets of liquid ethanol. In products with higher concentrations of unfrozen organic solvent, these solvents will be present throughout the frozen constituents, thus giving the appearance of a semifrozen mush. Organic solvent is also likely to be displaced to the top of the cake as ice crystals, which have a larger volume than liquid water, form. This may result in a layer of organic solvent on top of the semifrozen mush that will contain some of the solute.

There is little that can be done to facilitate freezing, as the ultimate temperature is governed by freeze dryer performance. Freezing of the product outside the chamber, (e.g., in liquid nitrogen), will have little effect, as the material will rapidly warm up. It must also be remembered that, in order for freeze drying to progress, the condenser temperature must be below product temperature. Therefore, additional product cooling will not help unless accompanied by an equal drop in condenser temperature. At temperatures where ethanol will be frozen, freeze drying will progress at a very slow rate, resulting in long drying times.

The presence of the liquid phase becomes apparent in primary drying. As the system pressure falls, the liquid phase will boil and froth will form that, in extreme cases, will spill out of the container. The freeze dryer condenser temperature (typically –70°C to –85°C) will condense the organic solvent vapour as a liquid, but will not immobilise it as a solid. The liquid phase will reflux from the condenser chamber base to the condenser coils, whilst applying an appreciable vapour pressure. It should be noted that there is not a large drop in SVP as a substance freezes; organic solvents often have high vapour pressures as they are processed at a temperature far away from their freezing point.

Therefore, it is unlikely that a cosmetically acceptable cake will ever be obtained from a feedstock that contains appreciable amounts of unfrozen organic solvent. However, an advantage may be taken from the characteristics of solvents within the freeze-dried cake. If skin formation is apparent, then the inclusion of a nonfreezing solvent within cake, and therefore, primarily within the skin, will leave discontinuities within the skin once the solvent has evaporated. This disruption to the skin will allow vapour to escape from below and may allow freeze drying to proceed as if the skin were not there.

Once primary drying has ended, there should be little organic solvent left in the system. Frothing and solvent voiding should no longer be issues. Organic solvent that is still present may be associated with the product. Elevated temperatures during secondary drying may result in undesirable chemical reactions between this solvent and the product.

Organic solvent vapours will pass into the vacuum pump during processing. Freeze dryers are usually equipped with twin stage oil seal rotary vacuum pumps. Organic vapours will condense in the oil and cause a breakdown in lubrication, which will cause accelerated wear and premature failure. The ultimate vacuum of the pump will also reduce as the organics come out of the oil during operation. The vacuum pump can be protected by the use of a liquid nitrogen trap. The trap should be piped into the vacuum line downstream of the vacuum valve. It should be valved in such a way that it can be used without the freeze dryer condenser to trap the organic solvent. Once the organic solvent has been trapped, it can then be valved out of the system after the freeze dryer condenser has been switched on.

If the freeze dryer is not equipped with a solvent trap and the process is nonsterile then another possibility is to trap the organic solvent, as a liquid, in the condenser shell, using the freeze dryer condenser then to break vacuum, drain, and restore vacuum.

If feedstocks containing organic solvents are dried in nonsteam sterilisable freeze dryers, then the acrylic doors will "craze", reducing visibility and, in extreme cases, structural strength.

Other considerations that must be taken into account when organic solvents are used in the freeze drying process are flammability and the environment. Many organic solvents are flammable, and the risk of explosion must be taken into account. The vacuum sensors in most freeze dryers are of the hot wire resistance variety (thermoelectric, Pirani, etc.). These sensors must be placed in direct contact with the vacuum in the chamber and, therefore, are in contact with the organic solvent. It is recommended that hot wire resistance vacuum sensors are replaced with a capacitance manometer-type diaphragm gauge. The output from the vacuum pump will contain these organic solvent vapours and the necessity of operating in an explosion-proof environment, including the use of explosion-proofed electric motors and cabinets, must be assessed.

Dependant on the solvent used, the disposal of waste from the process must be considered. The organic solvent will either collect in the condenser as a solid or a liquid or be passed through the vacuum pump as a vapour. The environmental impact and the current regulations concerning the disposal of waste must be addressed.

CONCLUSION

Freeze drying was once a technique poorly understood. There is little that is complicated within the process; most of the complications are found in the formulation of the product to be freeze-dried. The last decade has witnessed a wider appreciation of the physics of the process, and how this is translated into a practical freeze drying cycle. It is now the case that an increasing number of commercial freeze drying cycles has been optimised on a scientific, rather than an intuitive, or empirical, basis. The ancillary activities, and the materials handling techniques, have also undergone a close scrutiny. The result is reflected in an improved product quality that meets the demands of modern pharmaceutical production.

2

THE FREEZE DRYER AND FREEZE DRYER DESIGN

Kevin Murgatroyd

Biopharma Process Systems Ltd.
Winchester, United Kingdom

The freeze dryer (Plate 2.1) is the machine that converts the theory of freeze drying into the reality of the production of a freeze-dried product. The freeze dryer is an unusual item of equipment; it is not generally understood, and it is usually the bottleneck in production flow. Whilst there is little of a highly technical nature within the machine, it incorporates many technologies, thus making maintenance, repair, and spares holding as well as procurement, unusually difficult. Nevertheless, most pharmaceutical companies utilise freeze drying as a production technique for at least one of their products.

The principles of freeze drying are now more readily understood in more detail, and the scientific method is starting to be applied to the optimisation of freeze drying cycles. The implementation of these cycles is made possible by the degree of control that is available with a modern freeze dryer. Shelf temperatures are now controlled to within less than a degree Celsius; vacuum control has equal precision. Sophisticated computer control systems mean that the cycle is always reproducible, and can be automatically documented to the standard now required by both the regulatory authorities and the user's internal requirements.

There have been many milestones in the development of freeze drying design, all of which have had a great impact on the freeze-dried product that have resulted in a product quality and reproducibility

Plate 2.1. Typical pilot freeze dryer.

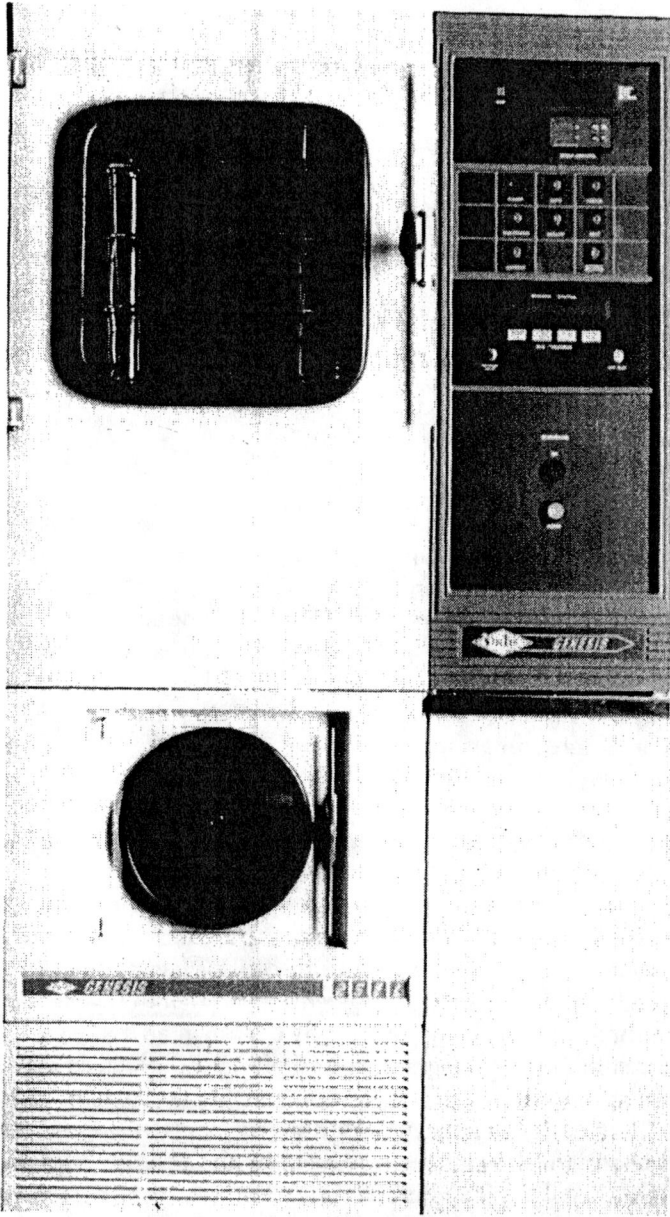

Reproduced by kind permission of the VirTis Company.

that was impossible 20 years ago. Possibly, the biggest step was made in the late 1970s, when the advent of shelf thermoregulation by the circulation of silicone oil, or originally trichloroethylene, made close shelf temperature control possible. Shelf hoses, that had previously carried refrigerant, needed to be rigid as the freon was evaporating within them. Silicone oil made the use of flexible hoses, to and from the shelf, possible, which led to the ability to move the shelves, and, hence, to stopper in the chamber without using bladders.

The early 1980s led to steam sterilisation and the almost universal manufacture of freeze dryers that were constructed from AISI 316L stainless steel, or its local equivalent. The rigours associated with the requirement for the freeze dryer chamber to be a coded pressure vessel ensured the quality and good design of this chamber, the main item of the freeze dryer.

The availability of computers and, to a certain extent, programmable logic controllers (PLCs) had the greatest impact on freeze dryer design and construction. From the mid-1980s on, the degree and sophistication of control became as it is today; actions taken by the machine in the case of alarms and datalogging were important incorporations. The electronic age is here and the technological advances that seem to occur almost daily are incorporated into the freeze dryer control system. Systems are now totally user friendly, often will link with other popular software packages for data handling, and can interface with other parts of the process or the building management system. Networking and modems mean that it is now no longer necessary for the operator to be by the plant. Whilst it is not desirable to attend to a problem on a freeze dryer at 3 A.M., it is preferable to do it through a modem link on a laptop computer rather than going to the plant to diagnose and rectify the problem.

In the late 1980s and early 1990s it became necessary not only for a product to be of high quality, which was already achieved, but also to have the paperwork to prove it. Specifically, this was a time when some of the onus was transferred to suppliers, because the pharmaceutical industry had already been performing these tasks. Freeze dryers were no exception; it was difficult for a manufacturer of what were virtually "one-offs" to produce the quality of paperwork that was now necessary. The major freeze dryer manufacturers responded to the challenge and the documentation that is supplied with the plant is now of a high standard and gives all the necessary information.

The Montreal Protocol was, at this time, addressing the depletion of the ozone layer. Many of the refrigerants used in freeze dryers, notably R13b1 and R502, were no longer available for use. Europe phased out R13b1 by the end of 1993 and R502 by the end of 1994, the other signatories of the Montreal protocol followed a year later. The refrigeration industry, after a slow start, is now producing alternative refrigerants, but the intervening years were difficult. The freeze drying community still demanded the low temperatures, on both the shelf and the condenser, which they had previously enjoyed. Liquid nitrogen was investigated as an alternative and is a viable proposition for many plants. Hydrofluorocarbons (HFCs) now seem to be the way forward.

Development is concentrating in many areas, and it is difficult to see what the next major design step will be. Loading systems, end point determinations, new materials, and energy saving are some of the likely candidates.

THE PHARMACEUTICAL FREEZE DRYER

As there are many different varieties of freeze dryers, there are also many opinions on pharmaceutical freeze dryer design. In fact, there are usually as many opinions on design as there are parties to the discussion. This chapter and the next chapter will consider the pharmaceutical freeze dryer—its components and systems. The most common designs will be discussed for each, and the advantages and disadvantages of each shown. There is not a design that is better in all aspects for all freeze drying protocols. There are many different components or systems designs; the choice can be made by the user as to which configuration suits the proposed use.

It is an often heard complaint that freeze drying courses give little information that is of use when specifying a freeze dryer. This chapter is not intended as an authoritative work, but is an unbiased assessment of the minimum requirements within a freeze dryer—their function and a comparison of some of the more common options.

Most freeze dryers are composed of two chambers: a drying chamber and an ice condenser (Figure 2.1). It is possible to combine both of these functions within one chamber. Both chambers can be subjected to a vacuum by a vacuum pump(s) that is usually connected to the ice condenser. The freeze dryer operates subliming water from the product within the drying chamber to cooled coils within the ice condenser, leaving the dried product in the drying chamber.

The drying chamber has a door, which usually occupies the complete front face of the chamber, through which the product is loaded for freeze drying, and then withdrawn after drying. This door, on a sterilisable freeze dryer, usually opens into the clean area. The door surround is sealed to the clean area wall, becoming an integral part of the area. Providing that the inside of the freeze dryer has been

Figure 2.1. The freeze dryer chamber and condenser.

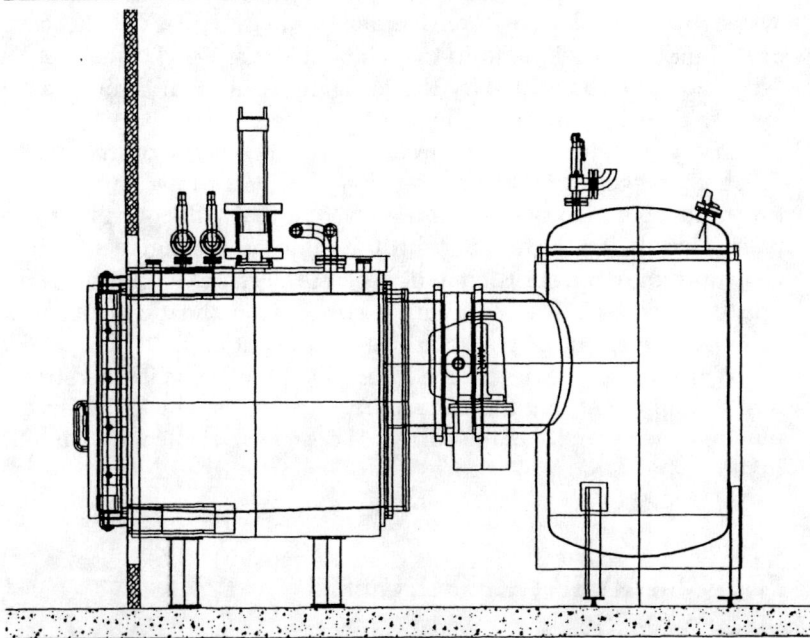

Reproduced by kind permission of Usifroid.

sterilised, this arrangement allows the facility to process the product under sterile conditions. The parts of the plant that would be difficult, if not impossible, to sterilise, or are moving and, therefore, generating particles, are outside the clean area.

The drying chamber contains product shelves upon which the product is dried. These shelves have at least two characteristics: they are level and flat and they have the ability to be accurately controlled in temperature by the circulation of a thermoregulated fluid within them. The shelves on most freeze dryers have a third characteristic in that they may be moved together to effect vial closure by pressing a partially inserted stopper into the vial.

The ice condenser contains one or more coils that are cooled by direct expansion of a refrigerant within them. Designs are possible where plates are used rather than a coil. At the end of the drying cycle, the coils must have a method of removing the ice that has condensed upon them. This is usually achieved by a water spray, or by steam as part of the sterilisation cycle.

A refrigeration system will supply cooling to both the shelves and to the condenser. The condenser is cooled directly by the refrigeration system by the expansion of refrigerant within the coils. The shelves are cooled indirectly by the fluid that circulates through the shelves. This fluid can either be cooled by the refrigeration system through a heat exchanger or may be heated by electrical resistance.

In order to function, the freeze dryer requires a control system. This may range from a simple set of manually operated switches and timers to a sophisticated computer system that will control, produce batch records, and interface with the building management system. Generally, the control system will generate electrical impulses that will operate solenoid valves, allowing the use of a pneumatic system to operate the valves on the plant and, hence, to control it.

Whilst the above describes 95 percent of the plants in operation today, it is apparent that there are many exceptions. This only serves to illustrate the diversity of the variety of designs possible within a freeze dryer.

FREEZE DRYER COMPONENTS

The Drying Chamber

The purpose of the drying chamber is to allow the support of product shelves within a drying, vacuum, and sterilising environment. Drying chambers that form part of a steam sterilisable plant are designated as pressure vessels and must be built according to a national pressure vessel code. In the United States this is usually ASME; but in Europe there are codes for each nation (e.g., BS5500 in the United Kingdom, TÜV in Germany, CODAP in France, and ISPESLS in Italy). The United Kingdom will accept most codes, but other European nations and their insurers demand their country code; America usually demands ASME.

It must be recognised that although sterilisation should occur at 121°C, not all of the chamber will reach this temperature when subjected to the equivalent steam pressure. It follows that there should be some latitude to allow the bulk of the chamber to be at a higher temperature in order to enable the chamber cold spot to achieve sterilisation temperature. A reasonable minimum specification is for the chamber to be rated at 2.5 bar_a which would relate to 127.5°C on the steam tables. This would indicate a maximum operating temperature of 125°C to allow for an operating band for a slight temperature overshoot without actuating the pressure relief system.

There are two usual chamber geometries: rectangular and cylindrical. Cylindrical chambers are less expensive to manufacture;

however, as all the shelves located within the chamber are generally of the same width, they are wasteful of chamber volume as the full diameter cannot be used, except in the case of a single shelf. It is for this reason that cylindrical chambers are usually only used for freeze dryers with small (<3 m^2) shelf areas. Plants containing shelf areas greater than this usually utilise a rectangular chamber as the more common design. The additional chamber volume within a cylindrical chamber is only detrimental in terms of the space required in the installation; the additional time required to pump the chamber to vacuum is trivial; once the chamber is at vacuum, there is no additional effect. There is less welding in the manufacture of a cylindrical chamber, which explains the lower manufacturing costs, but it is rare that a weld will leak or fail.

A difference between the two geometries is apparent in the chamber drain. A drain is necessary to clear condensate from the sterilisation cycle or wash water from cleaning or CIP. When a drain is fabricated into a cylindrical chamber, there is a tendency for the weld to pull the chamber out of shape as it cools. Although good manufacturing techniques will avoid this, it is possible that this distortion may result in a weir, a few millimetres high, that will prevent adequate condensate clearance during sterilisation. It is also difficult to obtain a slope to the drain on a cylindrical chamber. A rectangular chamber is easy to slope to a drain by slightly tilting the floor. A dished floor with the drain in the centre is aesthetically pleasing, but will give poor access to the flange and drain valve beneath the chamber. A better solution is to drain to a corner, thus allowing good access.

The chamber is usually manufactured from AISI 316L stainless steel or its local equivalent. Nonsterilisable plants may be made from AISI 304 or 304L. Chambers have been manufactured from fibreglass at one end of the scale to highly corrosion resistant nickel alloys at the other. Chamber reinforcement is external and is usually manufactured from corrosion-protected mild steel. The chamber is insulated to prevent condensation and corrosion. Armaflex™ or polyurethane foam is normally used for nonsterilisable plants, and rockwool or some other nonshedding material for sterilisable plants. The insulation is then usually clad with either stainless steel or aluminium cladding. At least one manufacturer will cover the top of the chamber with an aluminium plate to allow the plant to be stood upon for maintenance or other work. Provision should be made for lifting points on the top of the chamber in order to facilitate installation.

The chamber finish is usually satin; there appears to be a tendency for the market to move away from a mirror polish, as it is difficult to fully clean and marks easily. Although the finish is normally described as 240 grit (or whatever is in the specification), this is not a good guarantee of the surface; it merely means that the final polish was done with an abrasive of this specification. A better indication is a Ra value that will indicate surface roughness and, therefore, some of the cleaning characteristics. A Ra value of around 0.5 μ is acceptable. All welds should be ground smooth, radiused, polished, and then passivated to prevent corrosion. This specification applies to all the product contact parts within a freeze dryer, including but not limited to the chamber, condenser, condenser coils, shelves, and inlet pipework.

In order to allow the freeze dryer to operate, there must be many breaks in the integrity of the chamber; the pipework system attempts to limit the number of these lead-throughs, but the number is still large. The breaks within the chamber may include but are not restricted to the following:

- Door
- Flanged back plate
- Vacuum duct to the condenser
- Chamber inlet
- Chamber drain
- Pressure relief valve port(s)
- Inlet and outlet for the thermoregulation fluid
- Stoppering actuators
- Pressure equalisation valve
- Vacuum probe port
- Temperature probe lead-throughs
- Validation port(s)
- CIP ports
- Illuminated viewport(s)

Sterilisation is dealt with in chapter 6 but the important feature of the design is that all dead legs within the chamber wall are free draining and are as short and wide as possible in order to facilitate steam penetration. Most dead legs are in the chamber roof, but those that are situated within the chamber wall must have a definite slope with no ridges which would retain condensate.

In addition to the above, the chamber will incorporate mounting brackets for the shelf support system and the thermoregulation fluid distribution manifolds. A chamber with an internal condenser will also require mounting points for the condenser coils, inlets and outlets for the refrigerant cooling the condenser, and a vacuum duct to the vacuum pump. A plant with an internal condenser will also require a polished radiation shield to be mounted in order to prevent direct line of sight between the condenser coils and the product, which would cause irregular drying of the product on the shelf edges.

Although it is not strictly necessary, a good design is to have the back face of the chamber flanged in both the cylindrical or rectangular formats. This allows good access if maintenance or modification work must be performed in the rear of the chamber. In extreme cases, it would be possible to perform work from the rear of the chamber and, by sterilising prior to opening the door, not compromise the clean room sterility. This design also facilitates pass-through freeze dryers that can be unloaded from the rear to linearise material flow.

Pressure relief valve ports are flanged so that relief valves may be replaced or removed for testing. Relief valves are incorporated to protect the chamber from an overpressure if a fault were to develop with the steam delivery system during steam sterilisation. The valves are usually of a soft seat spring-loaded type, and the relief flow contact parts should be manufactured from stainless steel. Hard-seated and weight lifting types work well as relief valves but are often difficult to seat, to the leak tightness required within a freeze dryer, once they have lifted. Bursting discs may be used and can be expected to give a good leak tightness. The perceived objection to the use of a bursting disc is often concerned with the impossibility of nondestructive testing and being able to assess their ageing, especially after many steam cycles, and the effect that this has on the blowoff pressure. These concerns are largely emotive, but are a real barrier to the widespread use of bursting discs.

The pressure equalisation valve is sometimes fitted to ensure that the pressure within the chamber is equalised with the clean area to allow the door to open. The valve should not be operable if the pressure differential across it is greater than 50 mbar to avoid steam escaping or a disruption of vacuum. This valve is not required if aeration at the completion of the freeze drying cycle is from the cleanroom side. As many clean areas are at a positive pressure, any aeration from the plant area would be of an insufficient pressure and the door could not be opened. This would be the major objection to plant room air that, for a steam sterilisable plant, would be sterile as it must pass through the freeze dryer's sterilising filter, although in this case the filter would have a heavier challenge and could blind.

The validation port should be of a sufficient size that it would accept all the probes necessary for validation. This may amount to over

30 thermocouples, corresponding to 60 wires. A large port that will accept a variety of lead-throughs is essential. If the freeze dryer has many shelves, and the use of more than one data logger is envisaged, then thought should be given to equipping the chamber with more than one validation port.

Viewports are of debatable value, but are usually specified. The important aspects are that they provide illumination and that they are in a position where they can be accessed after final installation. Their view should not be obscured by shelf supports, the stoppering mechanism, or flexible hoses, for this reason, most are fitted to the rear of the drying chamber.

The chamber closing plate, often called the bioseal or the bezel, bridges the gap between the chamber and the clean area wall. It is usually attached to the chamber, overlaps the clean area wall and is then clamped to the back of it. The final seal is usually made with silicone; this plate then becomes an integral part of the cleanroom wall. The plate should preferably be one piece and, as it is not a contact part, could be made from AISI 304 stainless steel. Many users specify, and manufacturers supply as a standard, AISI 316L stainless steel.

The closing plate is used as a support for the clean area freeze dryer controls. These controls should be kept to a minimum. The strategy should be to operate the plant from outside the clean area and to only perform minimum operations within the clean area. The usual controls are as follows:

- Stoppering, but only to change shelf interdistances

- Pressure equalisation valve across the door (if required)

- Sterilisation and cycle indication lights

- Chamber pressure gauge

There are always exceptions. Some door mechanisms require a vacuum to enable the mechanism to be operated; therefore a vacuum pump start switch would be required. A plant with an inflatable gasket will need a control to deflate the gasket prior to unlocking. A non-sterilisable plant would be operated in a different way—the entire control cabinet may be present next to the chamber. However, if the plant is operating in a clean room, it is difficult to justify other controls within this area.

If a loading cart is used, then docking points, which will be fixed to the chamber or chamber frame, will usually pass through the closing plate.

It is becoming more popular for the chamber to have a cooling jacket to allow forced cooling after sterilisation. The cooling medium is usually a silicone oil that is cooled by the freeze dryer's refrigeration system. Water is a poor choice. It is simple to pass chilled water through the cooling jacket, but this would have to be completely drained to avoid cracking of the cooling jacket or chamber during freezing.

The Chamber Door

The chamber door is the means by which the drying shelves are loaded and unloaded; it faces into a clean area. The door in a steam sterilisable plant must resist a pressure gradient from within the chamber during sterilisation, and from the clean area when the plant is under vacuum. Therefore, it is necessary to interlock the door to prevent opening when the chamber is at a positive steam pressure. There are at least five types of door locking mechanisms and three types of door hinges with many minor variations on each. On a large freeze dryer, the door may weigh several tonnes, but must be closed, and locked, often by a single operator in sterile area clothing. The door can, therefore, be seen as a major component of the freeze dryer. It has been the subject of a great deal of engineering design and development effort.

Some freeze dryers have two doors on opposite ends of the chamber to facilitate a good material flow. This design usually results in two clean areas, with a corridor between them within which the freeze dryer chamber sits. The condenser then must be offset, and access for maintenance becomes difficult. Another design has a subdoor, or a loose-fitting door with a loading slot, within the main door to allow constant height product loading on cold shelves without frosting the chamber by condensation from the atmosphere.

The door for a small nonsterilisable freeze dryer may be made of an acrylic plastic, this will allow a clear view within the chamber. Unfortunately, a transparent door will provide additional heat input, by radiation, to the front of the shelves, which may cause the product situated there to dry at a different rate as compared to product further back on the freeze dryer shelves. The door may be dished outward for structural strength. The use of solvents may cause a plastic door to craze (i.e., become covered in small stress fractures), which will weaken the door. Larger nonsterilisable plants will have stainless steel doors as the strength of an acrylic door limits its size.

A nonsterilisable plant is not envisaged as ever having a positive pressure within it; so a locking mechanism is not required. The fastening mechanism is usually a simple screw bolt or swing bolt that will place the door in position so that a vacuum can be pulled. The vacuum then holds the door in place. If a positive pressure is ever achieved, for example, by allowing the plant to warm up after aeration, then the excess pressure will spill out past the door seal. Many operators will pull a slight vacuum (a reduction in pressure of about 100 mbar) in order to seat the door at the start of a cycle. This prevents the possibility of the control system starting the vacuum pump at the start of primary drying, the door not sealing, and air being dragged into the chamber until the problem is noticed.

The door on a sterilisable plant is manufactured from the same material as the chamber, usually AISI 316L stainless steel. During the steam sterilisation cycle, the steam is at a positive pressure within the chamber, and the door must be positively locked into place. An additional necessity is that the door (un)locking mechanism cannot be operated at a positive chamber pressure, and that the steam inlet valve is not enabled until the door is closed and securely locked.

There are a diversity of door/steam interlocks. The operating criteria are that the door must not only be in the locked position but must also has be closed. Microswitches usually perform the steam inlet valve interlock function. One microswitch will be situated on the chamber face and is actuated when the door shuts against it; the other will be switched on as the locking mechanism is operated. The door closed microswitch often has a secondary function to prevent stoppering with the door open for operator safety considerations, especially when the plant stoppers automatically or can be operated from the plant area. The pressure generated by the steam inside the chamber will usually ensure that the locking mechanism is prevented from operation because of friction; additionally, a diaphragm can be used to insert a locking rod into the door locking mechanism when the chamber is under pressure. Systems that use inflatable gaskets can be locked in place by the pressure of the gasket, the gasket will only be allowed to deflate when the chamber is not at positive pressure.

The door sealing gasket is one of two types, static or inflatable. Static gaskets are usually made of silicone and are of a "D" section. They can be situated on the chamber face or on the door; there is little difference between the two locations. The static gasket gives good vacuum sealing characteristics, but is relatively incompressible. Inflatable gaskets (Figure 2.2) are usually situated on the chamber face and, when deflated, will allow the door to move slightly. They are usually supplemented by a static gasket for vacuum sealing, although this is not strictly necessary. The question arises as to the effects of the inflatable gasket bursting, which could result in steam escape. The actuality is that the gasket is constrained; bursting rarely, if ever, occurs. The gasket is kept under a constant flow of compressed air; small leaks would not affect gasket performance, but would be noticeable. During freeze drying the inflatable gasket is flattened and vacuum sealing is performed by the static gasket. The design is such that the static

Figure 2.2. The principle of the inflatable door gasket.

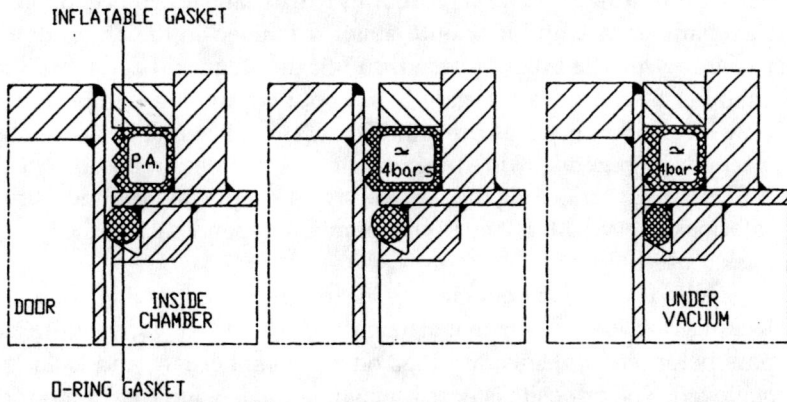

INFLATABLE GASKET

P.A. | ~4bars | ~4bars

DOOR | INSIDE CHAMBER | UNDER VACUUM

O-RING GASKET

Reproduced by kind permission of Usifroid.

gasket is positioned inside the area bound by the inflatable gasket so that any nonsterile, compressed air leakage would be to the clean area and not into the drying chamber and, ultimately, to the product.

A third, and trivial, door gasket is possible. The chamber wall is extended past the chamber face and a U-shaped gasket is fitted over it; a flat door fits, and seals, against this. This design is used for many laboratory freeze dryers and is rarely found in cGMP plants, mainly because the inertia of the door can cut the gasket if the door is shut with a lot of force.

Door locking designs are dependant on the type of door gasket used. In order to avoid metal-to-metal contact, forcing the door to be shut against the gasket, most static gasket door locking systems depend on a vacuum being drawn to pull the door onto the chamber face prior to locking. This results in the requirement to have a vacuum pump control on the clean area fascia, and an operative to be in the clean area at the crucial times during the sterilisation cycle. It is not necessary to lock the door fully for freeze drying as the vacuum holds the door shut. Many static gasket systems have a two-position lock, the first position (drying) will nip the door shut and can be operated at atmospheric pressure; the second (sterilisation) fully locked position requires a vacuum in the chamber for operation. Some systems do not incorporate this, and a large force must be applied to lock the door. Wear is rapid. The question of particle generation within the clean area also arises. An inflatable gasket door locking system does not have these constraints and can be locked and unlocked at atmospheric pressure.

The simplest door locking mechanism is one, or several, swing bolts that may be hinged on either the door or, more likely, the chamber surrounding the door (Figure 2.3). The usual method is to hinge on the chamber face and lock onto a slot machined in the door edge. A variant is for the bolts to pass through the door and screw into the chamber face. This last variant is not popular and is a bad design for cGMP considerations, as the blind screw thread cannot be adequately cleaned. In general, swing bolts are not a good design because of the difficulty in interlocking them to the steam supply and the necessity to interlock every bolt. Swing bolts operate independently of the type of gasket used.

Cylindrical chambers may be locked by rotating a door-mounted locking ring, usually by one-sixteenth of a turn. The lugs on the ring pass behind complementary lugs on the chamber face and locking is achieved. The opposite is possible, where the locking ring is mounted on the chamber. This method of locking is often termed *bayonet locking* (Figure 2.4). A door utilising an inflatable gasket is locked prior to the inflation of a gasket. Normally, a door fitted with a static gasket is locked, and unlocked, under a partial vacuum.

The most common method of door locking is by the use of pins (Plate 2.2; Figure 2.5). This method can be used for both rectangular and circular doors. These pins are usually 25–35 mm in diameter and spaced approximately every 30 cm around the periphery of the door. They can move from either the door onto a raised locking plate fitted with location sockets and welded at right angles to the chamber face, or can be hydraulically inserted from the plant room into a recessed door. If the locking mechanism is in the door, it may be actuated by a single locking handle working through a series of levers and pushbars or through a chain or belt. Alternatively the pins can be hydraulically operated. The use of hydraulic locking necessitates a flexible hydraulic line being attached to the door. In the latter case, and in the case where the pins move from the chamber face into the door, care must be taken to ensure that hydraulic fluid and dirt is not introduced into the clean area when the pins move. This is usually achieved by the use of a rubber bellows connecting the hydraulic cylinder to a noncontact part of the pin, or by a wiper seal. The same rules regarding locking and unlocking that apply to the bayonet lock apply to this mechanism.

T-shaped lugs, passing through the chamber face, and locking onto slots or holes in the door periphery by rotation are the fourth method of door locking (Figure 2.6). The T pieces are spaced in a similar way to a pin and are usually motorised, being rotated by levers or chains in the plant area. The lead-throughs into the clean area only undergo a rotation, and sealing is not as critical as if movement was lateral. This mechanism is particularly suitable for inflatable gasket systems. A static gasket system would require a radial bevel on the T

Figure 2.3. Multiple hand-wheel locking door (swing bolt).

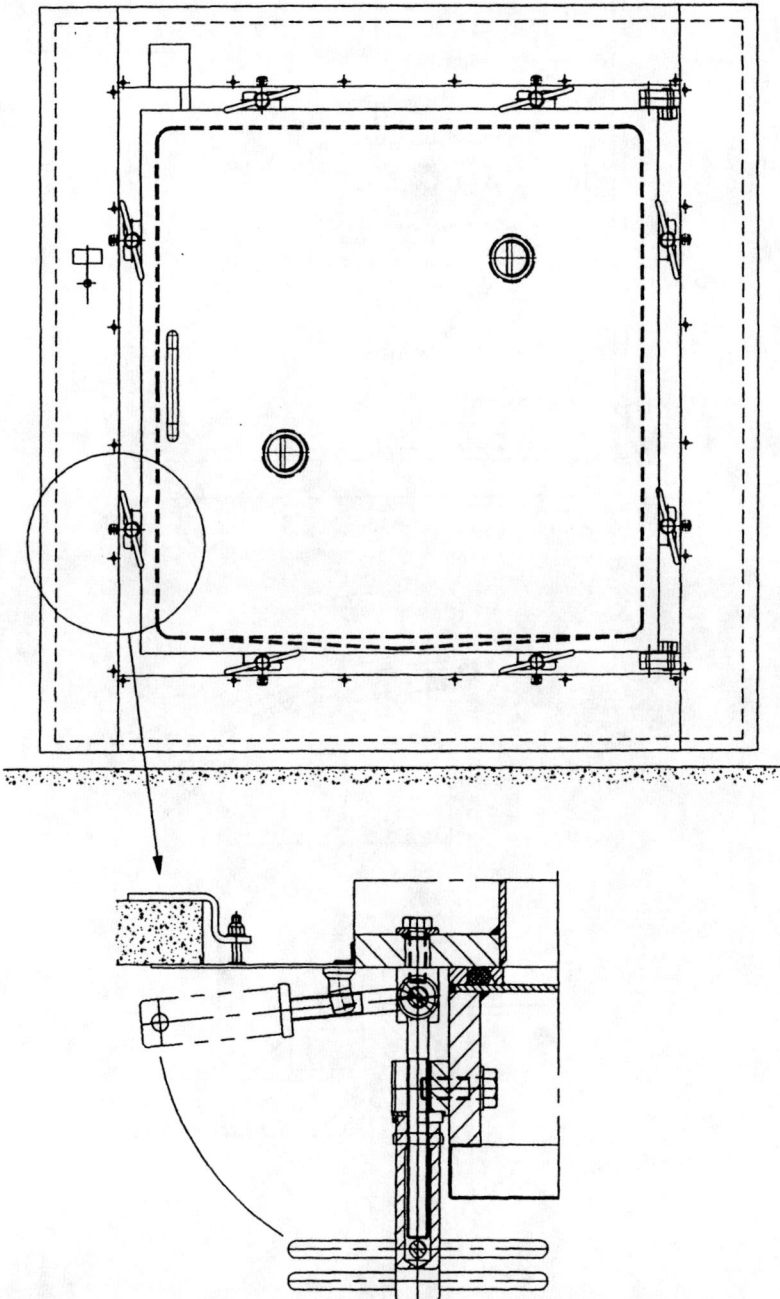

Figure 2.4. Bayonet locking door for cylindrical chambers.

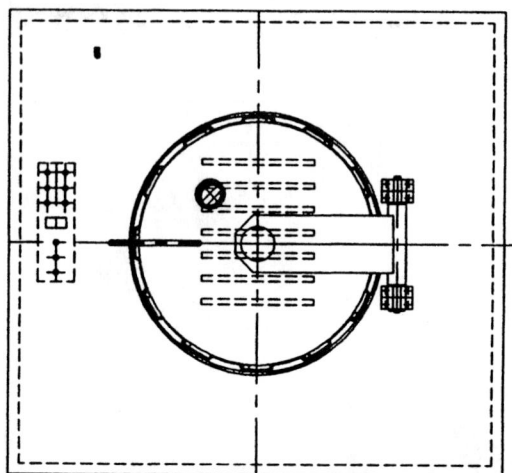

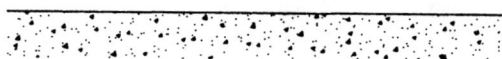

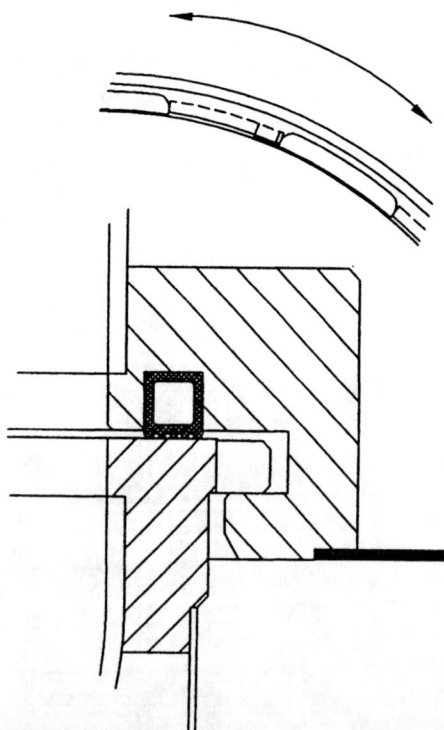

Plate 2.2. Multiple pin centrally locking door seen from the sterile area.

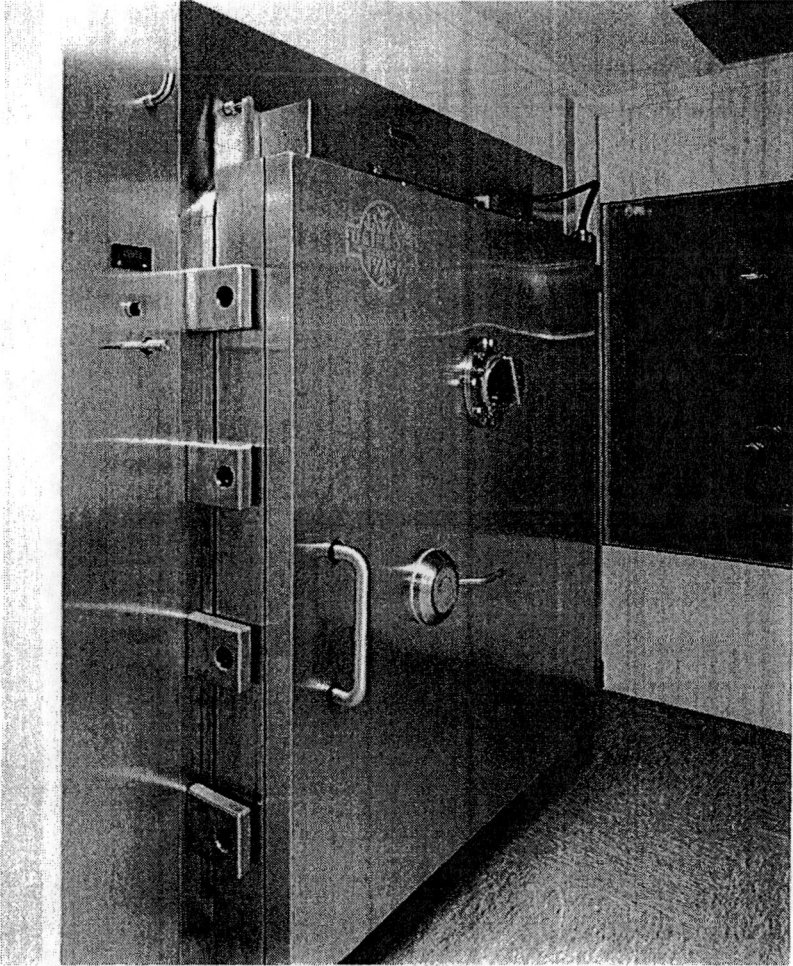

Reproduced by kind permission of Usifroid.

piece contact surface in order to clamp the door down tightly, which accelerates wear and generates particles. Systems do exist where the T pieces will rotate and then pull backwards to lock the door, but these are expensive and not common.

The final method is that of a sliding door mechanism (Figure 2.7). The door slides under a locking bar that encompasses half the circumference of a circular door or three sides of a rectangular door. A

Figure 2.5. Centrally locking door using multiple parallel pins.

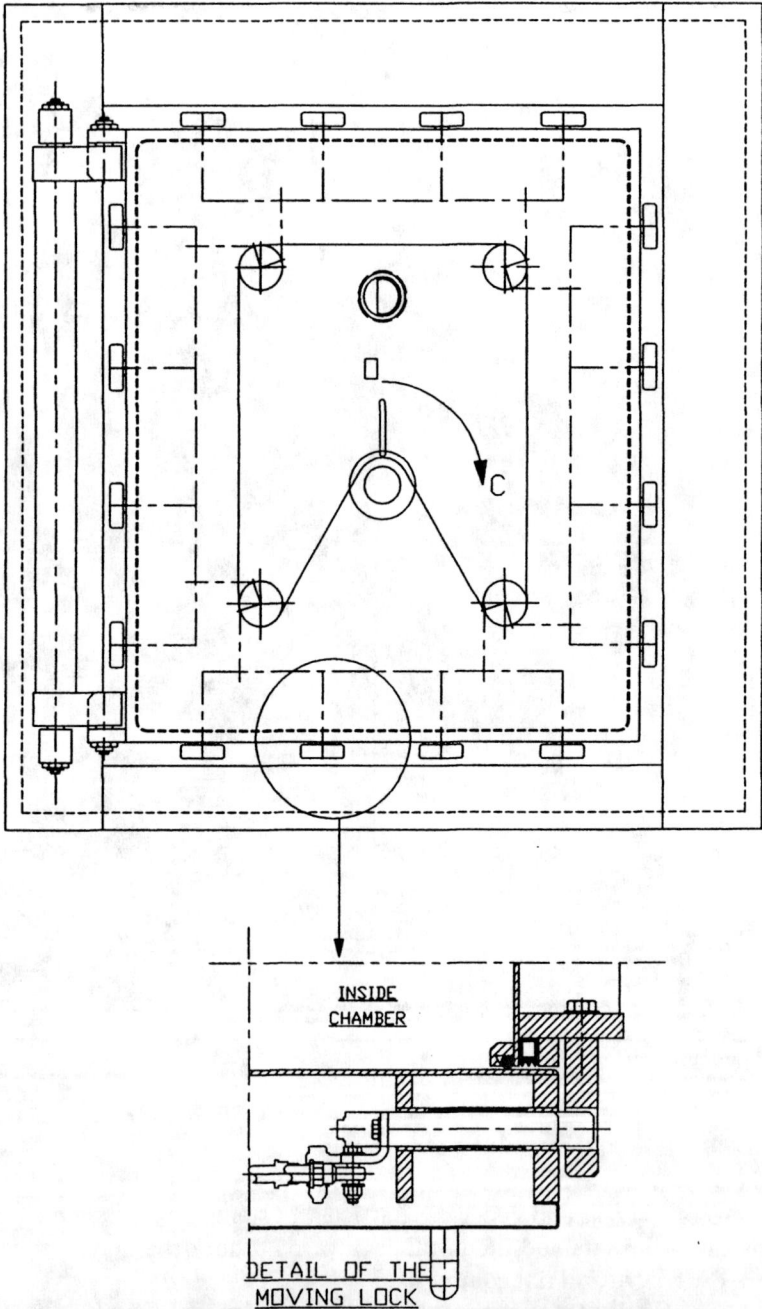

INSIDE
CHAMBER

DETAIL OF THE
MOVING LOCK

Figure 2.6. Powered peripherally locking door.

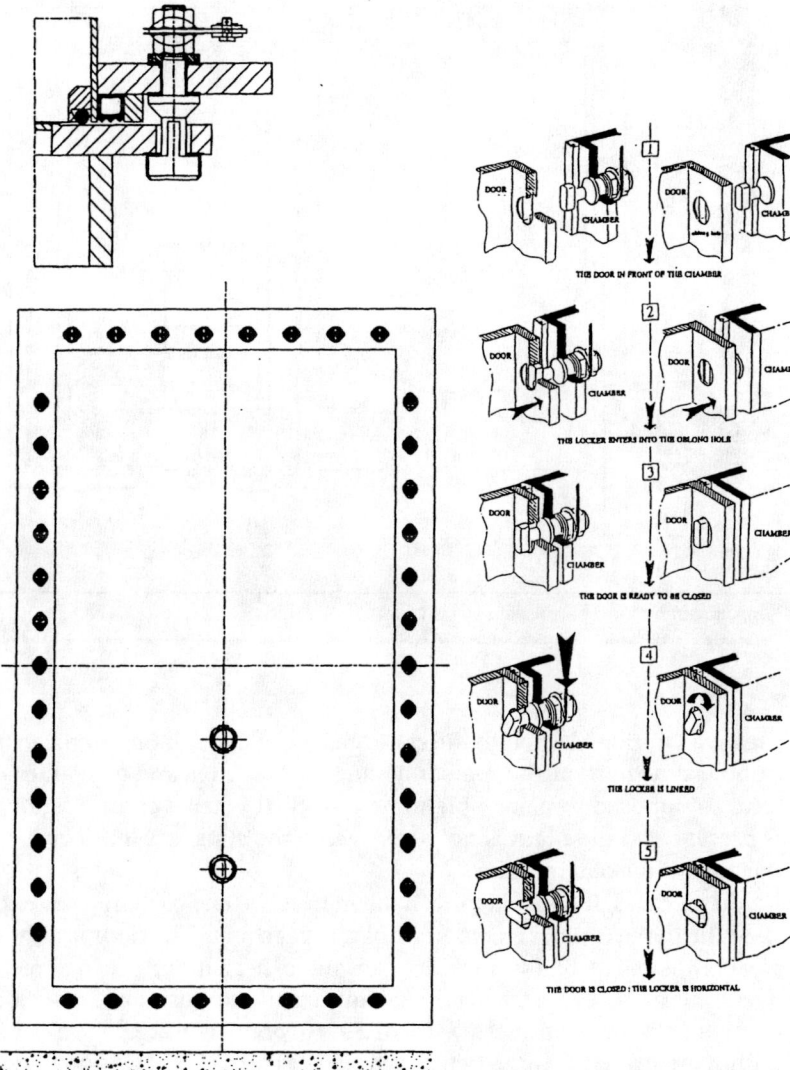

Reproduced by kind permission of Usifroid.

swing bolt may be used on the other half of the circle or on the fourth side. This mechanism would be difficult to design using a static gasket, and is normally only used with inflatable gaskets.

Whilst it can be seen that the inflatable gasket is the most versatile of the two gasket types, this does not necessarily mean that it is the

Figure 2.7. Sliding door.

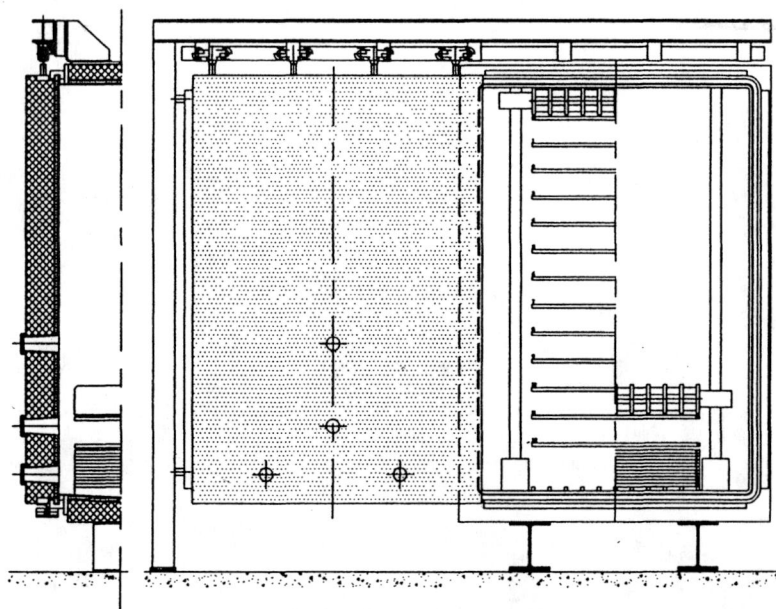

Reproduced by kind permission of Usifroid.

preferred option. Although the static gasket has limitations, and can be troublesome in requiring personnel in the clean area and a vacuum to lock, as opposed to being able to be unlocked whenever an operative is present and the plant is not at pressure, the static gasket does have the advantage of simplicity.

In all cases, the locking mechanism must be enclosed in a cover to keep the moving parts shielded from the clean area. The door is almost always insulated below the cover to avoid heat input during freeze drying and for operator safety during steam sterilisation. A sealed, foam insulation is preferred in order to prevent microbial growth within the insulation and, hence, within the clean area. The door cover is usually made of the same material as the door and chamber although AISI 304L would normally be sufficient.

An interesting variant is to have a subdoor built into the main door. This design will allow shelves to be loaded at constant height; shelf indexing to a constant height is achieved by the shelf stoppering mechanism. This method of loading has the advantage of loading heat labile product onto a cold shelf, soon after vial filling, without constantly opening the main door and frosting up the inside of the chamber. Constant height loading is also useful when bulk liquids are to be loaded. This design also allows a nitrogen blanket to be put over the product through the aeration system.

Thought must be given to the subdoor hinge and locking designs. Hinges that are situated on one end of the door will be under a terrific strain. The potential also exists that if both doors were to be opened at once, then the edge of the subdoor would circumscribe a large arc. The weight of the subdoor presents problems if the door is hinged on its upper or lower edges. Most subdoors are hinged on the side, as the alternative is a powered door, but this design is not optimal. Subdoors are usually locked by swing bolts and are, therefore, not interlocked to the steam supply, although a microswitch to ensure, at least, closure is often incorporated.

An alternative is a loosefitting inner door with a slot cut into it at the height of constant loading. The main door is left open and loading proceeds through the inner door. This inner door must, by necessity, not be gas tight, and plays no part in the pressure integrity of the chamber and the main door.

Door hinges come in three varieties—all are high quality and usually rotate on ball bearings rather than bushes. The first variety is the simple hinge, similar in principle to one that would be found on a domestic door. The disadvantage of this hinge is that the door will nip the door gasket at the hinge side, causing premature wear.

The second type of hinge is a development of the first type and has a double action that allows the door to seat against the hinge, parallel to the chamber face, thus avoiding wear on the hinge side of the gasket. This double action is achieved by having two pivot points in the hinge so that the hinge appears to have a chain link built into it. This type of hinge is now the most common.

The third type of hinge is to mount the door on a gimbals. In its simplest form it is composed of a C-shaped mounting that pivots, through a vertical plane, on the base of the C. The door is mounted on the bottom of the legs of the C and can also pivot through a vertical plane. This mechanism has the advantage of offering the door to the seal parallel to the chamber face. The swing of the door is only half its width. This is of particular interest if the freeze dryer is connected to an isolation bubble, although the best door mechanism for an isolation bubble is not a hinged door but a sliding door.

The freeze dryer door is balanced, and is built with minimum friction in the hinges, to allow the door to be closed easily by a single operative in clean area clothing. It is possible to build a friction device into the hinge, or spanning from the top of the door to the chamber face, to prevent the door from slamming. A door may weigh several tonnes. Repeated slamming will not only damage the gaskets but could actually move the freeze dryer and challenge the integrity of the clean area. Powered doors have been developed, which are usually closed hydraulically. The use of these doors is not popular because of the necessity to have a hydraulic piston within the clean area.

Doors often incorporate illuminated viewports; like the chamber viewports, they are of limited value but are almost always specified. The requirement for illumination results in a flexible, shielded electrical cable running from the closing plate to the door—another potential dirt trap. The important consideration is that the viewports are at the correct height for viewing the contents of a shelf.

Like the chamber, the door can include a cooling jacket for post-sterilisation, forced, cooling. This should utilise silicone oil, or an equivalent, to avoid freezing problems during the drying cycle. Door cooling will necessitate two flexible fluid lines from the chamber closing plate to the door and a cleaning regimen for the external surfaces of these must be devised.

The Chamber Isolation Valve

A freeze dryer with an internal (i.e., in-chamber), condenser does not have a vacuum duct to the condenser, but instead to the vacuum pump. In addition there are inlets and outlets for the refrigerant pipework to the condenser coils or plates.

A freeze dryer with an external (i.e., separate), condenser often has a chamber isolation valve in the vapour duct between the chamber and the condenser. This is often termed the *main valve*. Large freeze dryers may have a main valve up to 1 metre in diameter. This valve may be one of three types: a quarter swing (butterfly) valve, a mushroom valve, or a gate valve.

There are many arguments for the inclusion of a main valve, but the only valid reason to fit one is to enable the pressure rise test. The arguments for cleaning, defrosting whilst the chamber is being loaded, sterilisation of the chamber only, and the ability to cool the condenser before loading do not stand up to modern operating practices.

The butterfly valve is the most common type and is often modified so that a vacuum is pulled behind the seal to keep it flat against the valve body to prevent scuffing when it operates under vacuum. The valve is of the balanced type and can, therefore, hold a pressure differential either way, and can easily open against a pressure differential. The main disadvantage of the butterfly valve is that the vapour duct must be long enough to accommodate the valve when it is open, thus increasing the length of the plant.

A mushroom valve is usually operated from, and seals to, the condenser side of the vapour duct. It is not a balanced valve and must operate under a high pressure to keep the seal when subjected to a pressure differential from the chamber to the condenser, or to open the valve if the pressure differential is the other way around. The actuator rod passes through the condenser and must be protected to prevent ice crystals from damaging the actuator seals, although this phenomenon only occurs when the condenser is overloaded. The actuator area could be protected by a bellows as "the insertion of a nonsterile rod into a sterile area" argument that is well known for stoppering actuators applies, but the bellows would be inaccessible for cleaning. In addition, as the valve must be open for sterilisation, the bellows will be contracted and steam penetration would not be guaranteed. Another disadvantage is that as the actuating mechanism passes through either the length of a horizontal condenser or the diameter of a vertical condenser, then the condenser coils must be designed to avoid it. The valve is also difficult to remove and seal replacement can be difficult, especially in plants without a stoppering mechanism to move the shelves to gain access from the chamber. An advantage of the mushroom valve is that it causes a spreading of the vapour flow, especially if it is composed of one or more concentric rings around a central disc. This will spread the vapour load around the complete condenser rather than impacting it on the part of the condenser coil immediately behind the vapour duct.

Gate valves of the size required are very expensive. Their main advantage is that they require little room to actuate. They are not normally used unless plant length is critical for installation. These valves suffer from most of the drawbacks of the mushroom valve and have many working parts.

At least one manufacturer uses the bottom pressure plate of the stoppering mechanism as a main valve, thereby doubling up on the duty of the actuator. This is an elegant design that suffers from the disadvantages of the mushroom valve. It is only useful when the condenser is situated below the drying chamber, it may require a pit to accommodate the hydraulic cylinder.

The Ice Condenser

The ice condenser condenses water vapour evolving from the product and immobilises it, thus protecting the vacuum pump. It is important to realise that the vacuum pump will make little or no contribution to the removal of water vapour during the freeze drying process. To pump the amount of water vapour evolved during a freeze drying cycle, and generated at the pressures found within the cycle, the vacuum pump would have to be larger than the freeze dryer. The relatively inexpensive twin-stage oil sealed rotary pump could not be used, as the water vapour would condense in the oil, destroying the lubricating properties of the oil and causing premature vacuum pump failure.

The ice condenser consists of an ice condensing surface and is usually one of two types—coils or plates. In either case they should be made of the same material, and surface finish, as the chamber. The use of plates has declined and most modern freeze dryers use coil condensers. The coils, or plates, are cooled by direct expansion of refrigerant within them and, depending on the refrigerant used, may obtain temperatures between -50°C and -90°C. It is worth noting, to avoid confusion, that the freeze dryer's ice condenser is the refrigeration system's evaporator.

Alternative sources of condenser cooling are liquid nitrogen or a thermoregulated oil. The use of the liquid nitrogen is a topic of current interest and can have many advantages. The cooling capacity is constant throughout the temperature range, and peak loads can easily be condensed. An oil circulation method can give some advantages in the rapid cooling of the shelves by diverting the oil to the shelf circuit. It can be argued to have a greater heat sink capacity when subjected to peak load but the design is complicated and is not as effective now that the available refrigerants are less powerful (i.e., post-Montreal).

There is a third type of condenser design, that of a drum with refrigeration coils wound around the outside of the drum, or a double skinned, quilted drum carrying the refrigerant. This geometry is used mainly in laboratory- and pilot-scale freeze dryers and is rarely found in production units.

The sizing of the ice condenser is critical to the operation of the freeze dryer and is based on two criteria. The absolute ice-carrying capacity must be defined. This is calculated as an ice covering on the coils or plates to a certain thickness and is not the volume of the condenser shell. Ice condensers are usually sized so that at an ice thickness of between 11 mm and 15 mm, the capacity is equal to that of a 20 mm product depth on the shelves. In simpler terms, about 20 kg per square metre of shelf area. This measurement is not time dependant.

The condenser must also condense the initial high vapour load at the beginning of primary drying without a large rise in temperature. The absolute vapour trapping capability is dependant on refrigeration capacity and the surface area of the condensing surface. Vapour trapping capacity is usually defined for a given time. A 20 horsepower compressor, with 5 m^2 of evaporator (ice condensing) surface and utilising one of the usual freeze dryer refrigerants, will trap around 5 kg of ice per hour at -50°C. The same system will trap almost double that amount of ice at -40°C. If the load on the ice condenser is greater than it can condense, then the temperature of the condenser will rise in temperature to accommodate the increased load. This is a common occurrence at the commencement of primary drying.

The condenser may be external or external to the drying chamber. Internal condensers (Plate 2.3) are usually situated below the shelves, although they may be at the side. In either case, they are usually separated from the shelves by a heat radiation shield.

External condensers (Plate 2.4) are located within their own chamber that is usually situated to the rear of the drying chamber, although designs with the condenser at the side, above, and below have been frequently made. A pass-through system with double doors cannot have the condenser at the rear of the chamber. Irrespective of the condenser chamber position, it is common to have a heat radiation shield to prevent direct line of sight between the shelves and the condenser coils. The heat radiation shield is usually a louvered plate made from highly polished stainless steel of the same grade as the rest of the construction.

There is only one reason for an external condenser, because an internal condenser is certainly cheaper. If the plant is fitted with an

Plate 2.3. Internal condenser coils in the bottom of the drying chamber.

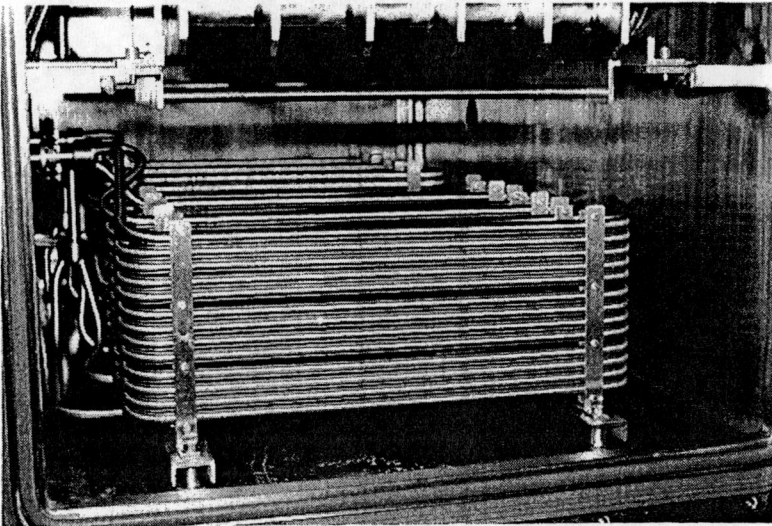

Reproduced by kind permission of Usifroid.

Plate 2.4. Condenser coils for a 300 kg external condenser.

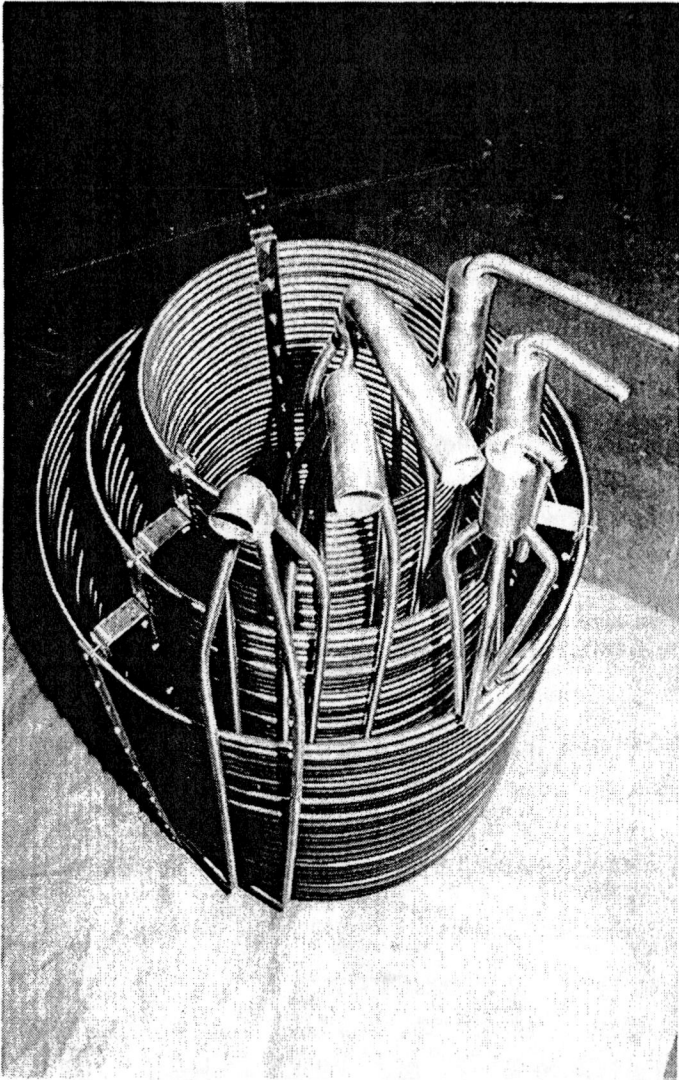

Reproduced by kind permission of Usifroid.

external condenser and a chamber isolation valve, then the pressure rise test is possible. Should a pressure rise test be necessary in a fully automated, reproducible, and validated freeze drying cycle? All other arguments regarding cleaning, defrosting whilst loading, and contamination are not valid. Similarly, an internal condenser is not better "because the vapour path is shorter." For a production unit that is not required to perform the pressure rise test, there is no real reason to specify an external condenser. An external condenser is often specified for the reasons of tradition and a perceived quality of machine. It is the user's choice.

The shell of an external condenser should be made of the same material, and have the same internal surface finish, as the chamber. It is usually insulated and clad in the same way as the chamber, or has a polished radiation shield between the condenser coils and the shell. The condenser should be sterilised with the chamber. All dead legs within the shell should be sloped to drain, without ridges, and be as short and wide as possible.

The breaks within the condenser shell may include but are not restricted to the following:

- Flanged access plate

- Vacuum duct to the chamber

- Condenser steam inlet

- Condenser drain

- Pressure relief valve port(s)

- Inlets and outlets for the condenser coils

- Vacuum duct to the vacuum pump

- Defrosting water inlet

- Vacuum probe port

- Temperature probe lead-throughs

- Validation port(s)

- CIP ports

- Illuminated viewport(s)

The criteria applying to the corresponding breaks in the chamber will apply (see discussion beginning on page 66).

A vacuum probe point is optional. Most freeze dryers will have a second probe, if fitted, between the vacuum pump and the vacuum pump valve in order to dead-head test the pump. A condenser vacuum probe is relatively rare.

Defrosting is usually now achieved by steam as part of the steam sterilisation cycle. If water is used for defrosting, then this should be filtered, externally to the condenser, to remove particles prior to entering the condenser spray bar. Defrosting was discussed in detail in chapter 1.

The external condenser may have vertical or horizontal condenser coils. Vertical condensers contain a true coil and are considered to be the most compact and efficient in terms of vapour trapping, as the coils tend to be closer together. A vertical coil also simplifies the return of oil, which has been carried over from the compressor, within the refrigeration circuit because they are self-draining. However, a space-saving solution is to place the refrigeration compressors below a horizontal condenser; a vertical condenser will need a separate frame for the compressors. A separate refrigeration skid, if well placed, does make maintenance simpler.

There will be increased deposition of ice at the bends in a horizontal condenser, which is caused by increased turbulence of the refrigerant gas within the condenser coil at this point. Even deposition of ice is largely a nonissue. Unless ice deposition is very uneven, to the extent that it could block the vapour or vacuum ducts, the important criterion is that no vapour passes the condenser and condenses into the vacuum pump oil. Even ice distribution would indicate an overloaded, or inefficient, condenser. Under high water vapour loads, ice will condense on all cold surfaces; under low water vapour loads, at the end of secondary drying for instance, ice will migrate to the coldest part of the condenser. In effect, this is freeze drying within the condenser and is entirely predictable. A condenser coil will have a temperature gradient down it; the coldest point will be at the top of the coil, just after the expansion valve.

The use of baffles and a vacuum duct collector pipework within the condenser ensures that water vapour must pass over the majority of the condenser coils before it can enter the vacuum duct and is, therefore, condensed. It does not guarantee even ice distribution.

The condenser coils should be manufactured from seamless tubing and preferably flanged to stubs leading through the condenser shell. This method of manufacture ensures that coil replacement is possible, although their lifetime would be expected to be that of the machine. They should not be welded to a frame, but be lightly clamped. A condenser coil may experience temperature differences of over 200°C, and some allowance for thermal movement must be made.

The temperature shown on a condenser coil temperature probe will reflect the position at which the probe is placed on the coil. A point halfway down the coil will give the fairest indication of the average condenser temperature. A probe placed near the expansion valve will show the minimum temperature within the condenser. Probes are usually fed into tubes that pass through the condenser shell and are welded to the condenser coil in order to give a good thermal contact. These tubes may be filled with an oil to improve the thermal contact even further, but this is not common. Several of these tubes are usually fitted, but not normally used, as an aid to validation.

If the freeze dryer is to be used to dry product that contains small amounts of solvent, then it is possible to have the coldest part of the coil at the bottom of the condenser to act as a solvent trap. If the drain has two valves in series, it is possible to drain off the liquid solvent as it preferentially evaporates and condenses in the ice condenser, without breaking vacuum. Another arrangement is to have the solvent drain into a trough that can be emptied under vacuum. Alternatively, a second condenser may be fitted that is cooled by liquid nitrogen and can be valved off.

The low condenser temperatures achieved by modern freeze dryers, and the greater understanding of the role of residual moisture with regard to shelf life, has resulted in the almost complete disappearance of the phosphorus pentoxide trap as an adjunct to the condenser.

The Shelf Stack

The purpose of the shelves is to support the product containers and to supply heat flow to freeze and to dry the product in a controlled way. The size of the shelf system also defines the size of almost all of the other components of the freeze dryer.

The shelf stack is composed of the product shelves, complete with their supports and the fluid distribution hoses and manifolds that are used to pass the thermoregulation medium through the shelves. The stoppering system, where the shelves are moved together to drive partially inserted stoppers into the vials, also comprises part of the shelf stack, but is dealt with in the section entitled "The Stoppering System". Product probes, if fitted, interact with the shelf stack.

The main characteristics of the shelves are that they are level and flat. They require sufficient structural strength to support both themselves and the product, containers, and trays, however, they also must be sufficiently flexible to withstand changes in temperature without distorting. If the freeze dryer is equipped with a stoppering system, then the shelf stack must also withstand the rigours of this. In addition, the shelves must be hollow, with an internal serpentine path to allow the passage of thermoregulation fluid.

Typically, the specification for shelf flatness should be a minimum of ±1 mm across any 1 m; ±0.5 mm is now more common. The temperature variation between any two points on the shelf surfaces should not exceed ±1°C under steady state conditions, and at any temperature within the controlled range, although ±0.5°C is usual for a modern freeze dryer. Steady state should be defined as a measurement after holding a given temperature for 10 minutes. The controlled temperature range will be defined by freeze dryer design and specifications, but will typically be from -55°C to 70°C.

The degree to which the shelves need to be level is of more interest in bulk applications in order to avoid a variation in product depth across the tray; the effect is not as marked in vial applications. However, it is good practice to have the shelves level. The manufacturer will build the machine so that the shelves are parallel to the machine frame, but the freeze dryer is usually levelled with respect to the shelves during installation. This additionally ensures, providing that the frame and shelves are parallel and the door hinge post is at right angles to the frame, that the door does not have a tendency to swing open or shut under gravity—a worrying and dangerous trend on a door that could weigh several tonnes.

The shelves are the nearest component of the freeze dryer to a direct contact part. They must, therefore, be built of the same material as the chamber, usually AISI 316L stainless steel, and must have their surfaces cleaned and then sterilised. The shelf surface finish is important for two reasons: cleanability and heat transfer. It is for these reasons that the shelves are almost never polished to a mirror finish. If the debate concerning the cleanability of a mirror finish is temporarily ignored, the fact still remains that a mirror finish has bad heat transfer characteristics. From an aesthetic viewpoint, a mirror finished shelf will rapidly become very badly scored as trays are pushed across it. This scoring is less apparent on a satin finish (but is still there), which gives better heat transfer. It is for these reasons that almost all shelves exhibit a satin, or bead blasted, finish.

In order to present the same heat input to all product, irrespective of the shelf on which the product is placed upon, a nonusable, radiation shelf is added to the top of the shelf stack. This shelf is especially necessary during secondary drying.

It follows that the shelves present more of an engineering problem than is immediately apparent. In order to obtain an even temperature across the shelf stack, thermoregulation fluid is forced down a serpentine path through the shelves with a sufficient velocity that the conduction of heat is not affected by standing layers within the system; thus under steady state conditions, the temperature gradient across any shelf is minimised. Fortunately these internal baffles, which create the serpentine pathways, can achieve two beneficial effects in that they can also be used to impart structural strength to the shelf. It is also important that the shelves are identical in order to avoid a preferred fluid flow through some of the shelves, which neglects others. The flow of thermoregulation fluid is approximately 1 m^3/m^2 shelf area/ hour.

The constraints on design are that the shelf should not be too bulky because this occupies chamber volume, but the requirement for structural strength is apparent. Shelves are usually 20–24 mm thick, but the stainless steel plates comprising the two surfaces have a thickness of 4 mm. This leaves little height for the fluid path, although the smaller in height the path, the higher the fluid velocity for a given pump flow, thus increasing the efficiency of the system. Unfortunately, it also increases the pressure drop across the internals of the shelf. Shelves have been made, on very large freeze dryers with a thickness of 15 mm, but these shelves had relatively little strength and could not be used for stoppering applications.

The thinner and lighter the shelf, the more energy efficient the freeze dryer. The heat reservoir within the stainless steel and the fluid within the shelf is large, compared to the heat sink caused by the evaporative cooling of the volatile product components during freeze drying. The thinner the shelf, and, therefore, the less fluid used, means that less energy is required to change the temperature of the system. The trend to thinner shelves is, again, constrained by the requirement for structural strength.

There are two main shelf (internal) serpentine pathway designs, although other minor designs exist. The most common is an up-and-down pathway, where the fluid flows in parallel paths up and down the shelf. The channels are approximately 100 mm wide. It is usual for the fluid inlet and outlet to be on opposite edges of the shelf. The second design could best be described as a double square spiral within the shelf. Fluid will spiral into the centre of the shelf and then escape by a parallel, but opposed, route. In this case, it is often found that the shelf inlet and outlet may be on the same edge of the shelf, although this is not strictly necessary. The "square spiral" will give a larger pressure drop, is more complicated to manufacture, and gives no process advantage, thus it is rarely used. The important characteristic is that there are no dead spots within the shelf. These would exhibit a different temperature from the rest of the shelf stack and may perform atypical freeze drying within this area.

The baffles that form the internal pathways do not have to be leaktight; they are only present to guide fluid flow. A certain amount of leakage across the pathways is allowed, as this infers that there will be a degree of flexibility in the shelf that will enable the shelf to withstand thermal stresses. It is important to remember that a shelf could experience temperatures between –60°C and 125°C during operation.

It is usual to manufacture shelves by one of three methods (Figure 2.8), but there are many minor methods. The most common method of

Figure 2.8. Main methods of shelf construction.

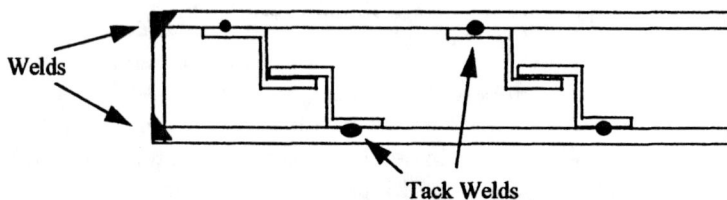

1. Modern, interleaved, tack-weld method.

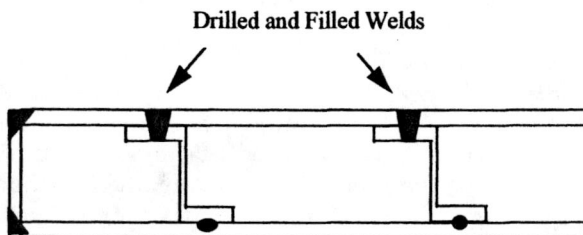

2. Older, drill and fill method.

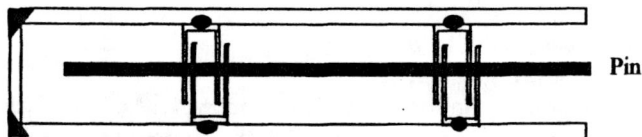

3. Pin method.

the recent past was to take one of the shelf surfaces and tack-weld U, or Z, shaped sections, along one of the open edges of the U, or Z, to form the pathways. The other shelf surface is drilled, in positions corresponding to the sections, and placed on top. The drilled holes are then filled with weld, welding the sections to this inner shelf surface. The welds are then ground flat. As with all of the following methods, the edges of the shelves are then seam-welded in place; the welds ground, polished, and passivated; and thermoregulation fluid stubs then attached. The shelf is, at some point in the manufacturing process, straightened on a point press. Whilst this drill and weld method gives a very strong shelf, it is relatively rigid and does not have the ability to "move" when subjected to thermal stresses. The large number of drilled and welded holes in one of the shelf surfaces will increase the possibility of leaks.

The second method, which is now adopted by most manufacturers, is to tack-weld U, Z, or right angled, shaped sections, by one edge, to both inner shelf surfaces and then interleave them. The edges of the shelves and the remainder of the shelf manufacturing process is then as above. This method has the advantage that the shelf outer surfaces are never compromised, and there is a sufficient flexibility to handle thermal stresses.

Shelves may also be assembled as a "sandwich", with strips of a low melting point alloy along the sections forming the channels. The whole shelf is then placed in an oven and the alloy solders the sections into place. The shelf is then finished by conventional means. This is an efficient method of shelf manufacture, although the flexibility must be questioned. The only drawback is the size of oven required for large shelves.

There are other methods of shelf manufacture. A U section may be welded on both shelf inner surfaces by the base of the U and interleaved. Pins, the width of the shelf, can then be pushed through predrilled holes in the sections along the axis of the shelf, locking everything in place. This method will give thin shelves but with a limited strength; therefore, they are unsuitable for stoppering. Alternatively, thermoplates can be used. Thermoplates are made by tack-welding two sheets of stainless steel, with dissimilar thickness, together and seam-welding the edges. Gas is expanded within the shelf and quilting occurs on the lower, thinner surface. Judicious placing of the tack-welds can give the required internal pathways. These shelves are lightweight, cheap, and thin. They are also variable and have little strength. The quilted lower surface, and the lack of strength, make them unsuitable for stoppering applications.

It is usual for shelves to possess shelf guides, on the side and back edges, to centre the trays, or vials, on the shelf and to prevent a tray overlapping the back of the shelves. These guides should allow free draining of the shelf during sterilisation or washing. They may, or may not, be removable. Pass-through freeze dryers have a system, composed of guides on the sides of the shelves and several vertical bars mounted on the inside of the back door, to act as guides for the back of the shelf.

Shelves that will comprise an element of an automatic loading system should have an accurately ground square front edge. In general, the docking of the loading system is the function of the loading system and not the shelf; however, the shelf must be very accurately positioned.

The shelves are connected to the thermoregulation system by shelf hoses, which are invariably flexible on modern dryers. A source of debate is the use of convoluted or braided shelf hoses. In actuality, a braided hose is a convoluted hose with a stainless steel braid laid over it. There can be no doubt that a braid makes the hose more difficult to clean; however, it also gives the hose more strength. A convoluted hose will lengthen slightly under internal pressure caused by fluid flow. Hoses are arranged and guided so that they will not be trapped by the shelves during stoppering. If the hose lengthens, then the probability of this occurring increases slightly. The probability of a hose becoming trapped is still remote, and convoluted hoses are the preferred option; but, as always, it is the user's choice.

Hose distribution manifolds can be placed either inside the chamber or external to it. It was fashionable to have an external manifold that gave the ability to measure the fluid inlet and outlet temperature of each shelf without having to pass the probe wires through the chamber wall. Unfortunately, this leads to many relatively thin tubes being welded through the relatively thick chamber wall. This is not an ideal manufacturing situation, and can easily lead to fluid leaks. An internal manifold, whilst making the incorporation of individual shelf temperature measurement less easy, can be flanged for easy removal. The lead-through can be the same thickness as the chamber wall, making manufacture easier. An internal manifold may require a slightly larger chamber but, by good design and because of the requirement for space for the stoppering system, the hoses, and the shelf support, the increase in size is minimal, if any.

Hoses can be screwed into the shelves and an internal manifold, or may be flanged onto lead-throughs from an external manifold; alternatively they can be welded. Welds are cleaner and cGMP prefers not to have screw threads whenever possible, because they are seen as dirt traps. However, the belief that screw threads can leak, or slacken, is untrue. It is a fact that hoses may work harden and leak, usually after a period of about 10 years, and especially on steam sterilisable plants. Once a single leak has developed, it is wise to replace all the hoses, as it is likely that another leak will develop in a short period of time. A screwed and flanged system makes replacement easy and makes the task of bringing the clean area back into operation sooner, as compared to replacing hoses that must be cut off and rewelded. The cutting, welding, grinding, and polishing that must take place in the clean area will cause widespread contamination, which must be cleaned out prior to being gassed. The welding is also difficult and in a confined space. Whilst there are no leaks, a welded system is probably favoured. If a long-term view is taken, then a screwed system is the best option. A system using Triclamps™, or the equivalent, is not good practice and should be avoided.

The shelf supports will vary depending on the presence, or not, of stoppering and the type of stoppering. They must be rigidly fitted to the roof and floor of the chamber and be constructed in such a way that they prevent fouling of the shelf hoses by the shelf stack. Alternatively, additional guards should prevent this occurrence. The base of the shelf supports should be such that they do not prevent the draining of condensate or wash water.

One important aspect of the shelf support system is that they should allow respacing of the shelves, providing the stoppering system is capable of achieving this. The supports should be manufactured of the same material as the chamber, with all welds smoothly ground and radiused. Polytetrafluoroethene (PTFE) inserts may be necessary to allow smooth running during stoppering. Care must be taken that product probe wires, if fitted, do not foul the shelf system and have sufficient free wire to accommodate stoppering.

An interesting variant is a double shelf stack, one behind the other, where the front shelves are cold and the rear shelves are hot. This system can be used when small volume products are to be processed. The product may be loaded, frozen, and then automatically transferred to the hot shelves for drying. Although this system is energy efficient, it is complicated and bulky and has not achieved widespread success.

Many food freeze dryers, in contrast to pharmaceutical freeze dryers, do not support the product on the shelf, but rely on the product being prefrozen and supported between shelves, where it is subjected to radiant heat at very high temperatures. Shelves heated by pressurised steam to over 150°C are not uncommon. The prefrozen product, monorail loading systems, lack of contact with the shelves, and the ability for the steam ejectors, which are used in place of vacuum pumps, to evacuate the system rapidly enable the shelves to be maintained at this temperature even during loading, thus obtaining high energy efficiency.

FREEZE DRYER SYSTEMS

The Stoppering System

The stoppering system is the means by which the shelves are closed together, effecting a final product container closure by means of driving a partially inserted stopper into the vial. This has the advantage of not only sealing the vials, as a preliminary to capping, under sterile conditions, but also under a controlled atmosphere. This atmosphere can vary from the freeze dryer vacuum to 900 mbar of an inert gas. The latter, or any regimen between that and a vacuum, is achieved by backfilling the freeze dryer with the requisite gas to the desired pressure prior to stoppering. A vacuum, or partial pressure, aids introduction of the diluent during reconstitution and prevents the stoppers from displacing once the freeze dryer has been fully aerated and the shelves relaxed to the drying position.

The stoppering system can also be used to assist in the changing of shelf interdistances, to allow the use of different sizes of containers. It is an aid to manual or automatic chamber cleaning by using its ability to move the shelves upward, out of the way of the operator or spray. Finally, it is the gateway to automatic loading systems.

Whilst the stoppering system is an invaluable asset to freeze dryer operation, it also produces problems of its own. Early systems introduced the piston from the hydraulic cylinder into the process chamber—hardly good cGMP. The system requires space within the chamber, and a hydraulic system requires additional height, either above or below the drying chamber.

The earliest stoppering systems were of the bladder type with a fixed shelf stack. Under each shelf, there was an aluminium platen that was supported on springs. Between the platen and the shelf, there was a bladder. The bladder was evacuated and, on completion of drying, was exposed to atmosphere with the chamber still under vacuum. The bladder would inflate, push the platen down, and stopper the vials. Unfortunately, many things could, and did, go wrong. The platens were thin to save weight, and would often bend and stick. If the bladder was not evacuated prior to chamber evacuation, then it would inflate, stopper the vials prior to drying, and leave a liquid fill, not a lyophilised product. Worst of all, the bladder could rupture. These bladders were filled with chalk to prevent the inside surfaces from sticking together. The effect on particle count can only be imagined! Fortunately, there are very few of these systems in operation today.

With the advent of flexible shelf hoses, it became possible to have a mobile shelf stack, and hydraulic systems were developed. These hydraulic systems, heavily modified from the original, are still the most prevalent form of stoppering actuation today. There are also cGMP screw and scissor mechanisms on the market today; most of which produce excellent, sanitary results. Systems that rely on cables or need lubrication should, in general, be avoided for obvious reasons.

The stoppering system will squeeze the shelves between the top and the bottom pressure plates. These plates are very rigid and usually of a webbed, or braced, construction with a flat plate as the surface that will touch the shelf. One of these pressure plates is fixed; the other is the surface that moves the shelf stack. Therefore, it can be seen that there are only two types of stoppering systems: a top stoppering system, where the top pressure plate moves down, and a bottom stoppering system, where the bottom pressure plate moves up. A system where both pressure plates move would be complicated and gives no advantage. There are, of course, many different methods of moving the pressure plates. The position of the prime mover, usually the hydraulic piston, is immaterial; it is the pressure plate that moves that defines the type of system.

Top-down stoppering systems involve the top pressure plate being supported by the actuating device. The top radiation shelf is suspended from the top pressure plate by stainless steel dumbbell-shaped rods. Each lower shelf is suspended from the shelf above. The bottom pressure plate is fixed to the chamber floor, it is not attached to the shelf stack, unless it acts as a base for the shelf guides. When stoppering is actuated, the top pressure plate moves down and the bottom shelf settles onto the bottom pressure plate. As the top pressure plate descends further, the second shelf from the bottom sinks until its lower surface rests on the tops of the stoppers of the vials on the bottom shelf. The supporting rods between the bottom and second to bottom shelves are now no longer under tension and slide through their attachment points; the shelf stack is kept in line by shelf guides. At this point, it is not important as to whether or not the stoppers have been inserted. Eventually, all the shelves are resting on the stoppers on the shelf below and all the support rods are loose. The shelf rods on different shelves must be staggered to avoid contact with each other. As the top pressure plate descends further, it pushes the stoppers fully home; some of the lower shelves may have already experienced stoppering because of the weight from the shelves above. When the stoppering mechanism is relaxed by raising the top pressure plate, the reverse occurs. The top two shelves open first, followed in sequence by the others.

Except in a specific case where it is possible to double the shelf interdistance by drying with pairs of shelves together, it is not possible to vary the interdistance between the shelves when using a top-down stoppering system. The exceptions to this are the replacement of the dumbbell support rods with a set of different length or the fitting of collars to the support rods. Fitting of collars can only reduce shelf interdistance (with no advantage), whilst the replacement of the support rods and subsequent shelf levelling could take a day. However, the top-down stoppering system has two advantages. It allows constant height loading and it gives easy cleaning.

Constant height loading consists of fully collapsing the empty shelf stack so that all the shelves are piled on top of the bottom pressure plate. The shelves are invariably cooled. The top pressure plate rises until the top usable shelf is stopped at a specific datum. This datum is usually the same height as the filling line, so a fixed height trolley can easily effect loading. After this shelf has been loaded, the top pressure plate rises again until the next shelf is presented for loading. This indexing of the shelves can be controlled in a variety of ways, including but not limited to, microswitches in the chamber, induction sensors in the chamber, sensors on the hydraulic piston, or the number of revolutions on an electric motor for a screw stoppering system. Constant height loading, in conjunction with a subdoor or inner door, is often used in automated loading systems, or where the product is temperature labile, as the shelves are loaded one at a time. The time between filling and freezing is minimised. The subdoor or inner door prevents the cold chamber and shelves from frosting, especially if a dry nitrogen blanket is introduced through the gas injection system. Unloading can also be achieved in the reverse shelf order; however, the entire shelf stack is often unloaded in one operation to minimise turnaround time between batches.

A constant height loading system has a dead volume within the chamber where the shelves are stored prior to indexing. For example, for a 12-shelf system, this volume would be less than 300 mm high, which is not usually of an overriding importance.

When all the shelves are collapsed to the bottom of the chamber, then the remainder of the chamber is available for cleaning, inspection, or repair. If the shelves are collapsed and then latched together, they can be raised to allow access to the floor of the chamber after an additional support has been placed under the raised shelf stack. Work should never be carried out under the shelf stack, unless there is an independent means of shelf support.

A bottom-up stoppering system (Figure 2.9) is the exact opposite of a top-down stoppering system. Bottom-up stoppering systems involve the bottom pressure plate being raised up by the actuating device. The bottom shelf is suspended just above the bottom pressure plate by pegs protruding from the side of the shelf that rest on the shelf support system. Each shelf is suspended in the same way. The shelves are not fastened to each other, but are constrained within the shelf guides. The top pressure plate is fixed to the chamber roof and is not attached to the shelf stack, unless it acts as a support for the shelf guides. When stoppering is actuated, the bottom pressure plate rises to meet the bottom shelf. As the bottom pressure plate ascends further, the bottom shelf rises until the tops of the stoppers of the vials push onto the bottom of the second shelf from the bottom. This lifts the

Figure 2.9. The principle of shelf repositioning to increase shelf interdistance.

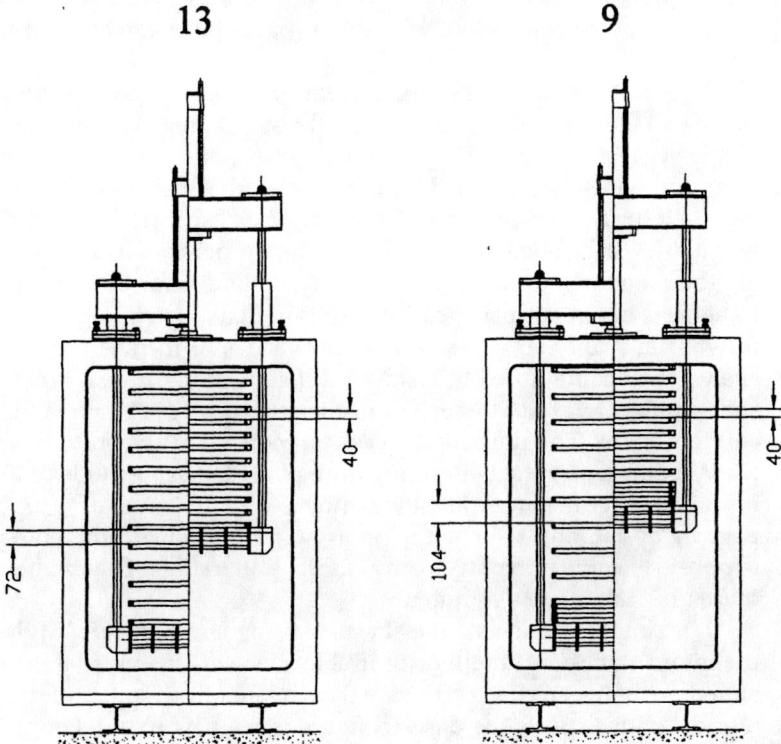

Reproduced by kind permission of Usifroid.

second shelf's pegs from their resting places; the shelf stack is kept in line by shelf guides. At this point, it is not important as to whether or not the stoppers have been inserted. Eventually, all the stoppers are pushing on the shelf above and the radiation shelf is pushing onto the top pressure plate. As the bottom pressure plate ascends further, it pushes the stoppers fully home; some of the lower shelves may have already experienced stoppering because of the weight from the shelves above. When the stoppering mechanism is relaxed by lowering the bottom pressure plate, the reverse occurs. The top two shelves open first, followed in sequence by the others.

Constant height loading is not possible with a bottom-up system but this system has a large advantage in that it can be used to vary the distance between the shelves, to accommodate different sizes of product containers. This is not without capacity cost, as the chamber has a finite size. It may, for instance, allow a freeze dryer that would normally have 10 usable shelves with a shelf interdistance of 72 mm to operate 8 shelves with an interdistance of 90 mm. The usable shelf area is reduced by 20 percent but vials up to 18 mm taller can be accommodated.

The bottom-up stoppering system achieves this conversion by raising all the shelves off their pegs. If the stoppering system is not full stroke because of ceiling height restrictions (i.e., the stroke of the actuating mechanism is insufficient to bring all the shelves together underneath the top pressure plate), then the use of spacers on the shelves will allow all the shelves to be raised. The support points for the pegs are then moved manually. The simplest method is for these supports to be slots cut into a plate, called a colison plate. By sliding one plate forward and another plate back, at both sides of the shelf stack, the shelves will come down to rest in a different configuration when the shelf stack is relaxed. It is usual for there to be three or four different configurations. The unused shelves rest together at the bottom of the chamber on top of the bottom pressure plate. Other methods of altering shelf interdistances are by removable complementary support pegs or by rotating the shelf support system to allow different shelf supports to come into play. In any case, the alteration of shelf interdistance only takes a few minutes.

It is simple to calculate the effects of using fewer shelves. Multiply the interdistance and number of usable shelves. This gives the available space between shelves. Divide the new, smaller number of shelves into the above space; the derived figure is the new interdistance. If a new freeze dryer is being contemplated, it is not possible to use the same formula to calculate the effect of adding, or subtracting, shelves to those present in the existing dryer, as the thickness of the additional shelves must be taken into account.

If the shelf stack is to be moved for cleaning, it can only be moved upward, and should be suitably supported before work commences underneath it. The lowering of all the shelves to the bottom is not possible, unless one of the interdistance options allows for it by having no supports.

Stoppering used to be a simple system. Top-down stoppering systems consisted of a hydraulic cylinder mounted on top of the chamber, with the hydraulic piston protruding through a vacuum seal and then attached to the top pressure plate. Bottom-up stoppering systems were similar, but underneath. They had the added complication that it may have been necessary to have a pit, beneath the freeze dryer, to accommodate the hydraulic cylinder. The advisability of introducing a non-sterile hydraulic piston into a sterile chamber when the product containers were still open was then raised. The ramifications of this observation have guided stoppering system design for more than the last decade.

The first design to attempt to overcome the above issue was saddle stoppering. Saddle stoppering consists of a yoke, or beam, that is supported over the chamber by either a single hydraulic cylinder mounted on the top of the chamber or two hydraulic cylinders mounted on the outside sides of the chamber. In the latter case, the hydraulic pistons are kept in synchronisation by microswitches. Lifting rods are attached to the yoke and these pass through the chamber roof to connect to the bottom pressure plate. This type of stoppering is, therefore, bottom-up stoppering, even though the hydraulic cylinder is situated on top of the chamber (or two on the sides). When the hydraulic cylinder(s) were actuated, they would lift the yoke, which would then withdraw the lifting rods from the chamber, thereby lifting the bottom pressure plate.

The system relies on the freeze dryer being sterilised prior to every batch. If sterile lifting rods are within the chamber and withdrawn from the chamber during stoppering, then there is no challenge to the sterility of the product. They are only reinserted, nonsterile, into the chamber once vial closure has taken place. An added refinement is to place stainless steel bellows around the lifting rods, attached to the chamber roof and the bottom pressure plate, so that sterilisation is not necessary for every batch. This bellows system is effective and sterile, as both the bellows and the shelf stack are in the relaxed (i.e., open), position during sterilisation.

An alternative was to extend the lifting rods and to pass them through steam chests so that they were sterilised with the plant and could also be steamed during reinsertion. The residence time of the lifting rod within the steam chests means that the lifting rods are only sanitised, not sterilised, during stoppering. Sterilisation is achieved when the lifting rods are steamed in conjunction with the rest of the plant. This solution is useful if the freeze dryer is not to be sterilised for every batch, as the lifting rods can be steamed independently in a static position.

The advent of saddle stoppering, as a means of bottom-up stoppering, effectively meant the end of systems that used a bottom entry hydraulic piston to achieve bottom-up stoppering.

Top-down stoppering is still frequently used, especially for constant height loading operations. In this case, the hydraulic piston is often surrounded with a stainless steel bellows that is attached to the chamber roof and the top pressure plate. There is a wariness, within the industry, of the effect of the bellows splitting. This is a remote possibility, since the bellows' manufacturers guarantee the bellows for an extraordinary number of operations. A bellows failure during a cycle would manifest itself as a vacuum alarm. A failure during sterilisation would result in condensate being trapped within the bellows, and an inability for the plant to reach vacuum as the condensate boiled off.

The point that is rarely noted is that if a top-down stoppering bellows is used, then the sterilisation exposure time must be doubled. If the bellows are open, then the shelf stack is closed, with the result that steam will not penetrate to the surfaces of the shelves. If the shelf stack is open, then the bellows are closed and steam will not penetrate the convolutions in the bellows. There is no halfway point, as this would involve some of the shelves still being closed. Therefore, it is necessary to steam the plant, operate the stoppering system whilst still at sterilising temperature, and then repeat the exposure time. The stoppering must also be operated during the drying segment of the sterilisation cycle. In this case, it is better to start the liquid ring pump with the shelf stack collapsed to dry the bellows, which have a small heat capacity. The shelves, with a large heat capacity, can be dried afterward.

The other item of concern is the cleaning of the bellows. However, this is of no greater magnitude than the problems experienced in the cleaning of flexible hoses.

Hydraulic systems still remain the most common method of actuating stoppering; however, other methods have been developed, including electrical drives, scissor mechanisms, cable mechanisms, and screw mechanisms. Of these only one is a viable cGMP alternative— screw stoppering.

Electrical drives that turn a screw thread, which in turn inserts a smooth rod into the chamber, are efficient, but suffer from the same drawbacks as a hydraulic system. Actuation is by the insertion of a nonsterile rod, which must be enclosed.

Scissor mechanisms also suffer from the nonsterile insertion problem, as they must be externally actuated, and have not gained widespread popularity. However, it should be possible to rotate the actuator to use a sanitary screw to open the scissors.

Cable and pulley systems are unsanitary and should be avoided.

A method of screw stoppering has been developed that does not involve the insertion of any part into the freeze dryer. Two high quality polished, stainless steel, helical screws are rotated, in synchronisation, by an electrical motor. The motor is mounted on top of the chamber, and the screws are mounted on either side of the shelf stack within the chamber. Where the screws pass through the chamber wall, they are smooth and the action is a rotary action only. Each screw passes through a carrier that may, in theory, be mounted on either the top or the bottom pressure plate. As the screws rotate, and as the carrier is fixed to the pressure plate, the carriers will move up or down the screw, depending on the direction of rotation. The movement of the carrier moves either the top or bottom pressure plate, so either top-down or bottom-up stoppering can be achieved. In practice, only top-stoppering systems are built in this way; there is no technical reason why bottom stoppering systems cannot be built.

With a screw stoppering mechanism, no part will enter the chamber, unlike a hydraulic system. There is no additional height requirement on top of the chamber, and there are no cleaning and sterilisation issues. The system has been shown to be fully sterilised and does not generate particles at a detectable level. The only disadvantage of the system is that it requires a slightly wider drying chamber to accommodate the screws. This system is capable of placing a shelf, during shelf indexing for constant height loading, to within a fraction of a millimetre and with no danger of "creep". The main inaccuracy, for a totally automated system, is the deflection of the shelf under load.

The operation of the shelf stoppering system should be smooth. This is of special importance for a constant height loading system, where unfrozen vials must be transported. An uneven stoppering action will cause the liquid to swill up the sides of the vial. This will look unsightly after drying; worst case would cause spillage or contamination of the stopper. A good test for the smoothness of stoppering is to balance a coin, on its edge, in a place on the shelf stack that will move but where it will not become sandwiched between two shelves. This is usually on the relevant pressure plate. If the coin does not fall over when the stoppering mechanism starts to move, then the action is acceptable.

The Fluid Circulation System

Older freeze dryers controlled the temperature of the shelf by having a series of parallel channels buried in the shelf that would carry two tubes containing a heating element or a space within which refrigerant was expanded. This system could produce temperature variations across the shelf of up to 10°C, even under steady state conditions. The product would therefore dry at a rate that was largely controlled by its position on the shelf; and in some cases it would collapse or melt. This unfortunate set of events gave the impetus to find an alternative system that would give better heat distribution, and so the fluid circulation system was developed.

The fluid circulation system (Figure 2.10), or thermoregulation system, is the system by which a temperature-controlled fluid is circulated through the shelves, thereby controlling the temperature of the shelves. This method gives tight control. The temperature variation between any two points on the shelf surfaces should not exceed ±1°C under steady state conditions, and at any temperature within the

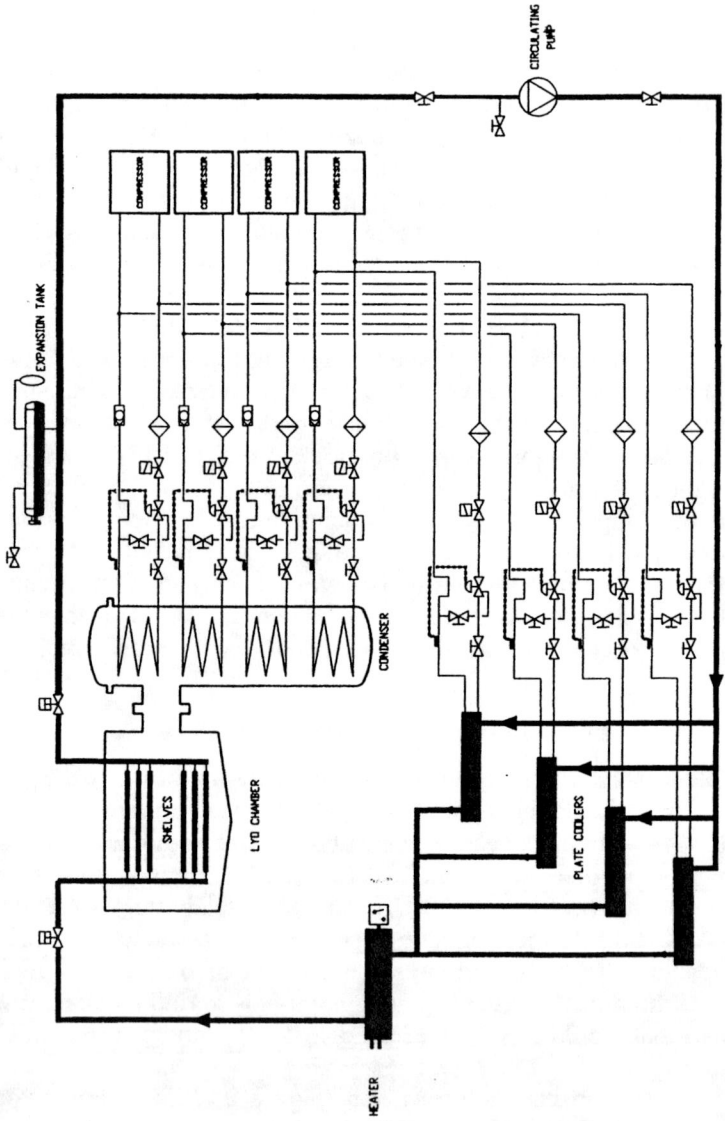

Figure 2.10. A typical refrigeration and fluid circuit P&ID.

controlled range. In practice, ±0.5°C is usual for a modern freeze dryer. Steady state should be defined as a measurement after holding a given temperature for 10 minutes. The controlled temperature range will be defined by freeze dryer design and specifications, but will typically be from -55°C to 70°C.

The fluid itself is, almost without exception in modern freeze dryers, a dimethylsiloxane silicone oil. These oils are graded according to their viscosity. The most commonly used is designated M5 which has a viscosity of 7.3 cSt at 0°C; it rises to 30 cSt at -50°C. Freeze dryers that are not steam sterilisable may use an M3 oil, which has a lower viscosity, but this is not recommended for steam sterilisable plants because M3 has a low flash point. These oils are inert and non-toxic to the skin, although in the light of recent court cases, in a totally unrelated industry, their systemic toxicity is suspect. Trichloroethylene and other halogen-substituted hydrocarbons have been used as thermoregulation fluids, but the Montreal Protocol now precludes their use. In any case, silicone oils are favoured because they have better heat carrying capacity.

The fluid circulation system, inside the drying chamber—composed of the shelves, shelf hoses, and distribution manifold—is concerned with controlling the temperature of the shelf by the thermoregulation fluid. The components outside the drying chamber are concerned with controlling the temperature of the fluid and are composed of the fluid transfer pipework, hot and cold heat exchangers, circulation pump(s), and the expansion tank.

It is normal for the pipework to be constructed in stainless steel, although mild steel could be used. The pipes are welded, although some elements, on larger plants, must be flanged to allow for installation. The fluid and, hence, the pipes can vary in temperature from -55°C to 70°C and, as the pipes may be several metres long, heavy insulation is required to prevent heat loss or gain. The insulation material is usually Armaflex™ or an equivalent.

The hot heat exchanger consists of a tube, through which silicone oil passes, containing several loops of electric resistance heater elements. These elements are very similar to those in a domestic electric kettle, although they may have a rating of up to 200 kW. In order to control the temperature of silicone oil closely, without temperature overshoot, these heaters are often split into several smaller elements within the tube. As the oil temperature nears the set point, the heaters will sequentially cut out. Alternatively, an electronic circuit that only allows current to pass to the heaters at adjustable phase angles may be incorporated. A third method of accurate control is to have a second hot heat exchanger with a low-powered element in it. The majority of freeze dryers contain only one hot heat exchanger.

The cold heat exchanger uses expansion of refrigerant, from the refrigeration group, to cool the silicone oil. Shell-and-tube heat exchangers were the normal design, until lately when they were superseded by plate-and-frame heat exchangers that are more efficient, carry less volume, and are smaller and lighter. It is normal to have one heat exchanger for each refrigeration circuit. The modern trend is to mount these in parallel, to reduce the pressure drop across the heat exchangers; many older plants fit the heat exchangers in series. All cold heat exchangers are utilised during freezing, but usually only one is used for thermoregulation during the sublimation and secondary drying sections of the freeze drying cycle. This control cold heat exchanger must operate during primary, and secondary drying, when temperatures above ambient are required, as the heat input from the circulation pump may cause the silicone oil to exceed the temperature set point, even when the set point is above the ambient temperature.

The entire cold heat exchanger assembly may be individually insulated, but most manufacturers will put them in a box and fill the box with insulating foam. Ideally the foam should not use a halogenated gas to form it, as the residual halogens make refrigerant leak detection difficult.

The hot and cold heat exchanger should be electrically interlocked to prevent them both operating at the same time.

The position of the silicone oil control and monitoring probes is a difficult problem, especially if there is a long length of pipe between the heat exchangers and the shelves. The control probe should be close to the heat exchanger outlets, to avoid temperature overshoot, whilst the monitoring probe should be in the proximity of the distribution manifold, to record the temperatures that the shelves are experiencing. No manufacturer places the probes in this position, and it is usual that a duplex probe is used to fulfil both functions. The rapid flow of silicone oil around the system makes this design satisfactory.

The probe is usually mounted in a pocket within the silicone oil flow; strapping the probe to the pipe is not acceptable. There have been reports that even a pocket may give erroneous readings. The most accurate method of measuring the temperature of the silicone oil is to have a glanded entry into the system through which the probe will pass. Again, this is not a usual method of manufacture, partially because probe calibration would become a messy operation.

Silicone oil is pumped around the system by an impeller pump. In order to increase product safety, it is usual to incorporate a second pump in parallel with the first. It is important that the pumps are independent of each other and do not contain a common body or motor. They should also be valved both up- and downstream to allow replacement, without having to drain the silicone oil from the system. A pressure measurement system is often incorporated to detect the failure of a pump; switchover from the duty to the standby pump may be either automatic or manual. Pump flow is calculated and set to between 0.75 to 1.0 m^3/m^2 shelf area/hour. A lower flow will result in uneven shelf temperatures.

The pumps will add heat to the system, which is balanced by the control system calling for cooling from the cold heat exchanger. Although the pumps are usually insulated, any bare metal will condense water from the atmosphere when the fluid is cold. For this reason, it is good practise to pack the pump motor terminal boxes with silicone grease or sealant.

The large range of temperatures experienced by silicone oil will result in large volume changes. Although M5 has a coefficient of expansion of approximately $1 \times 10^{-3}/°C$, it is possible that over 1 m^3 of silicone oil is present in the system. The requirement for an expansion tank is, therefore, obvious. Silicone oil will displace the air from the expansion tank as the silicone oil temperature rises and the oil expands, and allow air into the tank as the temperature falls. Silicone oil is mildly hygroscopic; any water that is adsorbed into the oil, from the air, will be carried around the system and freeze at the coldest point, which will be the cold heat exchangers, and, in extreme cases, may block them. This potential problem may be averted by placing an expansion bladder or a tube of silica gel on the expansion tank airway. Of the two methods, both are effective, but the bladder has the advantage of being maintenance free, until the rubber perishes. The silica gel system occupies less space. A moisture level of up to 60 ppm is acceptable.

Air entrapped within the system will invariably migrate to the top shelf; if for no other reason, that this is where it will do most harm. Other likely places of collection could be the hot heat exchanger, where it is inadvisable to displace silicone oil around the heater elements (There should be a thermostat fitted to cut power to the heater elements in this eventuality.) and in any position within the system where the feed is up and the drain is down. The correct method of filling silicone oil into the system is by pulling a vacuum and sucking the silicone oil in from the drain valve to avoid air locks. Topping of the system should not be necessary, but if it becomes so (e.g., after a pump mechanical seal failure), then it can be performed by pouring silicone oil into the expansion tank. The expansion tank will have a sight glass or level indicator; the tank should be half full when the silicone oil is at ambient temperature.

The Refrigeration System

There are two components within the freeze dryer that make use of the refrigeration system; the shelves and the condenser. The refrigeration system (Figure 2.11) cools the shelves through the cold heat exchanger

Figure 2.11. A simplified refrigeration circuit.

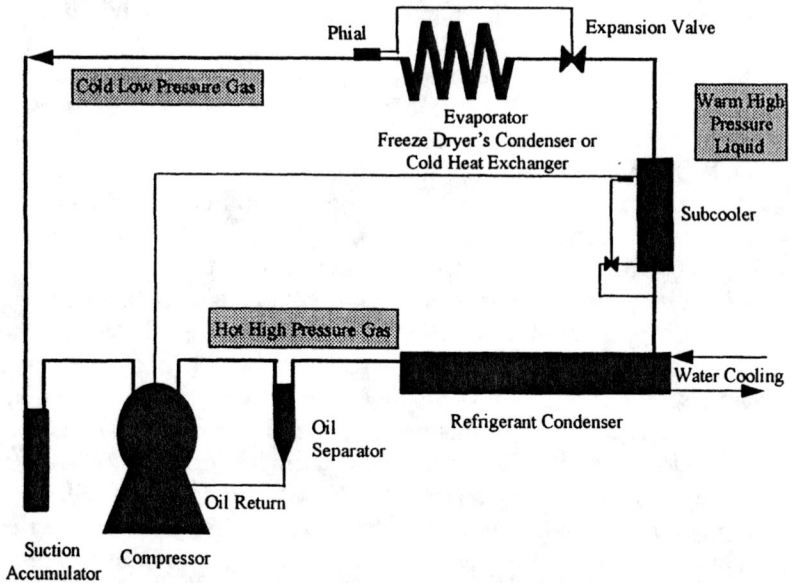

in the thermoregulation fluid circulation system; the condenser is cooled by direct expansion of refrigerant in the condenser coils.

The way that a freeze drying cycle operates dictates that the requirement for maximum cooling in these two components never occurs simultaneously. Condenser cooling is switched off during the product freezing steps of the cycle. There is usually little call for shelf cooling, except at low (below –30°C) shelf temperatures during primary drying when cooling is required for the condenser. The requirement for shelf cooling during primary and secondary drying is for control cooling to neutralise the heat input from the fluid circulation pump and any heat that leaks into the freeze dryer. These heat inputs are partially balanced by the sublimation of the product; every gram of water that sublimes removes 680 calories from the shelf system. External heat input is small as the system is operating under vacuum, and the chamber walls and fluid pipes are insulated. Nevertheless, shelf control cooling is required, even at the elevated temperatures during secondary drying, which adds complication to the design of the refrigeration system. At very low temperatures, the requirement for control cooling can be quite large.

It can be seen that an efficient refrigeration system design will utilise cooling from the same refrigerant system for both shelf and condenser cooling, whilst allowing flexibility to supply shelf control cooling without allowing the condenser temperature to rise. The system must also be able to maintain shelf temperatures when the condenser is initially cooled and the shelves are at their lowest temperature. This may be achieved in several ways, but in order to understand how this can be achieved, it is first necessary to describe how a refrigerant circuit works. A full treatise on refrigeration can be found elsewhere; only the basics are discussed below.

A refrigeration circuit is a closed loop containing a gas that will undergo a phase change to a liquid at the temperatures and pressures found within the circuit. This gas is usually called a refrigerant. These gases have contributed to ozone depletion and anthropogenic global warming, often named *the hole in the ozone layer* and *the greenhouse effect*. New gases have little or no effect on the ozone layer and a minimal effect on global warming.

The refrigerant gas is compressed by the compressor, causing the gas to become very hot. The gas passes through an oil separator that returns the oil droplets, which are suspended in the gas, back to the compressor. The high pressure, hot gas then enters a shell-and-tube heat exchanger where it is cooled, loses it latent heat of evaporation, and condenses into a warm liquid, which is still at high pressure because of the gas entering the heat exchanger. This heat exchanger is called the refrigeration system's condenser and should not be confused with the freeze dryer's condenser. Air-cooled systems use a fan-assisted radiator to perform the same function, and the high pressure, warm liquid collects in a liquid receiver. The incoming gas forces the liquid to the expansion valve through the liquid line. The expansion valve is merely an orifice, the size of which can be controlled by a temperature feedback mechanism. As the high pressure, warm liquid passes through the orifice, it experiences a drastic pressure drop and exits the orifice as a spray that evaporates in the reduced pressure. The latent heat needed to evaporate this high pressure, warm liquid to a low pressure, cold gas is absorbed from the surroundings. This removal of heat from the surroundings is the cooling effect that is desired from the refrigeration circuit, the area downstream of the expansion valve orifice is called the refrigeration systems evaporator. This evaporator can be either the cold heat exchanger in the fluid circulation system or, even more confusingly, the freeze dryer's condenser. At the distal end of the evaporator is a phial that is filled with the same gas as that in the refrigerant circuit. The phial is connected to the expansion valve by a narrow bore tube. The temperature at the end of the evaporator will alter the pressure within the phial; this pressure is transmitted to the expansion valve through the narrow bore tube, where it alters the size of the orifice accordingly, thus achieving feedback control. The gas is then pushed into the suction accumulator, which collects any liquid that has not evaporated, to prevent its return to the compressor, which would be damaged by it. Liquid passing through the compressor is named "slugging" and, in extreme cases, will hydraulically lock the compressor. Liquid collected in the suction accumulator will eventually evaporate, and is then scavenged by the compressor through the suction line, where the cycle starts over again.

The net effect of this continuous cycle is to remove heat from the evaporator (i.e., the condenser or cold heat exchanger), and to transfer it to the cooling water passing through the refrigeration system's condenser or to the air through the radiator.

Although this simplified description appears complicated, it operates in almost exactly the same way as a domestic refrigerator, freezer, or air conditioning unit. The difference between a domestic refrigeration system and that of a freeze dryer, apart from size and compressor type, is that a freeze dryer refrigeration system is usually water cooled, whilst a domestic system is air cooled. A domestic refrigeration system will use a hermetic compressor and the freeze dryer a semihermetic. A hermetic compressor has the compressor and electric motor completely enclosed in a sealed casing, whilst a semihermetic compressor can be dismantled. The electric motor in both types is cooled by the incoming cold refrigerant gas.

The compressor is usually a twin stage compressor that can achieve very low suction (incoming) line pressures. This increases the pressure drop across the expansion valve orifice and allows the attainment of lower temperatures. The attainment of these low temperatures can also be facilitated by cooling the high pressure, warm liquid upstream of the expansion valve by means of a subcooler. A subcooler works by taking some of the refrigerant liquid and expanding it through a second expansion valve and then into a heat exchanger that cools the liquid in the liquid line. This gas is scavenged into the interstage of the compressor.

The ability to split the liquid line gives an indication as to how control cooling can take place. Control cooling is the removal of heat to keep the shelf temperature stable at negative temperatures whilst the condenser is running. This ability is used in two of the three methods commonly used in freeze dryers.

1. The liquid line includes a diverting valve. If control cooling is required, the valve switches to supply refrigerant liquid to the cold heat exchanger in the thermoregulation fluid circulation system and is returned to the main suction line. This method

has the disadvantage of taking refrigeration duty from the condenser when control cooling is asked for, with the consequent and detrimental warming of the condenser.

2. A portion of the flow from the liquid line is passed through a small auxiliary heat exchanger in the thermoregulation fluid circulation system when control cooling is asked for by the control system. The return is through the compressor interstage. This method keeps the majority of the duty on the condenser and is an efficient method of control cooling.

3. A small auxiliary compressor is fitted that is dedicated to shelf cooling and separate to the main compressors. Whilst this method is preferable from the freeze drying cycle viewpoint, the auxiliary compressor is constantly switching on and off, which will accelerate compressor wear.

It is often the case, for example, where rapid freezing is required, that the refrigeration duty during freezing is greater than the condenser refrigeration duty required later in the cycle. The opposite could occur in a bulk application. Accordingly, there are three potential types of refrigeration circuits.

1. *Mixed.* The circuit can cool either the shelves or the condenser, and uses a diverting valve in the liquid line to switch duty; return is through a common suction line.

2. *Dedicated.* The circuit can cool only the shelves or the condenser and cannot change duty.

3. *Auxiliary.* A smaller compressor that operates during shelf freezing and when the system calls for control cooling.

Each circuit will contain a single compressor, and the circuits never mix gas. The reason for this is that in the case of a compressor burnout, the refrigerant gas turning acid, or a refrigerant leak, only one refrigerant circuit is affected, increasing the possibility of completing the cycle and reducing the cost of repair.

All refrigerant circuits may contain many other components.

•   A filter dryer to remove any moisture from the system that was not removed by the dehydration process prior to charging. Moisture will freeze at the expansion valve, blocking the system.

•   Optionally, an acid filter to remove any acidic components caused by the refrigerant breaking down at the high temperatures experienced at the discharge side of the compressor.

- A strainer to remove any particulates.

- High and low pressure gauges to enable system fault diagnosis. An interstage pressure gauge and a compressor oil pressure gauge are often included.

- High and low pressure controls to prevent system damage. For example, to turn the system over when it is idle and the suction line pressure rises due to leakage past the expansion valve. This will prevent the compressor from starting with a high inlet pressure and consequent strain during the compression stroke.

- A compressor crankcase heater to keep the oil viscosity low and to prevent refrigerant dissolving in it, thereby reducing its lubrication properties.

- Compressor overpressure, temperature, and oil pressure cutouts to protect the compressor.

- Refrigeration system condenser liquid-level sight glass.

- Refrigerant system condenser pressure relief valve.

- Liquid-line sight glass with moisture indicator.

The refrigerant system is connected together by refrigeration grade copper tubing that is brazed, or silver soldered, whenever possible, to avoid connectors that may leak. Brazing should be performed under an inert gas purge to prevent oxidation by-products of the brazing flux, which will catalyse acid formation from the refrigerant. The compressor should be mounted on mountings to reduce vibration; pipes connected to the compressor should incorporate flexible sections to prevent the copper tubes from work hardening by vibration and, subsequently, failing.

All pipework should be lagged to prevent heat ingress. Areas that are not insulated will collect an ice load, by condensation from the atmosphere, that will melt when the refrigeration system is switched off. These areas and the compressor should have a drip tray to collect and drain melt water.

It is usual to mount the refrigeration system on a separate skid from the chamber and condenser in order to facilitate installation and maintenance. This layout also gives flexibility when the freeze dryer is to be installed in a restricted space. Freeze dryers have been built with the refrigeration skid on a different floor to the chamber and condenser. In one notable case, a freeze dryer was installed in what had previously been an elevator shaft. Another approach is to mount the compressors and condensers under a horizontal freeze dryer condenser. This layout is elegant and economical of floor space, but makes maintenance difficult.

An alternative to mechanical refrigeration is liquid nitrogen. Liquid nitrogen was investigated as an alternative when it became apparent that many of the refrigerants in use in freeze dryers, namely R13b1 and R502, were to be banned from manufacture by the Montreal Protocol. Liquid nitrogen is used by the freeze dryer in the same way as a refrigerant liquid, but the heat exchangers and condenser coils are specially fabricated to prevent the buildup of an insulating layer of nitrogen gas on the heat exchanging surfaces.

In theory, a temperature approaching –196°C can be achieved with liquid nitrogen; in practice, the shelf temperature is limited by the viscosity of the silicone oil to about –70°C, and there is little point in having an extremely low condenser temperature. Liquid nitrogen does not exhibit the tail off in efficiency that occurs with mechanical refrigeration at low temperatures, and shelf cooling can be rapid. There is also no possibility of the shelf temperature rising when the condenser is first cooled. Peak vapour loads can be easily accommodated by increasing the flow of liquid nitrogen through the condenser coils. Consumption is approximately 15 litres of liquid nitrogen per kilogram of wet product, although the actual value will depend on the product and the efficiency of the freeze dryer.

The main advantages of liquid nitrogen are that space and maintenance are minimised as well as noise. Cooling water is not required. The disadvantages of liquid nitrogen are the need to store and pipe it to the freeze dryer, usually through vacuum insulated pipework, and the cost. The cost is significantly reduced if liquid nitrogen is used elsewhere on the site or the exhaust nitrogen gas can be used in some other process.

The Vacuum System

It has previously been stated that a vacuum is not strictly necessary for freeze drying to occur. The important factor is that the partial pressure of water vapour is less than the saturated vapour pressure of water at the temperature of the freeze drying interface. This lowering of the partial pressure of water vapour is achieved by the condenser. A vacuum facilitates freeze drying by allowing an easier migration of water molecules, as they will have a reduced probability of colliding with other molecules.

The vacuum system is often thought of as the vacuum pumping group; however, it is not only necessary to generate the vacuum but also to contain it. The vacuum system, therefore, consists of the pipework, chamber, condenser, and the pumping group.

The pipework must be leaktight and the valves within the pipework must be of a suitable quality. They must exhibit leaktightness in the order of better than 10^{-4} mbar/litre/sec, but they must also withstand the rigours of steam sterilisation.

The chamber, condenser, and pipework should be assessed as a working system. A typical specification for the whole system would be better than 5×10^{-2} mbar/litre/sec. This value is far less than would be expected from an autoclave. It is worth noting that freeze drying chambers are sometimes quoted as better than 10^{-4} mbar/litre/sec. This figure must be taken with suspicion, and almost certainly refers to the chamber and condenser with blank flanges on the ports. Thus it gives no information as to how the system will perform.

Whilst the chamber and condenser exhibit excellent leak rates, it is unfortunate that the requirements of cGMP and steam sterilisation will compromise their vacuum engineering. Screw threads will slowly leak under a vacuum. Blind threads would normally have a slot down the thread, or a hole bored through the male thread, to allow air to escape during evacuation. In the case of a freeze dryer, this would be a potential dirt trap and would also collect condensate. It is usual in a vacuum system to weld, for example, a continuous butt weld, on one side and an interrupted weld on the other side. This method of welding facilitates leak detection; otherwise a leak at one point would manifest itself at the nearest leak in the outer weld, and make the identification of the inner (and most important) leak difficult. The requirement to keep weight down, but still be strong enough to act as a pressure vessel for steam sterilisation, will mean that this method of manufacture is not always possible.

Although conductance of the vacuum system (a function of the ease of vapour flow through the system) will affect pump-down times, the requirement to pass the large volumes of water vapour is the most critical parameter. The size of the vapour duct between the chamber and the condenser is calculated on water vapour flow. The vacuum duct between the condenser and the vacuum pump is far narrower than the vapour duct. The tortuous path of the vacuum duct, which is usually from the bottom of the condenser to the top, through the condenser wall, and then down to the vacuum pump, indicates that the duct should have a significant diameter. The minimum specification is that the vacuum duct should have the same cross-sectional area as that of the vacuum pump inlet connection; usually it should be four or five times this value.

The vacuum duct geometry should be such that there is no danger of water entering it, either as condensate during sterilisation or as defrost water if a flood and flow method of defrosting is used.

The vacuum duct will usually contain two components. A valve that will isolate the vacuum pump and a gauge port. The vacuum valve has two functions. The valve will close if the vacuum pump is not running. The antisuck-back valve within the vacuum pump casing is neither reliable enough, nor leak-tight enough, to maintain the vacuum within the freeze dryer. The vacuum valve is especially necessary during a leak rate test. Many systems will start the pump and let it run to warm up prior to allowing the vacuum valve to open. Whilst this is desirable, it is not completely necessary with modern vacuum pumps. This warming up phase usually coincides with condenser cooling and does not delay the onset of sublimation. The second function is to protect the vacuum pump during sterilisation. Steam sterilisation would destroy the vacuum pump, if only by depositing condensate in the vacuum pump oil. The vacuum valve is shut during sterilisation, which results in the lower part of the vacuum duct not being sterilised. While this is not desirable, there is no design to negate this, and the issue is politely ignored.

A gauge port is usually blanked off, but will normally directly accept a vacuum gauge—a NW10 fitting is common. If a gauge is fitted and the vacuum valve closed, then, in the case of poor vacuum, it is easy to diagnose if the fault lies with the pump or if there is a leak in the system. A secondary function of a gauge port is that it will allow an easy connection to a helium leak detector.

There are three types of vacuum pumps that may be fitted to a freeze dryer. The most common is the twin stage oil-sealed rotary pump. The rotary oil pump may have a Rootes pump fitted, in series, upstream to increase pumping speed and to guard against backstreaming. The third type is a dry pump that is almost always preceded by a Rootes pump, as a dry pump does not have a suitably low ultimate vacuum low capability.

The most common system is two rotary pumps with control refinements that will turn one pump off once the desired pressure has been reached and will turn the standby pump on if the duty pump fails. Ideally, both pumps should possess a vacuum valve. There is product safety in pump redundancy, although modern vacuum pumps are extremely reliable. A single pump system is adequate for the task in small- and medium-sized freeze dryers. Large freeze dryers may have a Rootes blower preceding these pumps. A Rootes blower will decrease the ultimate vacuum by a decade and will significantly increase the speed of the pumping group, thereby reducing pump-down times. If the Rootes blower starts at the same time as the rotary pumps, it may damage the rotary pumps by feeding too much gas to the pumps, causing high pressures within the rotary pumps. To avoid this damage the control system may start the Rootes blower at a set pressure; alternatively, many Rootes blowers themselves will not start until they experience a preset, low pressure.

Dry pumps were developed for the semiconductor industry, where they often must pump aggressive atmospheres. The lack of oil and the temperature at which the pump runs will allow the gas being pumped to pass through the pump without condensing. The pump will, therefore, have significantly improved corrosion resistance. These pumps were offered for freeze drying systems because the lack of oil in the system makes it impossible for pump oil to backstream, and a potential source of product contamination is removed. This argument is marginal, as the incidence of backstreaming observed in practice is negligible. The dry pump has a poor ultimate vacuum and, in a freeze dryer, is almost without exception preceded by a Rootes blower, which boosts the performance to that equivalent to a twin stage rotary pump. The Rootes blower itself is a good method of stopping backstreaming by way of a physical barrier to the migration of oil molecules. Dry pumps are also very expensive when compared to a rotary pump. They are noisy and often need water cooling. Their only real indication is if there is a significant organic solvent element in the product.

The method of operation of these three pumps is well documented and full descriptions can be found elsewhere. Briefly, the pumps work in the following ways:

- The oil-sealed rotary pump has a rotor that rotates within a stator, but with a centre of rotation that is offset from the centre of the stator. Two diametrically opposed spring-loaded sealing blades, mounted on the rotor, sweep the stator in such a way that they induct gas from the inlet, seal, and then compress the gas, and finally discharge it through an oil-covered flap valve. Two of these pumping chambers are placed in series within the pump body, which enables the pump to have an ultimate vacuum of 10^{-3} mbar when rotating at a speed of about 1,500 rpm. The pump oil assists the blades to make a seal and to seal the flap valve.

- A Rootes blower consists of two rotating lobes, with a figure eight cross section, called impellers, which rotate in opposite directions and sweep the gas through the pump. The speed of rotation is between 1,500 rpm and 4,000 rpm. This pump gives a poor ultimate vacuum and is almost always used in conjunction with another pump.

- A dry pump uses a contra-rotating hook and claw rotor mechanism to displace the gas through the system. It is multistage and gives an ultimate vacuum of 10^{-2} mbar.

Although the oil-sealed rotary pump is the most common pump in freeze drying, it suffers from the drawback that if water builds up in the pump oil, it will reduce the lubricating properties of the oil and, ultimately, cause accelerated pump wear and failure. The condenser will remove almost all the water vapour, but a small amount will pass it. A rotary pump has a gas ballast that will allow a small quantity of air to be introduced to the pumping chamber during the compression stage of the pumping cycle. This air reduces the percentage of water vapour and prevents water vapour from condensing into and contaminating the oil. The use of gas ballast will reduce the ultimate vacuum of the pump by about a decade, which is still within the required range for sublimation. It is advisable to operate the vacuum pump under gas ballast during primary drying, and to optionally switch it off during secondary drying. This regimen is easy to automate. If a significant amount of water builds up in the pump oil, it will emulsify, which will be apparent in the pump sight glass. Light contamination may be removed by pumping the pump with the gas ballast on, but the general rule is to change the pump oil as soon as an emulsion is observed. Organic solvents will usually turn the pump oil black; the remedy, however, is identical.

The exhaust from a rotary pump should always be led outside the building because an oil mist is expelled from the pump. Small systems may utilise an oil mist filter that may return the oil to the pump. If the outlet is piped away, it should pass through a catchpot or a vertical T that can be drained. This will prevent oil and condensed water vapour from flowing back into the pump exhaust valve.

There is no advantage in having a large pumping system on a freeze dryer. A typical specification is that the pumping group can evacuate the freeze dryer to a pressure of 1 mbar in 20 minutes, although this is often improved on small freeze dryers. A more rapid pump-down will not give a significant advantage. The refrigeration system on an industrial freeze dryer is usually designed in such a way that the shelves will hold temperature during condenser cooling, so there is no detriment to the product. A saving of 10 minutes on a 20-minute pump-down time will require a large pumping group that is expensive both to purchase and to run. A saving of 10 minutes on a short, 24-hour, cycle is insignificant. Once the required vacuum level has been achieved, the pump must maintain vacuum against the air injection system, leaks, and outgassing from the subliming ice—a very low level of duty.

The Pipework System

The pipework system (Figure 2.12) is, in actuality, two systems: the inlet and the outlet, or drain. Both systems share many common features of design and fabrication. The overriding feature is to combine many

Figure 2.12. A typical freeze dryer pipework P&ID.

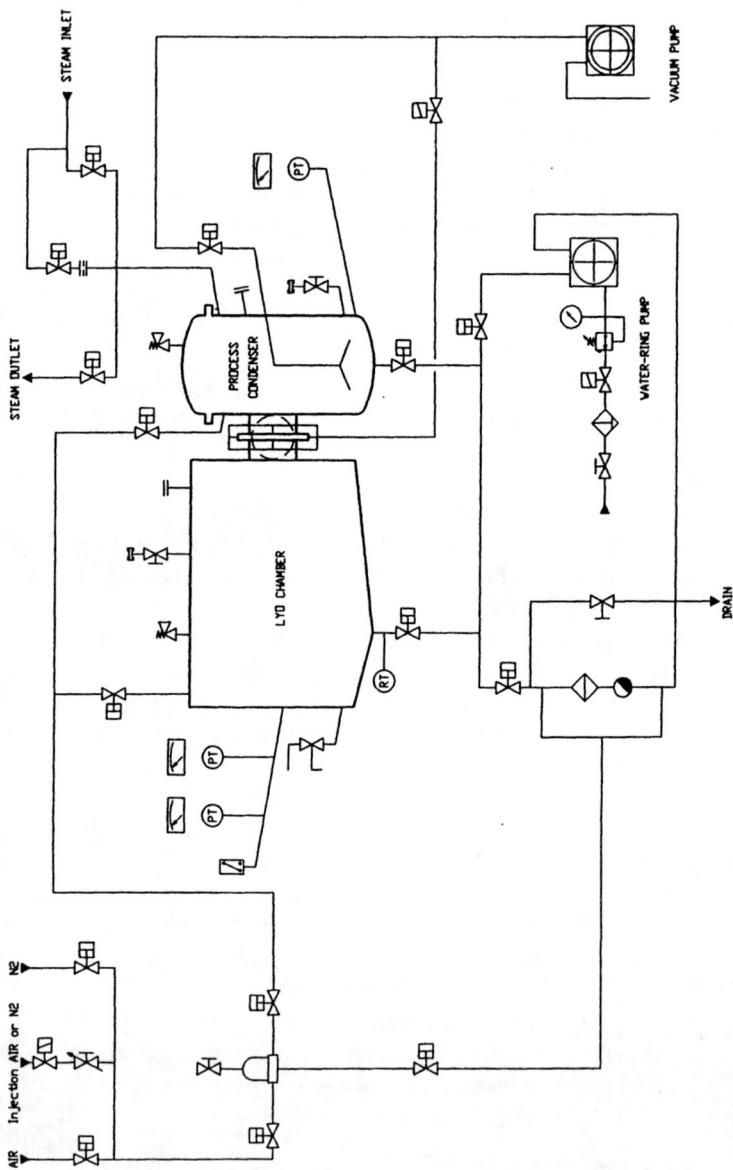

functions so that there are few breaks in the chamber and condenser walls. This is especially important in a steam sterilisable plant to ensure that the number of deadlegs, which would be difficult to sterilise, are kept to a minimum.

The pipework should be manufactured from the same grade of stainless steel, usually AISI 316L or the local equivalent, as the chamber. This is necessary because the pipework is a product contact component in the same way as the shelves or the inner wall of the chamber. The pipe should be smooth bored. Electropolish is often specified, but this is not strictly necessary. It is essential that the pipework is free draining.

The pipework should be welded into the minimum number of demountable sections, in order to reduce the possibility of leaks. The exceptions are the flange where the pipework is connected to the chamber or condenser and the sanitary fittings for the sterilising filter. It is common for valve bodies to be welded into the pipework and to become an integral part of it. The freeze dryer operates with gases being passed through the pipework, so a leak within the pipework, apart from reducing or negating vacuum level control, is a potential source of product contamination. It is for this reason that a leak test should be performed with the pipework included.

Welds should preferably be made by an orbital welder to reduce weld steps within the pipe that would prevent drainage of condensate. The pipework should be fabricated in such a way that it slopes to the drain and that there are no sections where condensate will accumulate. If the design includes sections that will not drain, then they should be valved and trapped at the lowest point.

It is not usual for the pipework to be insulated, potentially causing two problems. First, it is possible for plant room operatives to burn themselves during sterilisation. Second, the metal of the pipe is thin and has little heat storage capacity combined with a large radiative surface. Any condensate that is left in a pipe after sterilisation may not be totally evaporated by the liquid ring pump and may freeze under vacuum. Subsequent leak tests give erroneous results and time may be wasted looking for a phantom leak. Freeze drying would not be affected as the water in the pipe is, in itself, freeze drying. If ice forms in the pipe, then it is noticeable by the water vapour that will condense from the air and onto the cold section of the pipe. Should this phenomena occur, it can be managed by a variety of methods—heater tape, extending the liquid ring pump drying time, or lagging the pipe. A well-designed pipework system will not present this problem.

The tasks of the inlet pipework system (Plate 2.5) are as follows:

Plate 2.5. Gas inlet pipework with in situ integrity test ports. Note how all the pipework slopes to drain.

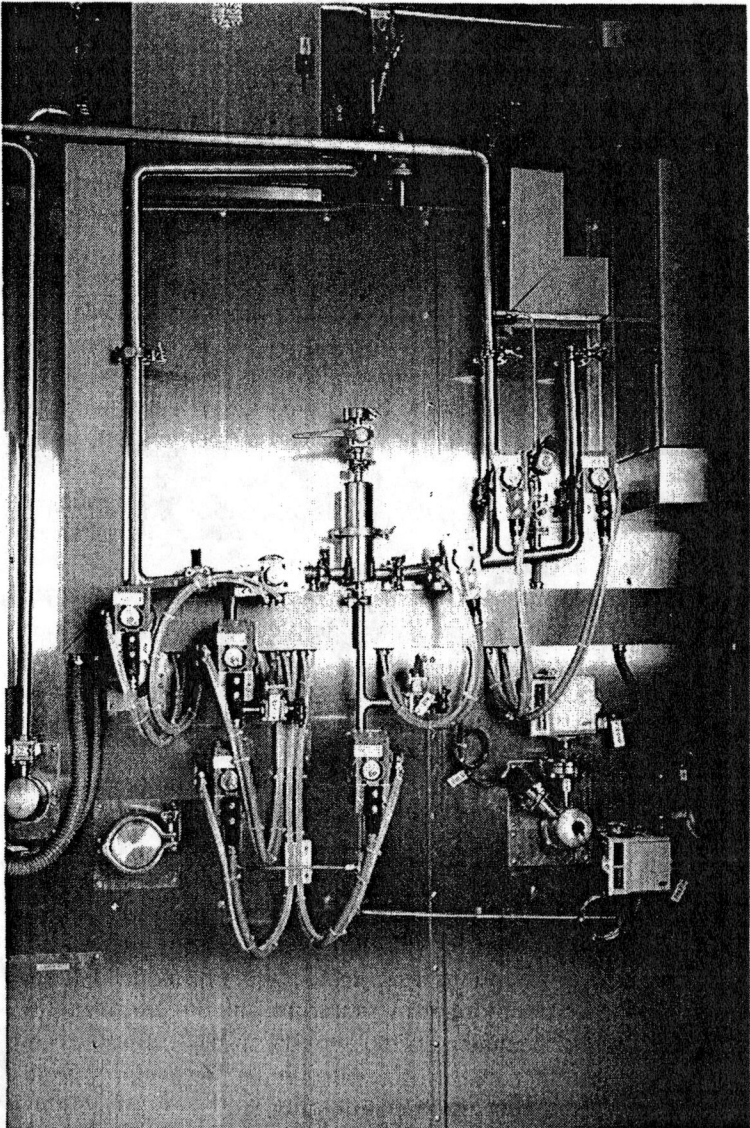

Reproduced by kind permission of Usifroid.

- Steam admission
- Incoming gas sterilisation
- Integrity testing of the sterilising filter

- Nitrogen admission for backfilling

- Air admission for aeration

- Air injection for vacuum control

Steam admission is controlled by either a modulating valve or a simple on/off valve that can be controlled by either drain temperature or pressure. The steam supply should preferably be pure steam produced from water of WFI quality. If pure steam is not used, then a filter, usually of stainless steel, should be incorporated into the spur off the main steam line. The use of factory, or boiler steam, will stain the internal surfaces of the freeze dryer, even with a filter incorporated. The steam supply should be trapped and reduced to a pressure of between 1.6 and 2.0 bar_g, unless the freeze dryer sterilises at higher temperatures, the steam pressure reducing valve should be of a stainless steel construction.

Most pressure vessel codes require that the vessel (chamber) incorporates a pressure relief valve. Some codes (e.g., TÜV) require the steam line to be relieved.

It used to be the case that the gas sterilising filter, which is sterilised at the same time as the plant, could be completely abused and steam entry would be through the filter. Modern filters have an identical specification as older filters, but will not tolerate a transmembrane pressure of 3 bars when they are rated at a transmembrane pressure of 300 mbar at 121°C! It is for this reason that steam entry will bypass the filter during the warm-up phase of the sterilisation cycle by either a simple bypass or by direct entry into the chamber and condenser. The steam then passes through the filter during the exposure time, when there is little pressure drop, or, alternatively the filter is backsteamed.

The gas sterilising filter is situated so that all incoming gases that enter the freeze dryer during the freeze drying cycle must pass through it. The filter, which is rated at 0.2 μm, is usually constructed of PTFE and is mounted in a stainless steel housing. The housing is usually connected to the pipework system by Triclover™ fittings to facilitate removal and filter change in addition for removal for integrity testing if this is not performed in situ. Surrounding the filter housing are the valves to permit in situ integrity testing, which is fully discussed in chapter 8. All manufacturers utilise a valving arrangement that will support both the forward flow and the water intrusion integrity tests. The filter housing is valved and steam trapped to remove condensate.

Both air and nitrogen admission lines enter the main inlet pipe upstream of the sterilising filter; these incoming gases do not need to be sterile, but they do need to be clean and dry. The lines are valved to prevent steam flowing up them. Nitrogen and air are conventional, but the systems will pass whatever gas is connected to them. If air is connected, then this should be connected to the clean area in order for the pressures to equalise between the chamber and the clean area to allow the door to open. Unfortunately, this will result in the pipe between the clean area and the admission valve being unable to be cleaned, although this does not create any problem because of the freeze dryer's sterilising filter. The clean area is often protected by a sterile grade filter that is placed over the pipework entrance into the area. Alternatively, the air can be admitted from the plant room, and the final pressure equalisation made by the use of a suitably interlocked valve on the chamber door.

Backfilling up to stoppering pressure is usually by nitrogen to lay an inert blanket of gas over the product, although vials may be stoppered under vacuum. The passage of gas during backfilling and aeration must be throttled to prevent the incoming air or nitrogen blowing product around the chamber and condenser. Typically, an aeration time will be of 20–30 minutes in duration; longer for large freeze dryers. Aeration to clean room pressure is by air. Although the atmosphere within the freeze dryer is predominantly nitrogen, there is little danger of operator anoxia during door opening because of the efficiency of clean room air handling units, although care should be taken not to reach into the drying chamber for extended periods.

The air injection system is a misnomer, as it is usually a nitrogen injection system; nitrogen is used to prevent oxidation of the product. The system works by flowing gas through a needle valve that is controlled by an on/off solenoid valve under the control of the control system. The volume between the two valves should be kept as small as possible; 10 mL of gas at atmospheric pressure becomes 100 L at 10^{-1} mbar and can cause pressure overshoot. Modulating valves are occasionally used. The gas injection system should be valved and placed upstream of the sterilising filter; designs that have the system downstream of the filter suffer from inadequate steam penetration and difficulty in drying after sterilisation.

The tasks of the drain pipework system are as follows:

- Sterilisation control

- Draining of condensate

- Steam removal

- Chamber drying

- Draining of wash or CIP water

The drain, or, more specifically, the drain valve seals and steam trap, are usually protected from broken glass and other foreign bodies by a strainer that is accessed from inside the chamber. A good chamber design will have the chamber outlet and drain valve accessible at the corner of the chamber.

Steam admission, during sterilisation, may be controlled either by drain temperature or by pressure, but the exposure time is governed by the drain probe temperature. The drain probe is invariably a duplex Pt100 temperature probe that is placed in a pocket protruding into the drain. This method of mounting ensures an easy removal for calibration. The pocket may be filled with a fluid for better thermal conductivity, but this is rare. The use of a duplex probe allows for one probe for control and one for monitoring.

During the sterilisation cycle, once the chamber pressure is above atmospheric pressure, the drain valve will open to allow the steam trap to remove condensate. Some manufacturers will place a nonreturn valve downstream of this valve, but this is not necessary because the drain valve should only open when there is a positive pressure within the chamber. Steam traps are usually of the float or thermostatic design.

When steam is released on completion of the sterilisation exposure time, it bypasses the steam trap and is usually allowed to escape freely until the pressure is just above atmospheric. In order to avoid filling the plant room with steam, this bypass may be throttled or a water spray incorporated into the tundish on the building drain. The freeze dryer drain should always enter the building drain through a tundish, to provide an air break to avoid suck-back when the steam in the freeze dryer drain condenses. Once the chamber pressure approaches atmospheric pressure, free escape of steam is stopped and the liquid ring pump switched on. The liquid ring pump is usually situated in the drain, although at least one manufacturer places it in the vacuum duct.

The liquid ring pump uses water to make its seal and, therefore, has a large capacity for water vapour. The freeze dryer is, internally, over 100°C, and any condensate within the freeze dryer boils off under the reduced pressure generated by the liquid ring pump. The ultimate vacuum of the liquid ring pump is governed by the SVP of the water at the temperature of the water making the seal. It is for this reason that a liquid ring pump cannot be used for the freeze drying cycle and obviate the requirement for a condenser. After drying, the plant is aerated through a sterile filter.

If the freeze dryer is used to dry a toxic product (e.g., a chemotherapeutic), the condensate is often collected to be assayed and, if necessary, decontaminated prior to disposal. In this case, the liquid ring pump feedwater should operate on a closed loop that can be drained and processed.

The requirement for large volumes of water to be removed if a CIP system is fitted to the freeze dryer requires the fitting of an oversized drain.

The most common, self-inflicted, source of a leak in a freeze dryer is the placement of a product probe across the door seal. The second most common, because it is often specified that product probes should reach the floor for calibration, is to allow a product probe to insert itself into the drain during sterilisation and to be trapped by the drain valve seal.

The Pneumatic System

The pneumatic system is the part of the freeze dryer that tends to be overlooked. There is little of contention within it but its function is of paramount importance, as it is the link between the electrical control system and the physical movement of the valves.

The majority of freeze dryers are constructed so that an electrical control signal will open, or shut, a solenoid valve, allowing pneumatic pressure to operate a valve, thereby controlling the plant. Most valve actuators will work at 6 bar, and the air required should be free from oil and particles. The use of a drainable trap upstream of the main distribution board regulator and downstream of the isolator valve is recommended. The usage by the freeze dryer is minimal and the freeze dryer can be operated from a nitrogen cylinder.

The solenoid should be capable of being triggered by a push button on the solenoid that allows a valve to be forced open, or shut, for maintenance purposes. The flexible pneumatic tubes should be neatly laid and fixed and, like the valves and solenoids, should be tagged in such a way that they can be identified from the electrical schematics and the pipework and valve drawings. The outlets from the actuators should be muffled.

The type of actuator should be chosen in such a way that, in the case of pneumatic or electrical failure, the valve will fail "safe". The perfect example of this is the steam inlet valve, which should fail in the closed position. Valves that are not critical for safety should fail in such a way as to protect the product whenever possible.

Valves should contain microswitches to show their position electrically for feedback to the control system. In this case, the control system should be programmed not to move to the next step in a sequence until the valve has been shown to move. This system will detect, and alarm, sticking valves or pneumatic leaks.

CONCLUSION

The pharmaceutical freeze dryer (Plate 2.6) has changed markedly over the last two decades in response to the increasing pressures which have been placed upon it by the necessity for reproducible, sterile manufacture of freeze-dried products. Many of these changes—the replacement of shelf cooling by direct expansion of refrigerant with a thermoregulated fluid circulation system or the replacement of bladder stoppering by hydraulic, or screw, stoppering—have resulted in an increased quality of freeze drying that has been reflected in the product that is produced. The advent of the steam sterilisable freeze dryer, and the subsequent design changes to ensure the complete sterility of the contact parts of the machine, have no bearing on the initial quality of the product but ensure that the product remains sterile and, therefore, remains of high quality.

The question remains of which direction will freeze dryer design follow next. There is a current debate regarding the replacement of ball

Plate 2.6. The sterile side of a cGMP freeze dryer.

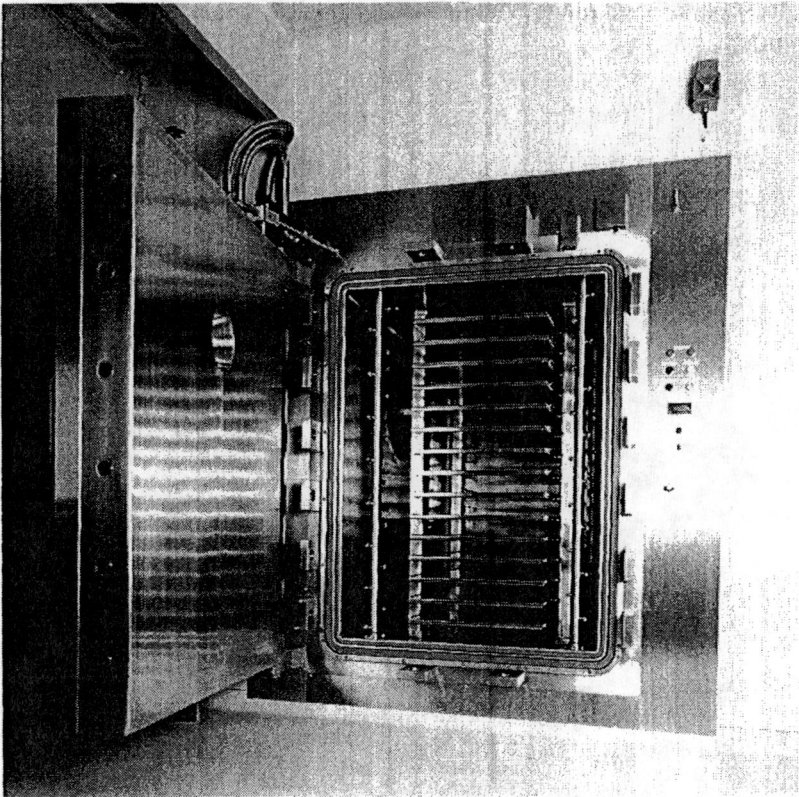

Reproduced by kind permission of Usifroid.

valves with diaphragm valves, a ball valve is vacuum tight but does not necessarily sterilise efficiently whilst a diaphragm valve is seen as easily sterilised but does not always have the vacuum tightness that is specified. Once this controversy is resolved then others will take its place.

The strategic development of freeze dryer design is likely to proceed along the direction of increasing the energy efficiency of the process by reducing the weight of those components that undergo the thermal cycle. The most noticeable development will probably be not in the freeze dryer, but in the development of loading and unloading systems. There are many loading systems that are available, but all have shortfalls and are expensive. The development of an efficient, trayless loading system, possibly associated with isolation bubble technology, could have the greatest impact on future pharmaceutical freeze-dried product production.

One thing is certain, although the evolution of the freeze dryer has progressed from the first, crude, commercially available apparatus to the sophisticated plant available today, this evolution has by no means ended.

3

FREEZE DRYER INSTRUMENTATION AND CONTROL

Kevin Murgatroyd

Biopharma Process Systems Ltd.
Winchester, United Kingdom

The freeze drying process is controlled on three parameters: time, temperature, and pressure. The ancillary valve switching functions within the cycle are also performed, as a general rule, by the freeze dryer control system. The control system will also perform other tasks associated with the freeze dryer; these functions are as diverse as the control of sterilisation to the production of batch records.

Of the three parameters, time is an absolute. A clock function is built into the control system. The accuracy of this clock guarantees that time measurement is not critical; a difference of a fraction of a second between actual elapsed time and the time measured by the computer will make little difference to a cycle segment that is several minutes, if not hours, long. In actuality, the measurement of time is more accurate than that of either temperature or pressure. The exposure time during sterilisation is critical, but as all sterilisation cycles have an exposure time longer than required, the likely error in time measurement is of no real importance.

The measurement of shelf and condenser temperature, and the measurement of vacuum, is more critical to the process. It is necessary to measure both temperature and pressure in order to control the process. The basis of control is to take an input (measurement), compare this with the set point, and then give an output to a device(s) that will change the actual value to that demanded by the set point.

INSTRUMENTATION

Pressure Measurement and Pressure Sensors

There are three types of pressure measurement required within the freeze dryer for the overall control of the freeze drying process and the ancillary tasks:

1. Vacuum during primary and secondary drying

2. Vacuum during backfilling and aeration

3. Pressure during sterilisation

It should be noted that the strict definition of an absolute vacuum is the complete absence of gaseous material. It follows that if there are traces of a gas present, then what is being measured is a pressure. For convenience, and to avoid confusion, measuring devices that measure pressures which are less than atmospheric pressure are termed *vacuum gauges* whilst those that measure pressures greater than atmospheric pressure are termed *pressure gauges*. The range of pressures to be measured within a freeze dryer can range from 10^{-3} mbar during the freeze drying process to 2.5 bar_a during sterilisation. Gauges will typically measure 3–4 decades of pressure, so at least two types of gauges are required.

The vacuum gauge will measure from 10^{-3} mbar to 10 mbar, although in most freeze dryer control systems it will normally come onto scale at 2 mbar. This gauge is used for the monitoring of pressure during the freeze drying cycle, and for control of pressure through the gas injection system. As it is unwise to use the same gauge for monitoring and control, then two gauges are often present. The types of gauges commonly used are the Pirani, the thermocouple, and the capacitance manometer (Figure 3.1).

The pressure gauge will measure, and control, pressure for backfilling, aeration and sterilisation and will usually operate in the 100 mbar to 4 bar_a range. Typically, piezoelectric or strain gauges are utilised.

Pirani gauges work on the principle of the thermal conductivity of a gas. An electric element is supplied with a constant voltage that will generate a heating effect within the element. The temperature of the element will be pressure dependant, but constant at a given pressure. The principle is that the element has a constant heat input that is

Figure 3.1. Sectional diagrams of the three gauge heads commonly used by freeze dryers.

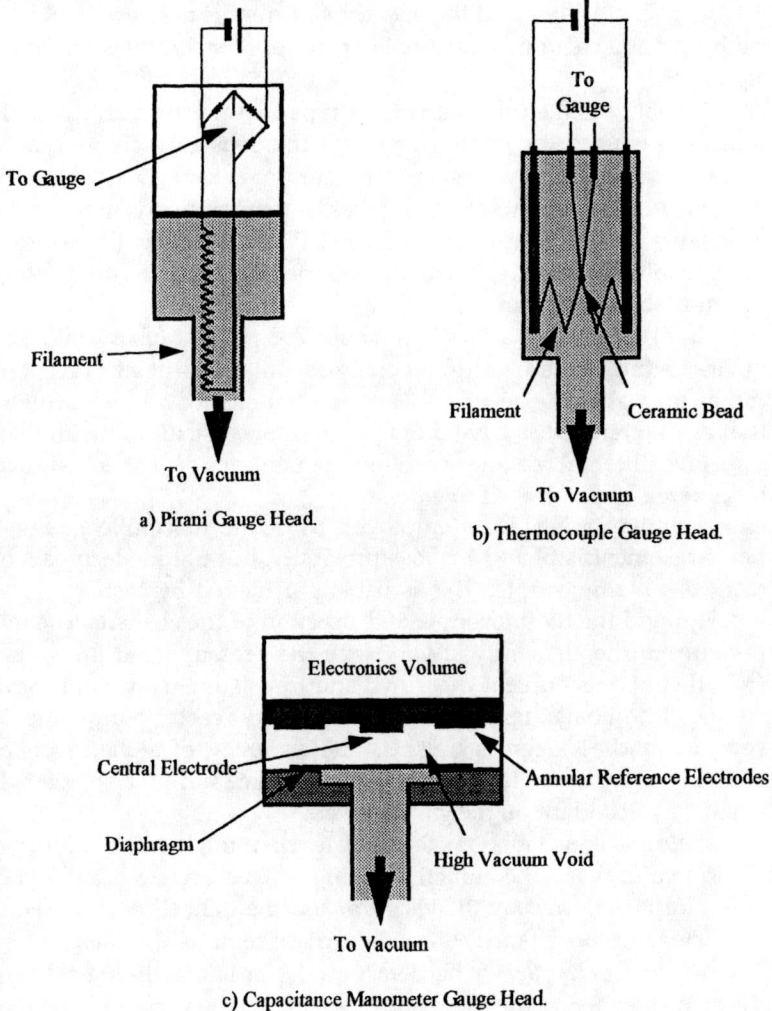

a) Pirani Gauge Head.

b) Thermocouple Gauge Head.

c) Capacitance Manometer Gauge Head.

challenged as gas molecules collide with the element and remove heat by absorbing energy. An equilibrium is rapidly reached where the element will exhibit a constant temperature at the given pressure. The more gas molecules that are present, the more collisions occur, and the lower the element temperature. The electrical resistance of the element increases with its temperature. As the electrical supply is designed so that the voltage across the element is constant, then the current that the element draws will alter with pressure. The element forms one arm of a Wheatstone bridge, and the balancing current is measured, which is calibrated as a vacuum scale. Analogue output for control is a 0–10 volt signal.

The above is the constant voltage type Pirani gauge; almost all Pirani gauges used for freeze dryers are the constant voltage type. A variant exists where the element temperature is kept constant and the variable voltage required to maintain this temperature is measured as a pressure scale. A constant temperature Pirani gauge will measure up to atmospheric pressure, whereas the upper limit of a constant voltage Pirani is about 10 mbar.

Pirani gauges are accurate to about 7–8 percent of reading. They are fast acting and are useful for control on the basis of a fast response rather than absolute accuracy. The disadvantage of a Pirani gauge is that as different gases have different thermal capacities, it will, therefore, give different readings as differing quantities of heat are removed by different gases at the same pressure.

A similar principle is employed by a thermocouple gauge. A heated element is placed in close proximity, but not in electrical contact, to a thermocouple. This is usually achieved by casting a glass bead around the thermocouple and a section of the element. The temperature of the element will vary with the pressure, and the voltage from the thermocouple is measured and translated to a vacuum scale. At low (10^{-3} mbar) pressures, the element may reach a temperature of several hundred degrees Celsius. The accuracy of a thermocouple gauge is approximately that of a Pirani gauge, and its response will, again, be dependant on the gas involved.

The capacitance manometer operates on a totally different principle to that of thermal conductivity gauges. This principle is that a diaphragm is deflected by the vacuum, and the deflection is sensed by the change in capacitance between the diaphragm and an electrode(s). The diaphragm has a very hard vacuum (approximately 10^{-7} mbar) in a sealed chamber on the reference side and has the vacuum to be measured on the other. There are usually two electrodes: a central electrode adjacent to the centre of the diaphragm, with an annular reference electrode around the periphery; the diaphragm is the final electrode. Alternatively, there may be an electrode at both sides of the diaphragm. The disadvantage of the latter model is that it is easily subject to electrode contamination. The capacitance manometer is accurate to 1 percent and is not sensitive to the gas it is measuring. The gauge is sensitive to temperature and is often thermostatically heated to over 100°C.

Of the three gauges, the Pirani and the thermocouple gauge are probably the best suited for a freeze dryer. These gauges may lack the accuracy of the capacitance manometer, but they are stable, easily calibrated, and have a fast response time. They are also substantially cheaper. Capacitance manometers work most effectively when they are subjected to a vacuum, calibrated, and then kept at vacuum. Allowing the gauge to return to atmospheric pressure, or, even worse, subjecting it to overpressure during steam sterilisation, can cause distortion of the diaphragm and necessitate recalibration. Older style gauges will experience baseline drift due to temperature changes, but this has been largely compensated for by constant temperature gauges. In practise, many users who have specified, and fitted, capacitance manometers have reverted back to a thermal conductivity gauge. The capacitance manometer is useful when a freeze drying cycle is transferred between freeze dryers; although if thermal conductivity gauges are present and correctly calibrated, this does not present a problem.

The main difference between the two types of gauges is the effect of the gas present; whilst the makeup of the gas is immaterial to the capacitance manometer, it has great effect on a thermal conductivity gauge. It is usual to calibrate freeze dryer gauges using air that is a relatively dry mixture of nitrogen and oxygen. During a freeze drying cycle, when the freeze dryer is operating at, for example, 0.1 mbar with an interface temperature of -20°C, the potential partial pressure of water vapour can be up to 1 mbar (the SVP of ice at -20°C). This pressure is never achieved because water vapour is removed by the condenser. If the freeze dryer pressure is below the SVP, under constant vacuum pumping of the noncondensable gases, then it is apparent that the majority of the gas within the freeze dryer is water vapour. Water vapour has a different thermal conductivity to dry air; therefore, the thermal conductivity gauge gives a different reading to what it would give at the same pressure in air. A capacitance manometer is calibrated in air, but will give the same reading in air as it would in water vapour. If a control pressure is set for primary drying, then this can be different depending on which type of gauge is used for control. For example, a set point of 10^{-1} mbar on a Pirani gauge will correspond to a set point of 6.5×10^{-2} mbar on a capacitance manometer.

Obviously, this fact must be taken into account if a cycle is to be transferred between two freeze dryers with different types of vacuum gauges. If the freeze dryer from which the cycle is being transferred has a Pirani gauge and the recipient freeze dryer has a capacitance manometer, then, if the set point is not altered, there will be a higher pressure of water vapour present during the cycle in the recipient freeze dryer. This will, in a pressure optimised cycle, slow down vapour evolution and evaporative cooling; in any case, there will be an increase in convective heat transport with the attendant danger of melting or collapse. In the opposite scenario, where the cycle is transferred from a freeze dryer equipped with a capacitance manometer to one with a Pirani gauge, the cycle will slow down as convective heat input will fall.

The vacuum gauge should be connected to the chamber through a short but wide, connector. This is ideally situated in the chamber roof to aid the removal of condensate after sterilisation and the prevention of damage by objects falling into the gauge. The gauge should be situated in such a position that incoming air from the inlet pipework, either from the gas injection system or during aeration, is not directed into the gauge head, as this could cause an inaccurate reading at best, and damage at worst.

If a second gauge is fitted, then this should be situated between the vacuum valve and the vacuum pump in order to diagnose the difference between a leak and a vacuum pump problem. There is little information that can be gained from a vacuum gauge that is connected to the condenser that cannot be gained by inference. The requirement for different sensors for control and monitoring can lead to the fitting of two gauge heads to the chamber.

Vacuum control is achieved, against a constantly running vacuum pump, by opening a valve that will allow gas to flow through a needle valve and into the chamber. The vacuum in the chamber is constantly challenged by small leaks, and by outgassing from subliming ice, which would raise the system partial pressure of noncondensable gases. An alternative method of vacuum control is to alter the conductance of the vacuum duct by throttling the vacuum valve and slowing down the removal of these gases. This latter method, and systems using a combination of the two methods, are rarely found in modern freeze dryers.

The pressure gauge controlling backfilling, aeration, and steam sterilisation is, naturally, of an accuracy more than sufficient for the purpose for which it is required. There is no preferred gauge. Piezo-electric gauges, strain gauges that measure electrical resistance in a semiconductor gauge attached to a diaphragm, or even capsule gauges can be used.

It is usual to fit a pressure gauge to both the chamber and the condenser. This requirement is especially necessary if steam is used for defrosting the condenser with the chamber isolation valve closed, or if the chamber isolation valve is not interlocked, in the open position, to the steam inlet valve. Pressure control is by an on/off valve for backfilling and aeration. Some steam cycles are controlled on pressure (but vetoed on temperature) but, again, control is usually on/off and modulating valves are rarely used.

Temperature Measurement and Temperature Sensors

There are four types of temperature measurement required within the freeze dryer for the overall control of the freeze drying process and ancillary tasks:

1. Shelf temperature

2. Condenser temperature

3. Product temperature (optional)

4. Sterilisation temperature

The range of temperatures that must be measured are from -100°C to 150°C. A condenser may reach an ultimate temperature as low as -90°C during secondary drying, when it has little load and hardest vacuum (which reduces heat ingress). At the other end of the scale, sterilisation is normally performed at 121°C, which may require temperatures of up to 125°C in the drain in order to achieve 121°C in the cold spot.

Freeze dryers may utilise two types of temperature sensors: the thermocouple or the RTD (resistance temperature detector, Pt100) (Figure 3.2). The thermocouple is small, inexpensive, simple, and self-powered, but is nonlinear in response, not very accurate, and can easily be damaged. The RTD is stable, linear, and relatively accurate, but is larger, expensive, requires a power source, and gives out heat. If the difficulties in integrating the two types of sensors into one system are ignored, then the ideal would be to utilise RTDs for machine functions and thermocouples for product probes. RTDs are less troublesome, and now that small RTDs—the size of a grain of rice—are available, most manufacturers will use RTDs as the standard build, but will fit thermocouples as an option.

The thermocouple works on the principle of the Seebeck effect (Figure 3.3). This was discovered by Thomas Seebeck in 1821, who found that if two wires, composed of dissimilar metals, were joined to each other at both ends, and the two junctions were at different temperatures, then a continuous electric current would flow around the circuit. If one junction was broken, then a voltage could be measured across the open ends. This voltage would depend on the metals used and the temperature of the remaining junction.

Unfortunately, temperature measurement is not as easy as measuring the voltage because as soon as a voltmeter is connected to the open ends, two new junctions are formed that generate a voltage. There are several ways of compensating for this. One way is to fix the voltmeter connections at a constant temperature by connecting

Figure 3.2. RTD (Pt100) temperature measurement circuits.

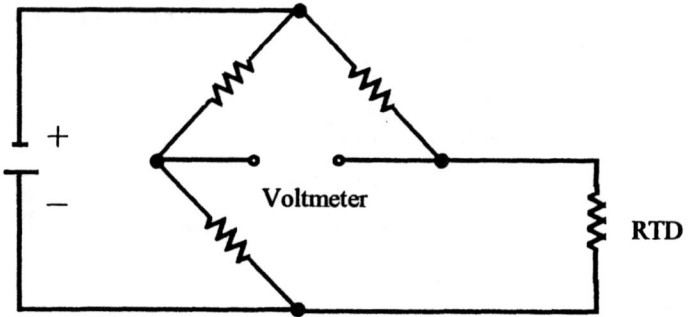

Two Wire RTD

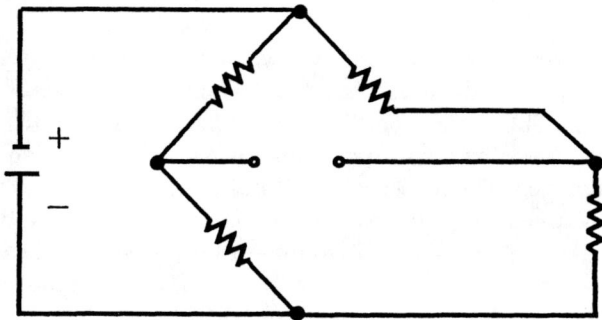

Three Wire RTD

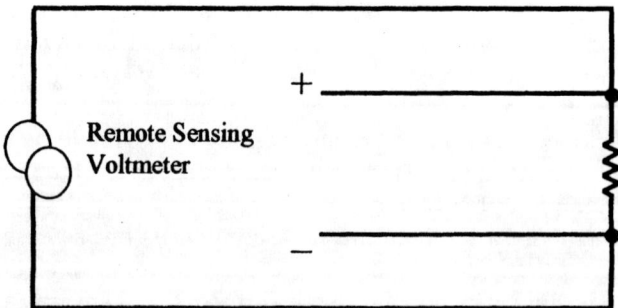

Four Wire RTD

Figure 3.3. The Seebeck Effect—the principle of the thermocouple temperature sensor.

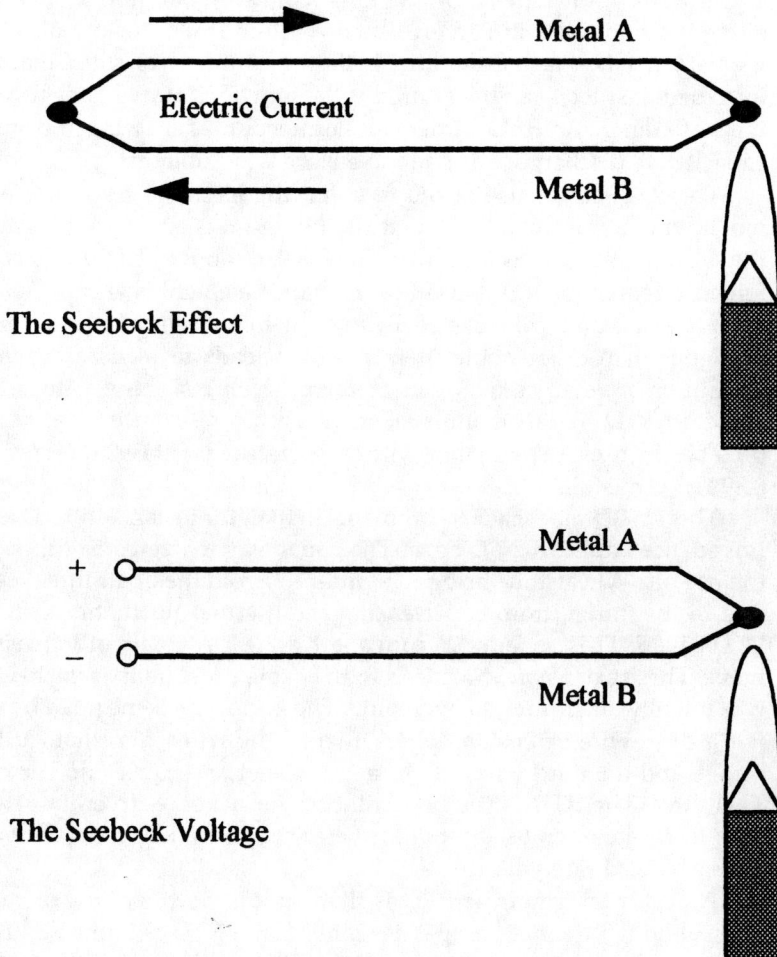

Metal A

Electric Current

Metal B

The Seebeck Effect

Metal A

+

−

Metal B

The Seebeck Voltage

them in thermal contact with a block of material with a high thermal capacity (i.e., at constant temperature), and to correct for the resultant voltage. Another method is to apply a voltage that will oppose that of the additional junctions on the block. The relationship between temperature and voltage is not linear and corrections must be made in order to have a linear output that can be used on a chart recorder or as a control input.

A thermocouple can be made by simply twisting two wires together; the first contact forms the junction. Soldering may be used; the solder adds a third metal, but as long as the temperature is constant along the soldered joint, an error is not introduced. The law of intermediate metals, one of the empirical thermocouple laws, states that the intermediate metal can be ignored if the junctions at both sides are at the same temperature. Commercial thermocouples are welded using a capacitative discharge technique to ensure weld uniformity.

The RTD makes use of the fact that the electrical resistance of a metal will increase with temperature. Platinum is often used because it has an excellent resistance to corrosion; on modern RTDs this is no longer a requirement because the resistance element is encapsulated. The other reason for the use of platinum is that its electrical resistance is higher than other noble metals, which leads to a more accurate measurement, or a smaller sensor for a given resistance value. The standard RTD has a platinum element with a resistance of 100 Ω at 0°C. The increase in resistance with temperature is 0.00392 $\Omega/\Omega/°C$ or 0.39 $\Omega/°C$ overall.

This small value leads to problems in that, for instance, a 10 Ω lead impedance implies a 26°C error. The usual way to overcome this is by the use of a Wheatstone bridge. In order to avoid the other three resistors in the bridge from experiencing the thermal fluctuations of the RTD, the RTD is separated from the bridge by a pair of extension wires. These extension wires lead to the same problem that the bridge was initially attempting to overcome. The issue may be negated by using a three-wire extension, where two of the wires form half of the bridge and the third wire acts as a sense lead and carries no current. This three-wire RTD is the best solution for a freeze dryer, but two-wire RTDs are often used for cheapness. Four-wire RTDs exist but are expensive and rarely used.

A disadvantage of the RTD is that, as it is powered, it generates heat, although the heat output is small. If the RTD is immersed in a thermally conductive medium, such as silicone oil or condensate, the heat output is dissipated and will not affect the media temperature or the sensor temperature to any large extent. The use of RTDs as product probes will cause minor problems in that they will supply heat to the product, although the amount of heat, and the effect, is small.

Ideally, the RTD should be sheathed in stainless steel. Duplex sensors are available that easily solve the issue of using different sensors for monitoring and control. The wires from thermocouples and from RTDs should be of the twisted pair type to avoid induced currents that would affect accuracy. Analogue output from temperature sensors is usually 4–20 mA.

With the exception of product probes, it is usual to place temperature probes in a thermowell. This is a pocket that protrudes into the area where the temperature is to be measured. The drain probes and thermoregulation fluid pockets are quite short, but those of the condenser may be over 1 metre long. It is also usual to have unused pockets in the condenser for validation. There have been reports of thermoregulation fluid thermowells causing inaccuracies, but the alternative is to place the probe into the silicone oil through a gland. This would make calibration and replacement a messy process, and is a source of an oil leak, so a thermowell is the accepted practise.

It is usual to specify probes that have long enough leads to enable all the probes to reach the floor at one of two points, one in the clean area and one in the plant room, as an aid to calibration. Although product probes are often fitted with plugs so that they can be removed, it is not wise to do so as this will negate the calibration. Instead, product probes should be specified that can withstand sterilisation.

THE CONTROL SYSTEM

The concept of the control system is twofold. The basic level is that the plant can be controlled in order to perform its functions at the correct time and at the correct temperatures and pressures. This is the essential element of the control system; you would not drive a motor vehicle if you could not control its direction and speed. The second element is that of automatic, or semiautomatic control. This will give the user the ability to give instructions to the plant and then to start it and leave it with the expectation that the plant will perform its instructions reliably and reproducibly. It is this reproducibility that is the key element in processing. It allows the product to be processed under the same conditions batch after batch. Providing that the batch from the processes upstream of the freeze dryer is of constant quality, it is then reasonable to expect that a freeze-dried product will be of the same constant, validated quality. The added bonus is that cycles do not have to be designed around working hours, and that human intervention (which is not validatable) is kept to the minimum.

The first semiautomatic control systems appeared in the 1970s and were hardwired systems that used simple feedback controls linked to a series of timers to control shelf temperature and little else. Alternatively, a shelf temperature profile could be cut onto a circular perspex cam, which was then followed by a cam follower linked to an arrangement to alter the heat input to the shelf. Unfortunately, these cams were notoriously difficult to cut. Later versions would use an optical line follower that had the facility to control vacuum and to switch key valves. Fully automatic electronic systems with proportional control began to appear in the mid 1980s.

It is fashionable to think of the modern control system (Plate 3.1) in terms of a complicated control panel with a computer screen giving an up to the minute readout of the status of the plant and the process. In actuality, control panels are not as complicated as they once were, largely because in a computerised system, the computer (PC) has taken over most of the functions. It must also be remembered that not all freeze dryers are controlled by a computerised system. Manual and microprocessor controlled systems exist and are frequently used; however most modern cGMP plants utilise the power of the PC, although they often have a hardwired, or wired through the programmable logic controller (PLC), backup system.

The complicated part of the control system lies in the software, where incoming data are processed and requisite outputs are then generated. The actual control of the plant is very simple and can occur in one of two ways: electrically or pneumatically. All motors are turned on and off through a relay, often called a contactor, that operates in a similar way to that of a motor vehicle starter solenoid. This relay is actuated by an electrical output from the control system. Valves on small plants are moved electromagnetically through a form of solenoid that is activated by the same method. Larger plants usually will use the control system output to activate a solenoid valve, which will then allow compressed air to actuate the valve being switched.

Manual Control Systems

The simplest manual control system involves a switch to control each component; in practise these systems are not produced and switches control a functionality. For example, the condenser cooling switch starts the compressor(s) and open the valves to allow the refrigerant to flow to the condenser coils. Another switch for shelf thermoregulation starts the circulation pumps and allows the manual temperature controller to interact with the shelf thermoregulation fluid temperature sensor, and use its control outputs to meet the set point by controlling the compressor(s). The valves allow the refrigerant to flow to the cold heat exchangers and the heating elements in the hot heat exchanger. This functionality methodology simplifies the manual control system by reducing the number of switches that must be switched on, thereby reducing the chances of error.

The usual array of functionality switches will probably include the following:

Plate 3.1. Interior of a typical freeze dryer control cabinet.

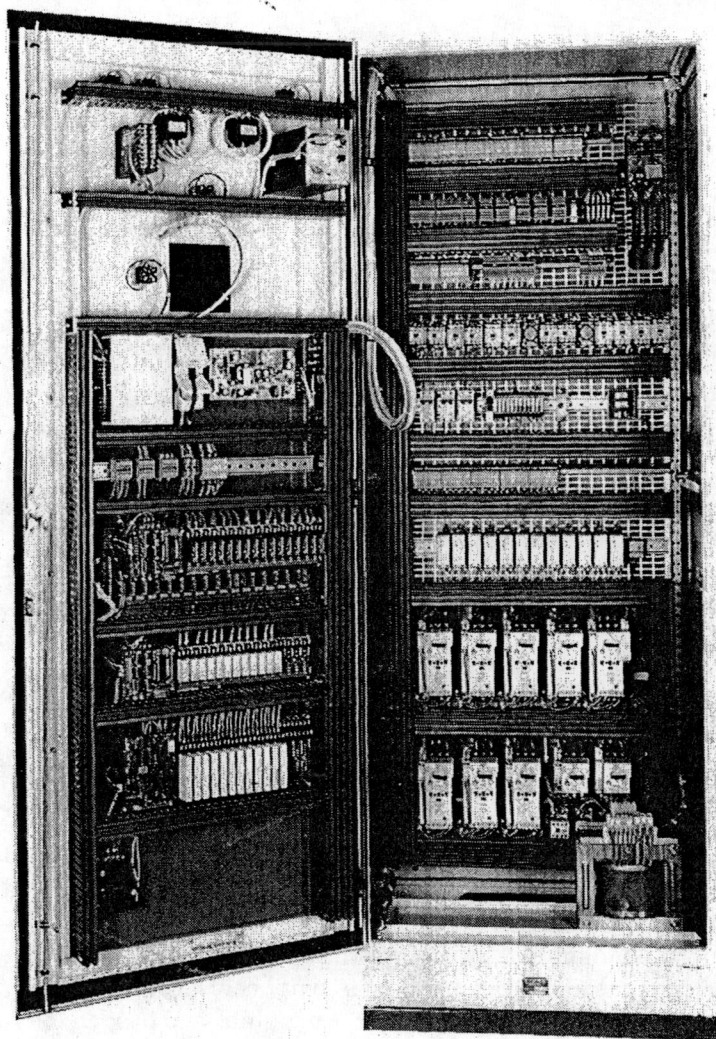

Reproduced by kind permission of Usifroid.

- Power on/off

- Shelf thermoregulation (alternatively, or additionally, there may be shelf heat and shelf cool)

- Condenser cooling

- Vacuum

- Chamber isolation valve

- Vacuum break/aerate

- Drain open

- Stoppering (up and down)

- Defrost

Manual systems that are fitted as a backup to an automatic controller will also have a manual/auto selector, which is usually a keyswitch.

The temperature of the shelves will be controlled by a shelf temperature controller. Multiple step controllers are available, but it is uncommon that they will have a temperature ramp facility. The shelf temperature will move to the set point as fast as the thermoregulation system will allow. The controller will include a temperature readout, usually as a liquid crystal display (LCD) or a light-emitting diode (LED) display. These controllers are now electronic; but in the past this function was performed by optical line followers or cams cut out of plastic.

Vacuum set point controllers are rarely incorporated into manual systems; or if they are, they are an expensive option. This is unfortunate, as the freeze drying cycle is most efficiently optimised by vacuum control. Vacuum will be shown, usually as a LCD or LED; if more than one gauge head is used, then this display will be switchable. The function of a vacuum level controller may be undertaken by the manual setting of a needle valve, but it is difficult to perform this function accurately by a manual method and the setting must be changed as the cycle progresses.

In addition to the switches, there will be hardwired interlocks to prevent damage to the plant or its components. For example, it should not be possible to turn on the vacuum pumps and to open the vacuum valve, which would normally be on the same switch, until the condenser was down to a preset temperature. Systems where it is possible to run the vacuum pumps without a cold condenser will risk damage to the vacuum pump by allowing water vapour to pass the warm condenser and to condense in the vacuum pump oil, causing reduced lubrication and premature wear or failure.

Manual systems may have audible alarm systems for vacuum failure and shelf overtemperature. The ability of the plant to autocorrect alarm situations is very limited and may not even include automatic freeze-down of the shelves.

As cycles cannot be automatically set, then a manual system must be closely monitored with a manual intervention every time a parameter must be changed. Thus, it is labour intensive. The switching of shelf temperature may be controlled by such vagaries as working hours or meal breaks, and the cycle cannot be claimed to be completely reproducible.

The inability to password protect the controls may lead to the fitting of a keyswitch to enable the power switch, but the system is always vulnerable to unauthorised intervention. The inability of a manually controlled cycle to be reproducible and the difficulty in preventing unauthorised intervention are the main reasons why a manual control system cannot meet cGMP. If unauthorised intervention is an issue, then the switches can be placed under a locked cover.

Sterilisation is never manually controlled, for obvious safety reasons. If present it will be initiated by a keyswitch. The sterilisation system may include a timer to control the exposure time and, more rarely, a drain temperature selector.

Hardwired Control Systems

Hardwired control systems were the first attempts to produce a semi-automatic control system. Whilst these systems now appear to be crude, it must be remembered that the age of compact devices capable of controlling a machine were not available until the early 1980s. It has been reported that, in 1969, the Apollo 11 lunar module had less onboard computing power than the engine management system of a modern family car, data was manually transferred from the command module to the lunar module. In many ways, these freeze dryer control systems were attempting to perform tasks when the suitable technology was not available and should be respected as such.

The first controllers achieved the programming of shelf temperature by a series of timers that had a simple feedback control to switch on an electrical current to a series of elements buried within the shelf for heating or to open a solenoid valve to allow freon to enter tubes within the shelf for shelf cooling. Sometimes, these timers were separate and sequentially transferred control from one to the other as the programmed time ran out; others were built into one chassis or unit and were the forerunners of manual shelf temperature timers and controllers that are used as a manual backup on modern plants. Valve sequencing was not achieved on these plants, and vacuum control, where it existed, was achieved by manually setting a needle valve.

An alternative to these electrical timers was a rotating cam that had the advantage of ramping up (or down) a temperature. These cams would rotate at a constant speed, usually 1 revolution in 24 hours. Cycles taking longer than 24 hours would presumably need a second cam that would be fitted during the cycle. The cutting of these cams was an art in itself because it was difficult to relate a cam profile to an exact temperature, and cams evolved rather than were manufactured. These cam systems would create a shelf temperature profile but nothing else; valve switching and vacuum control were manual processes.

Line followers were the last electromechanical systems before electronic systems. A photoelectric eye would laterally follow a thick, dark line on a roll of white paper that would scroll past the eye. The eye's position would be translated to the temperature at which the shelves were to be controlled. It was also possible to control vacuum. More advanced systems had a section on the scroll where the line was parallel to the scroll and would allow a valve to be switched on or off depending on whether the line was present or absent. Each cycle would require an individual scroll, and one advantage over the cam system was that the cycle could be as long as required, as the only time limit was the length of scroll that could be fitted onto the feed roller.

Although the absolute accuracy of these systems was suspect, they tended to be extremely reliable and some are still in use today. Line followers were extremely complicated, with a phenomenal clock-spring mechanism that was a triumph of the art of attempting to solve a technical problem, and succeeding, before a suitable technology existed.

These mechanisms are no longer used today; to a certain extent their passing could be viewed with nostalgia, and their use in modern manufacturing is precluded. However, the descendants of these timers exist today and are used as a manual backup and for the control of some laboratory and pilot plants.

Microprocessor Control Systems

Microprocessor-based control systems (Plate 3.2) are a true automatic control system for the control of the freeze drying cycle. They are capable of reproducibly controlling a freeze drying cycle, which has been recalled from memory, allowing the batch that the user wants to process to undergo the same freeze drying cycle as the previous identical batch, or one that was dried several years ago.

Plate 3.2. Typical microprocessor controls panel.

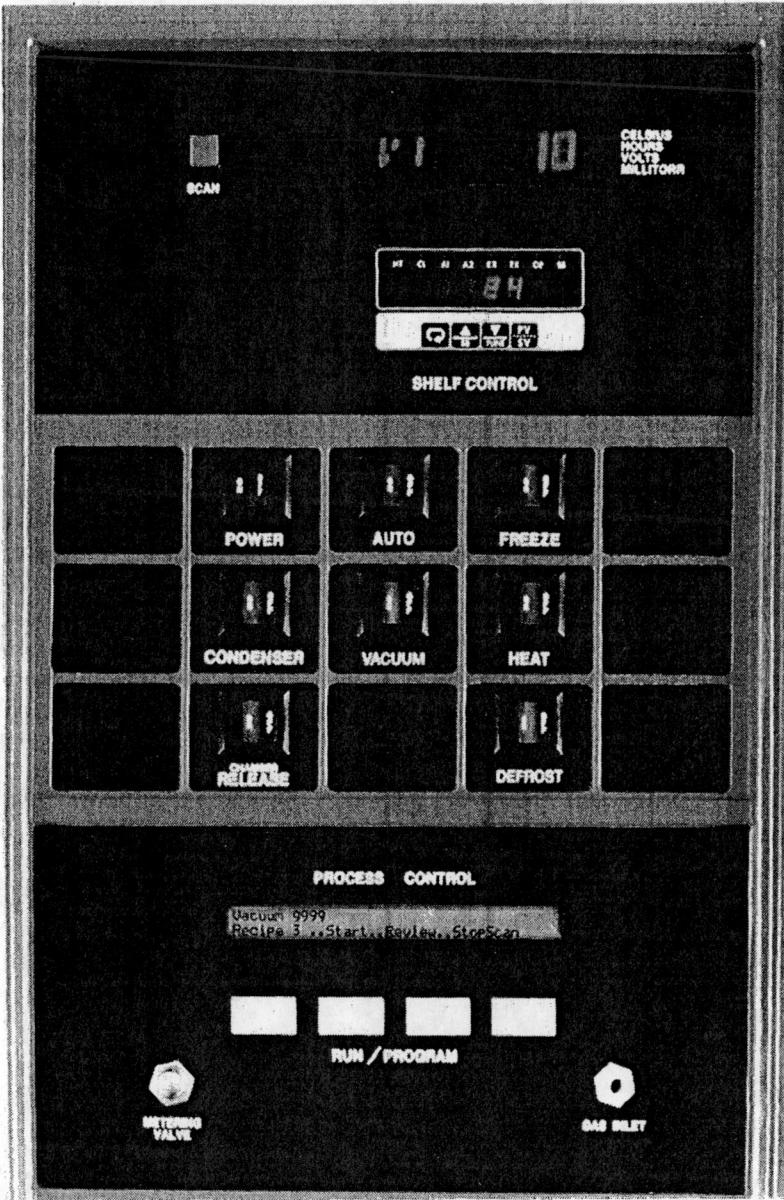

Microprocessor control systems are often seen as the inexpensive option for a freeze dryer control system. Most manufacturers market the PC–based system with a microprocessor system, often manufactured in-house, as the second string alternative. This is probably an unfair assessment of the microprocessor's capabilities. Whilst it is true that the user interface is less friendly, and the ancillary functions are limited, it must be stated that in terms of the important considerations of the control of shelf temperature and system pressure, when measured against a time base, the microprocessor is the equivalent of the more sophisticated PC–based systems.

Most systems are capable of multiple step freezing, primary drying, and secondary drying, and have the ability to perform thermal treatment during freezing, temperature ramps, and the pressure rise test during the two drying phases. Shelf temperature is automatically controlled, as is vacuum. The ancillary functions of stoppering, backfilling (preaeration) and aeration are included. Many systems include a sterilisation cycle, with the flexibility to control exposure time and drain probe temperature, and a defrost cycle.

The user interface, in any available freeze dryer microprocessor control system, can rarely be called friendly. The display unit is often a one line LCD or LED display. To exacerbate the confusion caused by minuscule data that can be displayed on this screen, the lack of an alphanumeric keyboard necessitates the need to scroll through menus in order to achieve anything, hopefully whilst still remembering where you are and what you have previously done. At least one system is programmed on only three buttons. Compared to many freeze dryer microprocessor control systems, the programming of a modern videocassette recorder pales into insignificance! There are systems that will give a multiple line display on a screen and have a minimum keyboard, but even on these systems the programming of a cycle is a tedious business.

Most systems have the capability to store several cycles in memory for recall. The number of cycles will depend on the available memory within the system, but will usually exceed 10. It is essential that the stored cycle parameters can be printed out to ensure that the correct cycle is being initiated.

The system will include several alarms and usually an alarm hierarchy, where it will allow the freeze dryer to perform several actions, of increasing gravity, to cancel an alarm state, before eventually attempting to freeze the product should these fail.

Data logging is rudimentary and is usually limited to a numerical printout of the main cycle parameters, with no graphical capability. It is usual for the print capability to include a cycle alarms list and the parameters for the current cycle. In general, batch records are not produced and a chart recorder is a necessary adjunct. There are systems that will transmit data to a PC, where it can be manipulated, or graphed, in one of the commercially available spreadsheet packages. If a PC is to be linked to the system, then the question must be asked, "Why is not the whole system put under the control of a PC?"

It is rare that a microprocessor system is fitted with an uninterruptible power supply (UPS); therefore, it is susceptible to mains fluctuations. Whilst these systems are reliable, they do not approach the reliability of a PC or a PC/PLC system.

It is wise to have a manual backup control system to a microprocessor system. These manual systems may take advantage of part of the microprocessor system or may be hardwired and independent, although they will share the same sensor inputs. The manual system is of special value during maintenance.

Whilst it is easy to show the shortcomings of microprocessor-based systems, it must be remembered that they are usually compared to a PC–based system, and that their control and processing power would be unsurpassed up to the mid 1980s. They represent a value for money option where a full PC–based system, is not required. Their cycle control is equivalent to a PC–based system and many control freeze dryers in FDA audited, cGMP manufacturing areas.

PC–Based Control Systems (Figures 3.4 and 3.5)

It is difficult to remember the times when PCs were not freely available, when letters (and books) were typed instead of produced on a word processor and calculators could be the size of the modern laptop computer, which is capable of performing millions of operations a second and having a gigabyte of memory storage. Freeze dryer manufacturers have taken advantage of this technological bonanza, and the power of the PC has been harnessed to provide the framework for modern freeze dryer control systems.

If modern systems are taken as a yardstick, then the first PC–controlled systems were extremely advanced. A modern PC that controls a freeze dryer probably has a minimum of a 486 central processing unit (CPU), 8 megabytes of random access memory (RAM), and works at a speed of 75 MHz. One of the first PC–driven systems, installed in the mid 1980s, ran 10 plants through PLCs and had most of the features incorporated today; this computer had the equivalent of a 8088 CPU (the XT type computer), 512 kilobytes of RAM, and probably worked at around 5 MHz. The increased power and speed of the modern PC is translated into the user graphical interface rather than

Figure 3.4. Block diagram of a typical PC/PC control system.

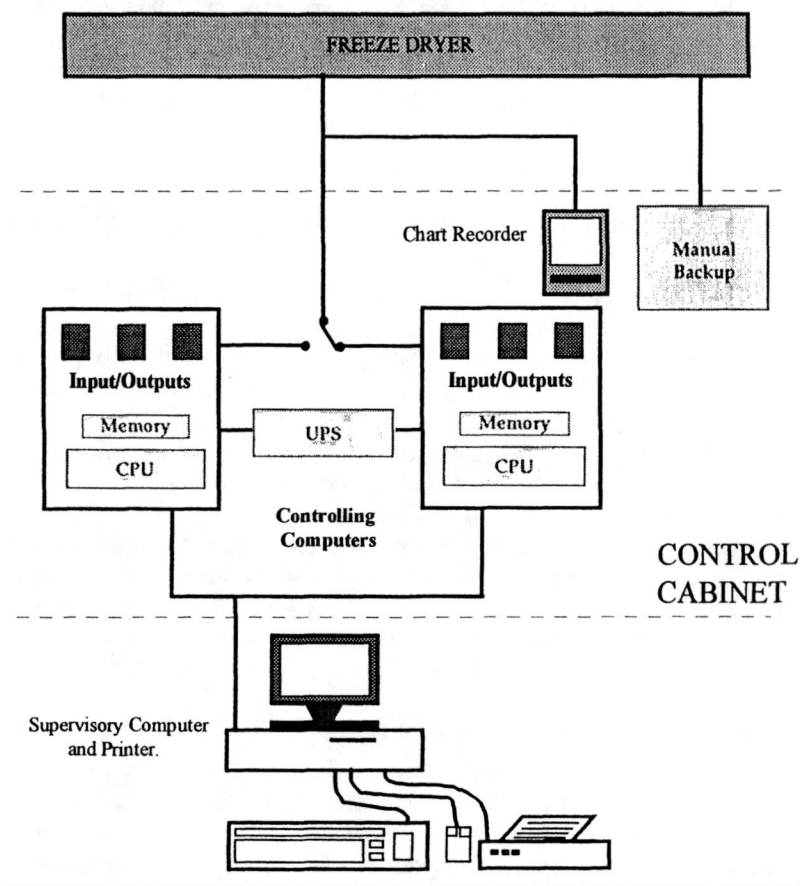

the control; many systems still use the same control software kernel that they did in 1985.

PC–based control systems operate in many ways. The majority of PC–based systems use the PC as the user interface and pass the cycle parameters to a PLC that then controls the freeze drying cycle. The PC remains linked, although this is not necessary for cycle control, and acts as the datalogger and the operator interface with the cycle. Systems were once developed using two PLCs in a master/slave relationship for security; the use of this configuration has now declined. Another system allows the PC to interface directly with input and output boards, often through optical links, whilst another type of

Figure 3.5. Block diagram of a typical PC/PLC control system.

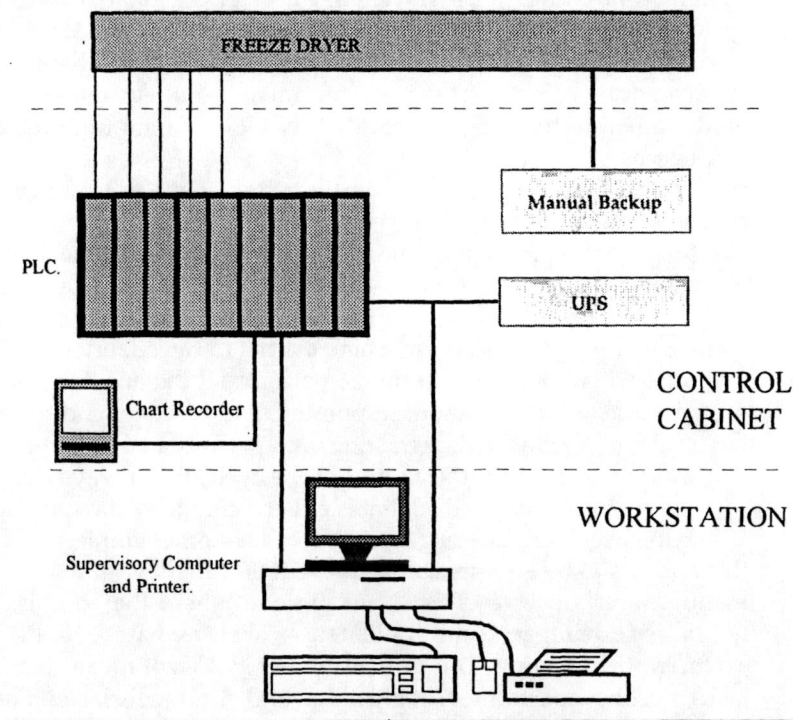

system will use a PC, but control the cycle through another PC as if it were a PLC. The advantage of using a control, or supervisory, PC to parameter another PC, or PLC, that actually controls the cycle is that this type of system will allow the supervisory PC to operate under a Windows™ environment, which enhances its user friendliness and graphics power, especially for comparing cycles. The parametered PC will operate directly under DOS, as Windows™ is not a sufficiently robust environment to entrust with direct control. A PLC will operate under its own operating system that is designed for the purpose. The system will include a keyboard, a visual display unit (VDU), and printer. The printer usually has a colour capability. The actual hardware configuration is not of particular importance; there may be slight advantages in both. A failure in a PC or a PLC is relatively rare; there is more likely to be problems with the software or the field devices.

The majority of PC systems can be seen to work in two parts. The first part is the supervisory PC, which acts to parameter the cycle for the controlling PC or PLC. The supervisory PC will then collect data and act as a viewport into the operation of the machine during the cycle. The controlling, or parametered, PC or PLC actually controls the cycle and cannot be directly interfered with by the operator without using the supervisory computer. Once a cycle has started, the supervisory computer has no part in cycle control and could be removed with no detriment to the cycle, except that the flow of data from the cycle would cease.

The parametered PC or PLC is, therefore, of little interest unless it fails to perform its tasks. The parameter PC or PLC will contain the plant logic; when it is given the necessary parameters, it will control the plant on shelf temperature and chamber pressure against time, handle the relevant actions in the case of temperature or vacuum alarms, and relay these and machine alarms to the supervisory PC. It will also, when instructed to do so, perform all the ancillary tasks of pressure rise test, preaeration, stoppering, and aeration, and the ancillary cycles of sterilisation, defrosting, and performance testing.

If a PLC is used for the control of the cycle, it is always tempting for the user to ask for the PLC that is either a company standard or one where the user's engineering department has some familiarity. Whilst this appears to be a reasonable request, it is fraught with danger. The manufacturer's choice of PLC will be one where the code is written, tested, debugged, and validated as well as having undergone extensive field testing. The use of another PLC will mean that these tasks must be reperformed, at great cost and effort, which could be adversely reflected in the reliability, the completeness of documentation and the ease of troubleshooting. Many manufacturers offer a choice of two, or more, PLCs, the safest course is to select one of these, or go to another manufacturer who can meet your request.

The supervisory PC is of far more interest. Its tasks are sixfold:

1. Parametering of the controlling device

2. Programming of cycles

3. Data acquisition

4. Data manipulation

5. Presentation of on-line cycle information

6. Batch documentation

The first thing that an operator should do if he or she wishes to access a freeze dryer control system is to enter his or her password and identity (ID). This security is necessary and a cycle initiation, or alteration, should show the ID of the initiator, automatically, on the documentation. Password systems are usually multilevel with tasks usually assignable to any level. This will allow the flexibility for the control system to work within the user's standard operating practices (SOPs). Top level passwords would normally have the facility to assign tasks to the lower password levels and to change these passwords should, as always happens, the existing passwords become compromised. Three password levels will usually suffice—operator, supervisor, and high level—although some users require more. Maintenance and engineering would normally require a top level password or a fourth level, where they have access to everything except password alteration. Once the user is in the programme, it is usual for it to ask for a password for every task; this is partly to make the software easier to write and partially to ensure that unexpected "back doors" do not exist in the software, where a low password level operator could obtain access to a higher password level function.

The following features could be expected to be present; others will exist and not all systems will have all of these features:

- *Cycle programming.* The expected capabilities would be to create and save a new cycle and to modify and save an existing cycle. There will also be trivial capabilities to view a cycle's parameters, delete a cycle, and to list all cycles. Cycles are usually programmed in segments. There are usually between 6 and 12 shelf temperature segments each for freezing, primary drying, and secondary drying. Each segment could either be a ramp or a soak or, in some systems, both. Step advancement between segments is usually by time, but some systems will use product probe temperatures. This latter system is useful for R&D freeze dryers, but is less useful for production machines. Most systems will also include vacuum control. Some systems will require a vacuum value for each temperature step; other systems allow vacuum to be programmed in segments but independent of shelf temperature. The functions of pressure rise, and so on will be programmed at the same time. Many systems are programmed to reject unsuitable values, such as a temperature outside the machine's range or a ramp that is unattainable.

- *Sterilisation, defrosting, performance tests, CIP programming.* These operations will have the same capabilities as cycle programming but the programming usually consists of a list of parameters where the values must be entered. For example, the parameters for a sterilisation cycle could be sterilisation temperature, exposure time, number of vacuum pulses, vacuum pulse minimum pressure, timeout for reaching sterilisation temperature, and liquid ring pump drying time. Prior to this, the operator may have had a choice between parametering the sterilisation cycle as a time and temperature cycle or as a drain Fo cycle; the latter would then show a different set of parameters on the screen.

- *Cycle initiation.* This would be similar for either the freeze drying cycle or one of the ancillary cycles. The capabilities would be to retrieve a cycle from memory; a list function would be present; and there would be the choice of starting the chosen cycle, aborting it, or modifying it. Whilst the latter should never need to be used in a production environment, it should be possible to alter a cycle as it is running, without altering the batch number on the documentation. The documentation should list all the changes. Before cycle initiation, the plant would ask for a password, ID, batch number, and product identification, and would print these, and the cycle file name, at the head of the batch records.

- *Data logging.* Most PLCs will not save cycle data; some parametered PCs do, but data logging is invariably performed by the supervisory PC. This, by preference, is into an encrypted file that will allow data to be copied from it for manipulation and analysis, but will not allow any value, within the file, to be altered. This ensures the integrity of cycle data. The data collected will be from all the sensors and any alarms at preset intervals, ranging from every 15 seconds to several minutes. Alarms, and their cancellations, are normally printed out as they occur, along with the time of occurrence, unless the printer can only print by page and not by line, in which case a time annotated list of alarms are printed out at the end of the cycle. In any case the alarms are always displayed on the VDU.

- *Data viewing.* Cycle data can be either viewed on the screen or printed. The presentation can be in either a numerical or graphical form. Numerical values can usually be exported into one of the commercially available spreadsheets for analysis. Most systems will not only graph the information but also automatically scale the graph so that the entire cycle is on screen or can be printed on a single sheet of paper. Many systems have the facility to "zoom" in on the part of the cycle that is of interest, right down to the level where individual data points are easily discernible. The flexibility to alter colours, graph selected channels, and to have a vertical cursor to give exact values at any given time are to be expected. Windows™-based systems will allow the cycle to proceed whilst the cycle graph is inspected, and, if necessary, compared with a previous cycle in another window or to compare the actual against the nominal. This latter function is also usual in DOS–based systems. The presentation of data is where a PC could be expected to excel, and the available graphics is only limited by what is useful and by the imagination of the software engineer who wrote the code.

- *Mimic screen.* This is often called the synoptic screen and is a pictorial representation of the plant on the VDU. Valves and components are colour coded depending on their subsystem (vacuum, sterilisation, shelf thermoregulation, etc.) and will contained a coloured flag to show if they are open or closed, or running or idle. These flags will change colour as the valve operates or a motor starts or stops. Boxes will give vacuum and temperature information and an area of the screen may show a current alarm list. Other information on the screen may include the segment of the cycle, elapsed time, date, time, and batch number. This screen is intended as a quick reference by which it is easy to monitor the status of the plant, but many systems will additionally use a mouse, trackball, cursor, or touch screen to switch valves or stop and start motors, providing that a suitable password has been entered. This is not intended as an emergency backup system, as any system failure will probably take down the synoptic screen; it is useful as a manual system or as an aid to maintenance and, initially, to validation.

- *On-line cycle information.* This feature varies tremendously between different systems, but will include a screen, or screens, that will show alarm status, where the plant is in the cycle, all the sensor outputs, a cycle graph to date, and a comparison of actual shelf temperature and chamber pressure against nominal values. Again, this is an area where a PC would be expected to excel and is only limited by what is useful and by the imagination of the software engineer.

- *Batch records.* Each user will have a different SOP for the presentation of batch records; it is usual to configure the system, during build, to meet this requirement wherever possible. It should be expected that computer-printed batch records should contain the batch number and date as well as all the relevant information. The chart recorder trace and a floppy disc copy of the cycle file can be added to this document. The floppy disc will ensure that a copy of the record can be printed out, or analysed, at any time in the future.

- *Other.* The supervisory PC will have many other capabilities that are not strictly necessary for the operation of the plant. These may include a facility to change languages, a context-orientated help screen, a maintenance log that will alarm if a component passes its maintenance time by a preset limit, calibration data and records, operating instructions, DOS shell or File Manager, and simulation. The latter will disconnect the supervisory PC from the rest of the system so that it can be used for training without operating the plant.

One disadvantage of a PC and a PLC is that the operating programme is in volatile memory; even a transient power loss or power surge will result in the loss of this programme, with the result that the system will have to be reinitialised, possibly under a different batch number, and advanced until the correct point in the cycle is reached. To combat this, most systems are fitted with smoothing circuits or filters, which will even out the incoming line voltage, and with a UPS that will keep the PC and PLC operating and data logging for a period of time, usually between 15 and 30 minutes. When power is restored after a break, the control system will take actions to control the alarm states that may have arisen and then continue with the cycle. The UPS should be constantly on-line and trickle charged; its main task will be to cover momentary brownouts and blackouts, and to cover the switch to an emergency generator and back to the mains once power is restored.

The ease by which a PC, especially now that large amounts of RAM and fast CPUs are available, can add features to a control package is obvious. It is not unusual for a prospective purchaser to look at the features of all the competitive control programmes available and to produce a functional specification that will encompass all of these features. Whilst it is desirable to have a system that exactly meets one's needs (or wants?), this is not always the wisest course. The end result would be to have a system where some of the code will not be extensively tested. A potential for disaster is then residing within the control system. It is better to select a package that is well tried and tested, and preferably can be proven to exist in areas that have undergone a regulatory inspection. A regulatory inspection does not prove that the software has been given a "seal of approval"; it does not even guarantee that the software has been looked at, but it will give a fair indication that the system is well used and, therefore, field tested and that the necessary documentation is in place.

It is an unfortunate fact that the PC control programme is usually the area that will give the most trouble during testing and commissioning. This situation is improving now that software life cycle validation documentation is a necessary element of the overall plant documentation; however, testing of all computer control functions is an essential part of the design qualification, factory acceptance testing, and commissioning process.

The advantage of the PC–based system is that it can be programmed to reproducibly run a cycle that is exactly what the user wants. The cycle can be initiated and no supervision is then necessary until the freeze dryer is unloaded and the batch record printed into the correct format.

Backup Systems

Even the most reliable control system should have a backup system. When the value of the product within the freeze dryer can, in extreme cases, be higher than that of the freeze dryer, it is unwise not to have a backup. These backup systems appear in many forms, and can range from a totally independent hardwired system to redundancy of the PC or PLC. The exception to this rule is if the plant is fitted with a manual system, a failure in this type of system can normally only be circumvented by the direct triggering of valves in the control cabinet.

The simplest backup systems are a manual control panel with switches controlling a functionality and a shelf temperature set point controller, many of which can perform sequencing. A chamber vacuum controller may be present. These systems may be fitted to either microprocessor- or PC–based systems. Care should be taken in assessing these systems, as many will work through part of the control system (e.g., the PLC), and if this fails, then the backup system fails also.

The next level would be an independent microprocessor system that, when used with a chart recorder, will be almost as effective as a PC/PLC system. Again, care must be taken that not too many components are common to the main and the backup system.

Systems that use only a PC and interface cards can be wired so that the interface cards can be triggered by a backup system. This is acceptable because if an interface card fails, it is one of many and only a few functions will be affected. It is, however, not as safe as an independent system.

The redundancy of PCs or PLCs will give some security; they should be linked and interfaced so that the backup unit is in synchronisation with the controlling unit. This system is acceptable, but will require a chart recorder as a backup method of data logging.

The specification of a backup control system is difficult. Unless you are an electronics specialist, it is difficult to assess how independent a system is and how easily an automatic backup system will take over control if the main system fails. Most people can intuitively grasp a mechanical system, but not an electronic system. The first decision should be whether the backup system will be manual or automatic and how a failure is brought to the operator's attention. If an automatic system is specified, the question that should then be asked is, "Can the backup system be expected to work in the likely failure modes of the main control system and have a reasonable probability of completing the cycle correctly?"

Chart Recorder

It is usual, even on systems that will data log, to utilise a chart recorder as a means of obtaining an alternative record of the cycle in a form that is easily read on-line. The minimum specifications for the recorder channels are as follows:

- Chamber vacuum
- Shelf thermoregulation fluid inlet temperature
- Condenser temperature
- Product probes (if fitted)

Plants that are steam sterilisable should also record the chamber drain temperature and, in the case of an external condenser, condenser drain temperature.

In order to avoid having different spans for the temperature probes and to expand the scale to the maximum, it is possible to utilise two chart recorders: one for process and one for sterilisation. The process chart recorder would typically record from -100°C to 100°C whilst the sterilisation recorder would have a span from 0°C to 150°C. The process chart recorder would record vacuum from 2 mbar down to 10^{-3} mbar; sterilisation pressure is not normally recorded. Most users tend to put all the data on one chart recorder. The relatively low cost of a six-point chart recorder, however, makes this a false economy.

Two 6-channel recorders will encompass all the relevant data, but 30 channel recorder systems are not uncommon. It is true that a temperature probe per condenser coil and shelf thermoregulation fluid outlet temperatures are useful data, but care must be taken in the selection of recorded measurements to ensure that the chart record is uncluttered and not covered with so much data that it is unreadable. This is especially true when the system is configured to record more than three product probes. In any case, the chart recorder must be calibrated.

Networks

PC control systems give the possibility of networks. The simplest network is the transfer of data from the supervisory PC to the parametered PC or PLC and the transmission of data back to the supervisory PC.

It is then a logical step to link another PC to the supervisory PC. The possibility then exists to have a supervisory PC on the plant and another PC in the production manager's office. If more than one plant is operating, then the supervisory PC of this plant could also link into the PC within the production manager's office. A network where several plants can be interrogated from a central PC can easily be set up. The difficulty is in the first plant, after that it is a simple matter of writing the software to switch between plants. The next step is to link the plants to the central building system; this step is more difficult, but only because it requires a joint effort between the manufacturer's software engineers and those of the user.

The technology to link computers separated by distance is now well understood and is not an obstacle to the setting up of the network system. It is possible to use a modem to interrogate the plant from almost anywhere in the world. This raises several interesting possibilities. A modem system can be used to ring for help if an alarm state that the machine cannot rectify is reached. The technology now allows the plant to call the operator out of bed at 3:00 A.M. without having to go through the intermediary of the night security guard. The difference is that, by using a laptop computer, the operator can interrogate to the plant and even attempt to remedy the situation without leaving his or her house. The plant can be connected to the manufacturer's factory where software can be debugged, expanded, or updated without the expense of the software engineer having to visit the plant. It could even be possible to diagnose mechanical faults if the relevant sensors are fitted to the plant. Cycles can also be transferred from one plant to another through a modem or network.

Interlocks

Irrespective of the perceived sophistication and reliability of the control system, there are certain areas that should, usually on safety criteria, never be entrusted to the control system. The most apparent area is that of door/steam interlocks. Almost all steam sterilisable freeze dryers will have interlocks that require the door to be in the closed and in the locked position before the steam inlet valve is enabled. This is usually backed by a physical immobilisation of the door locking mechanism when the chamber is under pressure. These interlocks should be hardwired into the plant electrical system and not be a flag in the control software. The simplest way of achieving this is to use microswitches to determine the position of the door and door lock, and to place these in series on the output from the controlling device to the steam valve solenoid. A similar argument and methodology should ensure that the door is shut before stoppering can take place, especially if stoppering can be initiated automatically or from the plant room.

Similarly, some safety devices should have a mechanical alternative. A software system may be programmed to release steam pressure if it rises above the specified limit; this limit will be below the safety relief valve lift pressure. This will prevent the safety relief valve operating; as if it does it may subsequently give sealing problems at high vacuum, or prevent the bursting disc from bursting. The fact that this controlled safety relief is present does not reduce the requirement for the mechanical system.

Although it is not strictly in the domain of the control system, it should be noted that electrical cabinets should not be able to be opened unless the power is switched off.

CONCLUSION

The purpose of a control system is twofold: to reproducibly control the freeze drying cycle and to relieve the operator of the necessity of being close to the plant throughout the cycle. The versatility of the electronic systems ensure that many regulatory, or operational, criteria are also met.

The degree of control has changed little since 1985, what has changed is the ability of the control system to present more detailed information to the operator, in an easily assimilated, and secure, form. It is likely that this trend will persist for the foreseeable future.

4

REGULATORY ISSUES: A EUROPEAN PERSPECTIVE

Peter Monger

Pharmaceutical Consultant
Dunnington, York, United Kingdom

THE LEGISLATIVE BACKGROUND

The manufacture and supply of medicinal products within the European Union (EU) is controlled by a series of directives that each member state is obliged to translate into national legislation, thereby achieving harmonisation.

Amongst the many such directives, three are particularly important:

1. 65/65 EEC, which made universal the requirement for a "Marketing Authorisation" (traditionally known in the United Kingdom as a Product Licence) for any medicinal product.

2. 75/319 EEC, which requires authorisation of manufacturers and for manufacturers to have available the services of a "Qualified Person" (QP) who meets very rigorous requirements for training and experience. This directive also made it a requirement for manufacturers to comply with the principles and guidelines of good manufacturing practice (GMP) that were to be provided in the form of a directive and detailed guidelines.

3. 91/356 EEC, which sets out the principles and guidelines of GMP in a series of articles covering general provisions and specific requirements regarding

- Quality management

- Personnel

- Premises and equipment

- Documentation

- Production

- Quality Control

- Work contracted out

- Complaints and product recall

- Self-inspection

Directives 75/319 and 91/356 refer to detailed guidelines on GMP that were first published in 1989 under the title, *The Rules Governing Medicinal Products in the European Community, Volume IV: Guide to Good Manufacturing Practice for Medicinal Products.* This first edition contained chapters corresponding to the Articles of Directive 91/356 (as listed above) and "Supplementary Guidelines" concerning the manufacture of sterile medicinal products. A second impression was published in 1992 that included some further supplementary guidelines and corrected some errors and mistranslations, but otherwise did not amend the text. The publication of supplementary guidelines has continued so that there are now a series of annexes to the guide concerning topics not covered, or not covered in detail, in the main body of the guidelines. These are as follows:

- Annex 1: Manufacture of sterile medicinal products

- Annex 2: Manufacture of biological medicinal products for human use

- Annex 3: Manufacture of radiopharmaceuticals

- Annex 4: Manufacture of veterinary medicinal products other than immunological veterinary medicinal products

- Annex 5: Manufacture of immunological veterinary medicinal products

- Annex 6: Manufacture of medicinal gases

- Annex 7: Manufacture of herbal medicinal products

- Annex 8: Sampling of starting and packaging materials

- Annex 9: Manufacture of liquids, creams, and ointments

- Annex 10: Manufacture of pressurised metered dose aerosol preparations for inhalation

- Annex 11: Computerised systems

- Annex 12: Use of ionising radiation in the manufacture of medicinal products

- Annex 13: Good manufacturing practice for investigational medicinal products

- Annex 14: Manufacture of products derived from human blood and human plasma

Member states were first asked to provide suggestions for a revised second edition of the guide in 1992. Progress on this has been slow however, and it was not until June 1995 that a draft revision of only Annex 1—Manufacture of Sterile Medicinal Products—was published for industry comment. A final version, for adoption, was produced in June 1996, but as of September 1996, it has not been officially published.

With this wealth of information on GMP, it might be expected that some substantial guidance would be provided for users of freeze drying processes and equipment. Regrettably, this is not so. The present (first) edition of Annex 1 of the Guide, which would be expected to be the most relevant section, makes no specific mention of freeze drying or lyophilisation.

Annex 5 (Manufacture of Immunoiogical Veterinary Medicinal Products) outlines some basic requirements for siting and sterilisation of freeze dryers and for decontaminating surrounding areas. The proposed revision to Annex 1 requires that the transfer of partially closed containers, as used in freeze drying, be done in a Grade A environment, or in sealed transfer trays in a Grade B environment; otherwise, there is no specific reference to freeze drying or lyophilisation.

This void has been noted, in the United Kingdom, at least, where the Parenteral Society established a working party in late 1991 that has since published several monographs on aspects of freeze drying, for example,

- Technical Monograph No. 5: Sterilisation of Freeze Dryers

- Technical Monograph No 7: Leak Testing of Freeze Dryers

- Technical Monograph No 8: Integrity Testing of Freeze Dryer Inlet Filters

A monograph on the validation of freeze dryers is also in preparation. These documents have been drawn up with the participation of the UK Medicines Control Agency (MCA), who might reasonably be considered to be in agreement with the content of the monographs.

The UK MCA's Medicines Inspectorate has over many years developed its own internal "Medicines Inspectorate Guidelines" (MIGs). These are designed to provide information to inspectors and to ensure a standardised approach to inspections, however, they are not normally available for publication. There is a guideline regarding the design, operation, and sterilisation of freeze dryers, which was written by this author.

One other significant source of guidance on freeze drying is the draft international standard on Aseptic Processing of Health Care Products (developed by ISO TC 198, WG9), which includes a specific section on lyophilisation. It is important to remember that adoption of any ISO standard is voluntary, but such authoritative guidance is likely to be widely used by regulatory authorities, therefore, users of freeze drying technology would be well advised to comply with the relevant sections.

PRACTICAL IMPLEMENTATION

Article 5 of Directive 91/356 includes the statement, "The manufacturer shall regularly review their manufacturing methods in the light of scientific and technical progress". This has been interpreted in the MCA to mean that consumers (i.e., the patient) should expect to benefit from improvements in technology, and there have been many improvements in the design and operation of freeze drying equipment in the recent past. On the other hand, the MCA is well aware of the very high cost of such equipment and its relatively long useful life, which leads to a considerable diversity in the age, design, and quality of equipment in use at any given time. This diversity makes the setting of appropriate GMP standards a difficult process, and one that must be continuously revisited.

DESIGN CONSIDERATIONS

Sterilisation

Undoubtedly, the design issue that has received the most attention in pharmaceutical freeze drying over the last 10 years or so is the ability of the equipment to withstand steam sterilisation. This includes the chamber, the condenser, vapour and vacuum lines, valves, gauges, and vent filters. It is a considerable testament to the engineering quality of freeze drying equipment that steam sterilisation is possible. Clearly, the extreme ranges of temperature (from -50°C to 121°C) and pressure (from near absolute vacuum to more than 2 bar) stress the equipment tremendously, but the equipment must be able to withstand these stresses with extremely low leakage rates. The inclusion of double door designs, vial stoppering mechanisms, clean-in-place (CIP) systems and other possible design enhancements all make this task more difficult, since more possible leakage sites are inevitably created.

Some equipment that cannot be steam sterilised is still in use, this may be acceptable in certain circumstances, although this is unlikely to be the case indefinitely. In these cases gas sterilisation may be possible. Historically, gas sterilisation this has been based on the use of ethylene oxide; however, recently, hydrogen peroxide vapour (VHP) has been proposed as a more acceptable alternate.

When no other technique is available, simple surface sanitisation is the only option. This is the least satisfactory of all techniques for two main reasons:

1.   The difficulty in accessing all parts of the equipment, particularly the condenser and pipework, especially where the condenser is located inside the chamber as in some designs

2.   The limited efficacy of the surface sanitising agents available

From a consideration of these factors, it can be seen that where it is possible, steam sterilisation is the method of choice. It is easy to validate using well-established physical techniques based on calculated cycle lethality, and the use of biological indicators is not normally required. The process is easy to control by simple time/temperature pressure measurements that can be readily documented.

In contrast, it is often difficult to control some of the parameters, such as humidity and gas concentration, which are necessary to ensure sterilisation by ethylene oxide or hydrogen peroxide. Furthermore, biological indicators are required not only to validate the process, but also to monitor each cycle, greatly increasing the problems of the process.

Steam Sterilisation

Steam sterilisation of a lyophiliser should be regarded as sterilisation-in-place (SIP) of a complex apparatus. Attention must be paid to the problems inherent in such processes. Some of the particular problem areas that have been identified by the MCA and other authorities include the following:

Steam Quality. High quality steam is an essential requirement. It must be remembered that product will be exposed in the chamber. Condensate should comply with water for injection (WFI) quality standards. Good steam supply practice is also necessary to ensure effective sterilisation. Detailed guidance on this subject can be found in Health Technical Memorandum (HTM) 2010.

The three most critical parameters are as follows;

1. A pressure reduction ratio of not more than 2:1 in a single stage (to prevent possible superheat)

2. A dryness fraction greater than 0.95

3. Noncondensable gases of not more than 3.5 percent

These parameters ensure the presence of dry, saturated steam at the required sterilisation temperature.

An issue that sometimes causes concern is the total loading on the steam supply system when all equipment connected to it is in use. The capacity must be sufficient to satisfy the maximum possible demand.

Equipment Design and Installation. Dead legs should be avoided wherever possible. Ports for temperature and vacuum measuring devices are particular problem areas. The aim, of course, is to ensure proper penetration of steam and contact with all surfaces. Any accessories or fitments that may interfere with this process should be avoided or at least treated with great respect. CIP systems and stoppering mechanisms are noteworthy examples.

There has been considerable discussion as to what represents an "acceptable" dead leg. It should be emphasised that what may be acceptable in a water system may not be acceptable for SIP. Orientation is very crucial. Young et al. (1994) have shown that, even in comparatively short dead-ended tubes, the time required to achieve a given reduction in bacterial spore concentration is increased dramatically over the time for sterilisation in saturated steam. The main reason for this is, of course, the presence of air. Air entrapment can occur even when dead-ended tubes are oriented only a few degrees from vertical (air is heavier than dry steam and will be displaced downward). The ratio of pipe length to diameter has been traditionally used to define a dead leg. For water systems, ratios of 4:1 or 2.5:1 have been suggested as "acceptable". For steam systems, anything greater than 1:1 should be regarded as a potential problem.

It should also be noted that temperature measurement cannot be relied upon to detect the presence of air. Even the presence of several percent of air will reduce the phase boundary temperature by only a fraction of a degree—and this temperature reduction will itself be masked by convection and conduction effects, especially in small bore tubes. The presence of this amount of air will, however have a significant effect on the energy transfer process that is the basis of thermal sterilisation. The magnitude of this effect can be appreciated by simple comparison of sterilising cycles at 121°C. For saturated steam, 15 minutes is accepted as overkill. The equivalent time for a dry heat cycle would be many hours.

All of these problems can, of course, be avoided with effective air removal, which can usually be achieved using the equipment's own vacuum system; what may be a more difficult problem to address is the removal of condensate. Freeze dryers are typically large, heavy pieces of machinery with high thermal masses. They are also operated at low temperatures; therefore, when steam is introduced, large quantities of condensate will result. (Indeed, this effect may be used as the basis for "clean-in-place" particularly where water soluble materials are involved. The large quantities of condensate produced when steam is introduced to cold equipment have been shown to provide an effective cleaning process in some cases).

If condensate is trapped, it may prevent free passage of steam or produce cold spots that do not achieve sterilising temperature. Experience has shown that this is most likely to occur when pipework is not appropriately sloped to allow condensate to drain away. This may occur when service connections have been installed that do not match the slopes on the equipment itself. Of course, the chamber itself must also be sloped to drain(and not produce a flood of water when the door is opened!

Steam traps are another area for concern. They should be of sanitary design, self-draining and should fail in the open mode so that the failure is self-evident. Full or partial failure closed may not be detected but could lead to a buildup of condensate and, therefore, failure to achieve sterilising conditions.

Steam sterilisation of membrane filters (such as those used on vent lines to allow introduction of vacuum break gases) is a particular problem. Air removal from the pore structure is extremely difficult, as is steam penetration. This problem is compounded by the fragile nature of the filters, which may be damaged if subjected to high pressure drops. (Filter manufacturers will typically guarantee integrity only if filters are exposed to pressure differentials of less than 300 mbar at 121°C.) Thus, air removal by creation of a high vacuum followed by the rapid introduction of high pressure steam is likely to lead to filter failure, and some mechanism must be established to avoid this possibility. One such method is to provide a steam bypass to allow the flow of steam to both the clean and dirty sides of the filter, thus allowing equalisation of pressure. When this is achieved, the bypass can be closed to allow the free passage of steam to facilitate air and condensate removal.

Gaseous Sterilisation

Ethylene oxide (EtO) is the most widely used gaseous sterilisation agent, although there has been considerable recent work using vaporised hydrogen peroxide (VHP) and other similar agents. These offer the significant advantage that they readily degrade, leaving nontoxic residues, unlike EtO and its decomposition products, which are both highly toxic.

Ethylene oxide sterilisation is difficult to control. It requires high humidity to be effective. This is difficult to achieve in equipment such as lyophilisers that do not normally have a mechanism for controlled introduction of moisture. EtO is also much heavier than air and is prone to stratification, clearly this could be a particular problem in a freeze drying chamber where multiple shelves are likely to contribute to this effect. Efficient sterilisation using EtO requires contact with all surfaces which would normally be achieved by circulation of the gas; this is also a facility not normally available on lyophilisers.

Monitoring the effectiveness of EtO sterilisation is a further problem; cycle parameters such as pressure, temperature, relative humidity, and gas concentration must be monitored for each run. While it is relatively simple to measure temperature and relative humidity, direct measurement of gas concentration (for instance, by gas chromatography or infra-red analysis) is difficult and not widely used. In practice, EtO concentration is usually derived from the simple measurement of the weight of gas withdrawn from the supply cylinder and into the equipment against the known equipment volume.

In the absence of direct measurement of sterilant gas and its uniform distribution, it is widely accepted that biological indicators (BIs) are also required to demonstrate the effectiveness of each cycle. These should be placed in locations where exposure is most difficult (as established during cycle validation activities). This is likely to be a difficult operation because of limitations of access to pipework and fittings. Furthermore, retrieval of the exposed indicator must not compromise the sterilisation process by exposing the system to nonsterile conditions. Of course, any use of resistant spores in a sterile product manufacturing facility is highly undesirable and must be rigorously controlled; in particular, contingency plans must exist to cover the actions to be taken in the event that all BIs are not recovered from a cycle so that product is not put at risk.

If results are to be meaningful, the handling and use of BIs must also be carefully controlled. Indicators with a population of at least 10^6 spores of *Bacillus subtilis* var. *niger* (ATCC 9372, CIP 7718, NCTC 10073), are generally regarded as suitable for verification of EtO sterilisation. The population and resistivity (D-value) of the indicators should be certified by the supplier. Population should also be verified independently, either by the user or a third party laboratory, for each batch of indicators. Some periodic verification of D-values may also be required, particularly for high volume users.

The indicators should be foil or plastics backed. Paper types are not acceptable since their porous nature may mean that sterilant residues can be retained and continue to provide a sterilising effect after the designated exposure has been completed, thus leading to a risk of "false negative" results.

The handling of BIs post exposure is also critical, and the time between exposure and incubation should be kept to a minimum to ensure the viability of any surviving organisms. Four hours would normally be regarded as an acceptable maximum time allowed for this phase. Of course results from the BIs will not be known for some time following the fumigation process; therefore any product processed in the equipment during this period is "at risk", which represents a further disadvantage of chemical sterilisation processes.

The sterilisation of filters is also a problem when using EtO because its compatibility with the filter medium must be established. The cycle, particularly the purging and "aeration" stages, must be designed to remove residues and toxic decomposition products.

As already noted, it may be possible to use other fumigants, such as formaldehyde and hydrogen peroxide. Formaldehyde would not be considered particularly suitable, largely because of the difficulty in the removal of residues. Hydrogen peroxide, on the other hand, does appear to offer some advantages to EtO.

- It is most effective in low humidity conditions that can be achieved in a freeze dryer.

- It decomposes readily to nontoxic residues.

- It appears to be highly effective and sporicidal in quite low concentrations.

A significant development effort has been put into the use of VHP by AMSCO and UpJohn, with the possible retrofitting of a number of existing nonsteam sterilisable freeze dryers with facilities for VHP gassing.

Surface Sanitisation

Surface sanitisation is the least rigorous method of freeze dryer preparation and is the least acceptable to regulatory authorities, such as the MCA. In general, it would only be acceptable where product is minimally exposed (i.e., in part-stoppered vials), even in these circumstances, it should not be regarded as a long-term option. Users of this technology can expect to come under increasing pressure from their regulators to adopt a more rigorous sterilisation approach, such as those already described. Surface sanitisation would not be regarded as acceptable where product is exposed during processing, for instance, in open trays or even in open ampoules, except where this is for the production, for instance, of an intermediate product that may then undergo further processing, including a sterilisation step.

Where this approach is used, however, then good practice in relation to disinfection must be followed. It is advisable to rotate disinfectants so as to avoid the possibility of a build up of a resistant strain. The disinfectant must not introduce contaminants (e.g., from nonsterile water used to dilute the disinfectant or from spores in alcohol). Correct concentrations must be used and materials should be freshly prepared. Containers should not be "topped up", but rather emptied completely, sterilised, and then refilled.

The effectiveness of the process must be demonstrated and this must be repeated at frequent intervals. Normal surface sampling techniques, such as swabbing, should be used. It would not normally be considered desirable to deliberately introduce contamination into the area (e.g., from spore suspensions) and then to demonstrate removal using this type of sanitisation technique.

The major limitations of this technique are, of course, the difficulty of access to all surfaces within the chamber, pipework, and condenser, and the reproducibility of the method. Even where surfaces can be reached, it is difficult to ensure that they are appropriately treated during each cleaning and sanitisation cycle, especially where this relies on purely manual techniques.

Sterilisation Frequency

Sterilisation of the freeze dryer before every run is clearly the most rigorous approach possible, and, as such, would not be questioned by the regulatory authorities. This would be the only approach considered acceptable for exposed product (for example, in trays or open ampoules).

It may be acceptable, however, for sterilisation to be carried out less frequently where there is a greater degree of product protection—for instance, in part-stoppered vials. This approach must be justified by suitable microbiological monitoring data, demonstrating that contamination is not significant over the relevant time interval. As a minimum, it would be necessary to carry out sterilisation each time there is a product changeover and/or the freeze dryer is cleaned.

Other Design Considerations

Valves and Gauges

It is essential that valves and gauges are of sanitary design to ensure proper sterilisation. This would normally mean the use of diaphragm types, where all surfaces can be exposed during the sterilisation process. This is in contrast to ball or needle valves that are not favoured since all surfaces cannot be sterilised; although, in practice these types of valves are often used since they provide a superior mechanical seal. This is clearly an area where there is a conflict between GMP and functionality. Under these circumstances, the acceptability or not of a particular valve type must be considered vis-à-vis the application.

Where diaphragm valves are used, the diaphragms may be damaged by repeated sterilisation or sanitisation (i.e., by exposure to heat or chemical agents), and failure of the diaphragm could cause contamination from leaking hydraulic transfer fluid or expose the product to nonsanitised surfaces. Thus, these items should be subject to regular planned preventive maintenance, which would normally include periodic replacement of the diaphragms. Corrective action must be taken in the event that a failure is found during use.

Vacuum Relief Filters

Vacuum relief filters are also items of some concern. They should preferably be sterilised-in-place (e.g., using EtO or steam) or may be presterilised and fitted to the lyophiliser under aseptic conditions. This is normally best achieved by locating the filter connection in the aseptic area, but is not recommended practice.

As already noted, if sterilisation-in-place is used, the compatibility of the filter with the sterilant (e.g., EtO, steam) must be established. For EtO, the filter should be monitored for the presence of residues, and if using steam, care must be taken to avoid exposing the filter to too great a pressure differential, which can be achieved in a variety of ways, such as by use of a steam bypass or by careful control of steam flow rate.

Since the filters used are typically hydrophobic, integrity testing is difficult. Conventional techniques require the use of a wetting agent, such as isopropanol or methanol, that would then normally be removed by passing a drying gas through the filter. This vapour-laden gas may have to be vented through the chamber and may present hazards due to flammability or operator exposure. Under these conditions, regulatory agencies may prefer users to fit two filters in series and carry out only a post-run integrity test.

Alternatively, the problems associated with the use of solvents may be avoided by using the water intrusion technique. This test relies on the measurement of the rate of water movement compacting the filter cartridge and possibly intruding into the membrane, which is not wetted by this process. Although developed several years, ago this method has only recently been promoted as a viable alternative to the diffusive flow tests more widely used, and data have only recently became available to allow testing to be performed.

It should also be noted that the use of the bubble point test is not normally recommended for large surface area filters, such as the cartridges generally used on freeze dryers. This is because there will be an appreciable airflow through such filters, which makes the determination of the bubble point subjective and not reliable.

Vial Stoppering

It is now common practice for vials to be stoppered inside the chamber before removal. This is normally achieved by closing the shelves together, thus pushing the preinserted stoppers home. There are two main variants of the closing mechanism. The first uses a hydraulic ram to push the shelves together directly; the second utilises a yoke arrangement so that rods connected to the shelves are withdrawn from the chamber to effect closure. Where a ram is used to push the shelves together, there is the disadvantage that during the closing operation a nonsterilised surface is introduced into the chamber, raising the possibility of contamination of the product. In practise, this risk must be regarded as quite small for various reasons:

- The vials are being closed as the ram is being introduced, thus limiting the opportunity for the transfer of any contaminants

- The ram surface would be expected to be cleaned by the wiping action of the hydraulic and vacuum seals necessary.

Nonetheless, various approaches have been used to overcome this potential problem. Probably the least successful of these has been the use of an extendable bellows arrangement to cover the ram. The bellows must, of course, be able to withstand sterilisation which is where problems have arisen. The more successful approach has been to reverse the mode of action of the closing mechanism. In this variant, the vial closing rod is connected to the shelves by a yoke or saddle arrangement and is withdrawn from the chamber to effect closing of the vials. A modification of this technique is to use threaded rods that are attached to the shelves by threaded lugs. The rods are rotated and, thus, the shelf positions are changed. This is said to offer advantages in the precision of shelf positioning when stepping motors are used. It does, however, appear to present surfaces that are difficult to clean and sterilise, and may lead to shedding of particles by mechanical action. While the use of a hydraulic mechanism attached to a yoke and effecting closure by withdrawal from the chamber is most favoured by the regulatory authorities, this often presents practical problems on-site because a significant height clearance (above or below the chamber) is normally required. Where closure is made by rod insertion, the degree of risk associated with this process should be established by surface monitoring of the ram.

Chamber Cleaning

The process of cleaning a freeze dryer chamber is often difficult; the size of the chamber and narrow intershelf distances may make it impossible to reach all of the chamber interior. There are two major design features that have been put forward as a way to overcome these problems:

1. Double door chambers

2. Use of CIP systems

Neither option has been particularly successful or widely adopted.

Double door designs allow access to the chamber from both sides and may allow a more rigorous cleaning regime to be applied from the "dirty" side. Unfortunately, the problems associated with sealing the second door (against leakage of "dirty" air) generally outweigh the advantage gained.

CIP systems generally involve a series of nozzles designed to provide spray coverage of all shelf and chamber surfaces. The complexity of freeze dryers generally makes this difficult to achieve, typically, some areas are "shadowed" so that they are not in direct contact with the cleaning agent. The CIP system itself also introduces considerable complexity into the freeze dryer and may present problems to the chamber sterilisation process. Another problem is the high volume of purified water typically required for such systems.

An alternative approach that is being used is to introduce steam into the chamber at low temperature and to allow the condensate to act as a cleaning agent. This has some obvious advantages over a complex CIP system. In both cases, however, care must be taken to ensure that water drains adequately from shelf surfaces. Although these should be perfectly flat, this is not always the case and "puddles" may be formed. In some freeze dryers, it is possible to tilt the shelves (via the vial closing mechanism) to facilitate this process.

Whatever cleaning process is used, however, one of the major concerns is broken glass, which can cause two particular problems:

1.   Blockage of the drain and, therefore, failure of the sterilisation cycle due to condensate buildup.

2.   Damage to the drain valve or door seal leading to leakage of air that may contaminate product

Therefore, particular attention must be paid to the removal of glass fragments from the chamber.

The required frequency of cleaning will vary from case to case. The chosen interval between cleaning should be justified, in particular with regard to product build up and microbial cleanliness. Inspectors will expect to see evidence that such an evaluation has been carried out.

OPERATIONAL CONSIDERATIONS

Freeze Dryer Siting and Work Flow

One of the most commonly encountered problems during the inspection of freeze drying installations is poorly designed work flow, particularly in the transport of filled containers to the freeze dryer and of the stoppered (but not sealed) containers to the crimping station. Indeed, this issue is of such concern that it has been addressed directly in the proposed revision to Annex 1 of the EC GMP Guide.

. . . Transfer of partially closed containers, as used in freeze drying, should be done in a Grade A environment or in sealed transfer trays in the Grade B environment . . .

The draft international standard (ISO TC 198) on Aseptic Processing of Health Care Products makes a more rigorous requirement in stating that such transfers should take place in a grade A (equivalent) environment.

Ensuring that conventional transfer containers are completely sealed is difficult and is likely to be regarded with suspicion by an inspector. If a grade A "pathway" (e.g., a curtained laminar airflow [LAF] area) does not exist between filling and the lyophiliser, then the use of transfer carts that provide a positive LAF is likely to be the preferred option. However, this is an area where the use of isolator technology may be appropriate, and the use of a dockable transfer system can provide a high level of assurance of environmental integrity.

It should, of course, be noted that these requirements apply either to partially stoppered vials or open ampoules or trays. What should not be ignored, however, is the transport of stoppered vials from the freeze dryer to crimping stations.

It is difficult to guarantee that a vial with a partially seated stopper will always be rejected by the crimper; for this reason these materials should be handled in the same way as vials being transported to the freeze dryer. This is an area where practice appears to differ significantly between Europe and North America. In the latter there is often an overriding concern to maintain "class 100" conditions at the point of fill; therefore, crimping, which may generate a high particulate loading, is often carried out elsewhere, sometimes in a completely noncontrolled environment. This is not regarded as acceptable by European authorities.

Loading and Unloading

The process of loading filled containers into the freeze dryer carries with it a high risk of product contamination, particularly when the loading process is performed manually. For this reason, automatic loading systems are preferred, but they are at present far from widely used.

Where a manual process is used, this should be carefully designed so as to minimise the risk of contamination. For instance, where trays are transported from filling to freeze drying using a transfer cart, the cart should be loaded from the top down, trays should be removed from the cart from the bottom up and placed in the freeze dryer chamber from the top down. This sequence of action will minimise the risk of contamination dropping into a vial during these various manipulations. A similar principle should be applied during chamber unloading (i.e. from the bottom up, etc.).

Leak Testing

The regulatory authorities are concerned to ensure that leak rates are not unacceptably high and do not present a hazard to the product from the ingress of contaminated air. It is important to distinguish between real leaks and virtual leaks. The latter may be due to outgassing of moisture or solvents from within the system, from elastomeric seals, and so on.

Leak rates are normally calculated in mbar litres/second, and a typical leak rate for a new, clean, empty freeze dryer would be 2×10^{-2} mbar litres/second. A simple calculation shows that for a cycle of around 24 hr this represents a total leakage of approximately 2 litres of air at 1 bar pressure. Since most of this leakage is likely to be of "clean" air (for instance, from the clean room through the door seal), the risk of microbial contamination being introduced by this mechanism is extremely low.

It would normally be expected that a short leak rate test be carried out after each sterilisation cycle. A longer, more rigorous, test should be performed after any significant maintenance activity is carried out.

Calibration and Maintenance

A freeze dryer is a complex piece of equipment and a system of planned preventive maintenance should be in place, together with a routine calibration system. The ppm programme should define appropriate maintenance intervals and state required actions. A list of critical devices for calibration is required. Calibration should be traceable to an authentic standard (e.g., NPL, NBS, etc.).

REFERENCES

Health Technical Memorandum (HTM) 2010. ISBN 0-11-321746-3. London: NHS Estates/Her Majesty's Stationery Office.

Young, J. H., B. L. Ferko, and R. P. Gaber. 1994. Parameters governing steam sterilisation of deadlegs. *Journal of Pharmaceutical Science and Technology* 48 (3).

5

REGULATORY ISSUES:
AN AMERICAN PERSPECTIVE

L. David Butler

Schering-Plough Research Institute
Kenilworth, New Jersey, USA

The U.S. Food and Drug Administration (FDA) recognizes that the technology associated with the manufacture and control of lyophilized dosage forms is complex. Their expectations for the manufacturing process of a commercial product can, however, be stated very simply. They believe that the process should be well defined, validated, and controlled. For example, the development work for the lyophilization cycle should be completed before the final process is written, appropriate process controls should be in place, and the process should be validated to demonstrate that it repeatedly achieves its desired results. The FDA also understands that there are many complicated factors involved in the task of successfully lyophilizing a pharmaceutical product; so in July 1993 they issued a *Guide to Inspections of Lyophilization of Parenterals* to provide guidance and information to investigators about industry procedures, and to discuss selected inspectional concerns associated with lyophilized products. The information in this chapter is derived mainly from the Guide and published observations from recent FDA inspections.

Of the myriad issues associated with lyophilization, the FDA continues to focus their attention on several specific aspects of the manufacturing process:

- Formulation of the bulk product

- Filling the product into partially stoppered vials

- Lyophilization cycle, controls, and validation
- Lyophilizer design and sterilization
- Finished product testing
- Finished product inspection

However, because inspectional guides are not necessarily comprehensive documents, this listing is not intended to represent all of the potential FDA concerns about lyophilization.

The reader should be aware that for the purpose of simplifying many discussions in this chapter, several sections refer only to solutions in vials. Nonetheless, it will be apparent that the concerns apply to other dosage forms and container types as well.

FORMULATION OF THE BULK PRODUCT

Bioburden Control

With regard to the manufacture of the bulk product, the emphasis should be placed mainly on minimizing the accumulation and growth of microbial contamination during the formulation and holding of the nonsterile product. The bioburden in the product should be maintained at very low levels, and the bioburden should be determined prior to sterilizing bulk solutions for filling. This means that the compounding of bulk solutions should be controlled up to the time that the solutions are filtered in order to prevent increases in bioburden that might result in the generation of endotoxins or excessive challenges to the filtering medium. Achieving this can be especially challenging for products that do not contain preservatives. Of course, if the product is a suspension or emulsion that is intended to be manufactured aseptically, and not subsequently sterilized by filtration or other means before being filled into containers for lyophilization, bioburden control during compounding and handling becomes more critical.

The FDA considers it good practice to conduct batch operations in sealed tanks in an environment where the levels of microbiological and airborne particulate contaminants are controlled. It is particularly important to monitor the bulk solution for gram-negative organisms, which are the primary source of endotoxin contamination in solutions. It should be recognized that water for injection (WFI) is not necessarily sterile; in reality, it frequently contains *Pseudomonas* species. When WFI is used in compounding, *Pseudomonas* can be expected in the presterilized bulk product. Therefore, storage of the solution for any length of time prior to sterilization should be discouraged.

Holding Times for Bulk Solutions

The FDA's *Guideline on Sterile Drug Products Produced by Aseptic Processing* (1987) emphasizes that there should be an "established maximum" holding time for bulk solutions. In recent FDA inspections, companies have been cited for not providing proper holding time limits. In one particular case, the FDA objected to the fact that a firm had assessed bioburden levels after holding the solution for less than 7 hours, while the company had established a holding limit of 1 day, which was defined as about 10 hours. Therefore, it seems prudent to expect that the FDA will require that holding times be established on the basis of real time experimental data, and will not accept conjecture or industry norms as substitutes for actual data from the product in question. In addition, the main reason for lyophilizing a product is generally its inherent instability in water. Therefore, when considering maximum holding times for bulk solutions, chemical and physical stability as well as biological activity of the product must also be taken into account.

FILLING THE PRODUCT INTO PARTIALLY STOPPERED VIALS

Filling and Transportation of Vials

Sterile injectable products can be lyophilized in vials, ampules, syringes, or trays. The filling of vials will be considered in this section, but the concerns addressed are similar for other containers. For vials to be lyophilized, the filling operation is similar to those employed for other sterile products, but the stopper is only partially inserted prior to loading the vials into the lyophilizer. After filling, the partially closed vials (frozen separately or not frozen) are transported to the lyophilizer and loaded onto the shelves for drying. In most cases, the stoppers are inserted the rest of the way into the vial in the lyophilizer at the end of the drying cycle, which may be several days long. Following drying, the stoppered vials are transported to a capping station where aluminum seals are applied.

Vials are subject to contamination until the time they are fully closed and sealed. This potentially lengthy exposure means that the validation of the filling process is more complex and difficult than it is for conventional aqueous products because it must also take into account the exposure time in the lyophilizer and during transport from the filling line to the lyophilizer.

Manual Stoppering

Some firms still allow operators to stopper filled vials manually. Even if sterile forceps are used for this purpose, the immediate route of contamination presented by the operator has made such hand stoppering operations generally difficult to justify to the FDA, especially in large-scale operations.

Environmental Monitoring

An environmental monitoring program for the filling area must be in place, as it does for any other aseptically filled product. The program should include an evaluation of the bioburden present on cleanroom personnel, garments, and gloves. In addition, critical surfaces and the air supplied to the area where the product is exposed to the environment during filling and transport to the lyophilizer should be sampled during filling operations. Regulatory difficulties have resulted when manufacturers have failed to conduct and document such monitoring of the environment and personnel properly.

Once vials are filled and partially stoppered, they are transported and loaded into the lyophilizer. This sequence is of particular concern to the FDA. It should be carried out under primary barriers such as laminar airflow transport carts or by extending laminar airflow hoods from the filling line to the door of the lyophilizer. Firms have been cited recently because their environmental monitoring program allowed agar contact plate counts from the carts used to transport filled vials from the filling line to the lyophilizer to be as high as 50 CFU/100 cm^2, and did not require sampling to be performed during every filling/transportation operation. The FDA has also required that airflow velocity and turbulence be evaluated at the working height of transfer carts during operations such as vial transfers and adjustment of stoppers and vials.

Experience concerning the level of environmental control required by the FDA during the transportation of stoppered vials to the capping machine and at the capper itself is somewhat variable. However, the FDA has required class 100 conditions for the transport of unsealed vials and the supply of class 100 air to the capping area in many instances. Requiring this level of air cleanliness seems justified due to the possibility that stoppers may rise partially out of the neck of the vial during transport. If the stopper were then reinserted by the capping machine after being exposed to uncontrolled air, the sterility of that vial would become questionable, and unless an operator noticed the exposed stopper prior to sealing, the potential problem would not be visually detectable and might not be detected by routine sterility testing. In this manner, the obviously undesirable event of a nonsterile vial reaching the marketplace could occur.

Media Simulations

Validation of the handling of partially stoppered vials should include media simulations. This brings us to another area of concern—the design of appropriate media simulations. Some manufacturers carry out a partial lyophilization cycle as part of their media simulations. This includes freezing the media in an effort to better simulate the process. Unfortunately, freezing the media can reduce the levels of some microbial contaminants. Since the purpose of the media simulation is to evaluate the ability to keep microbes out of sterilized product and containers during aseptic processing and handling, the freezing of media is not warranted.

With regard to the number of units to be filled, several firms have initiated expanded media simulations in which 9,000 or more vials are filled with media. The filled vials are then divided into three segments, where one-third of the vials is stoppered completely on the filling line; one-third is transported to the lyophilizer and stoppered; and the remaining third is loaded into the lyophilizer, exposed to the nitrogen flushing procedure used to relieve the vacuum at the end of the drying cycle, and then stoppered. This method helps to identify the portions of the process where contamination is most likely to occur. The sterilization of the lyophilizer and sterilization of the nitrogen system require separate validations, so the focus of media simulations should be on the filling, transportation, and loading operations. For the routine processing of less than 3,000 units, the number of units filled for the media simulation should be equivalent to the maximum batch size of the process. In the case of dual chamber vials, the media simulation should include filling media into both chambers.

Fill Volume Control

Another major concern is the accuracy of fill volumes. As in all products, a low fill volume may result in vials containing less than the specified amount of active material. But in the case of lyophilized products, this low fill volume may not be readily apparent after the product is dried, especially if the product contains only a few milligrams of active ingredient. Such subpotency may have serious clinical significance, so it is very important to monitor fill volume throughout the filling operation and to provide for the isolation of segments of the filled containers, so that appropriate action may be taken in the event of a high or low fill volume. In order to accommodate both high speed and low speed filling operations, the frequency of fill volume checks should be determined from the statistical analysis of filling machine accuracy and precision data, and not simply based on time.

As a general practice, filling operations must be tightly controlled. As an example of the FDA's expectations in this area, in published observations from recent inspections of manufacturing facilities, the FDA has objected when a firm's batch record described the method for adjusting fill volume if in-process assay results were outside the specification of 95–105 percent, but did not place a limit on how much the fill volume should be adjusted.

Bulk Drying

Finally, there are instances where solutions are filled directly into trays and lyophilized in bulk, rather than filling the product into vials or syringes before freeze drying. This practice has the procedural control difficulties inherent to increased product exposure to the environment during transport to and from the lyophilizer and the manipulations required to remove dried product from the trays. Therefore, drying in trays may be somewhat difficult to justify because alternative technology is currently available.

LYOPHILIZATION CYCLE, CONTROLS, AND VALIDATION

Cycle Development

There are two central concepts concerning the lyophilization cycle: (1) It should be well defined with appropriate process controls and (2) the cycle should be based on development work completed before the process is transferred to production. FDA inspectors expect to see a written report that clearly describes the steps in the drying process, and they consider it poor practice to fine-tune the system during production or use production runs to validate the cycle "on the fly."

The scale-up of lyophilization cycles has presented problems of many types. For example, the method and rate of freezing the product have been shown to affect the structure of the frozen cake as well as the physical form of the drug substance. Such changes can have a large impact on the drying rate, potency, and stability of the product. Under these circumstances, there may be poor agreement between research and production batches with regard to the time, temperature, and pressure profiles experienced by the product. The FDA views freezing times, sublimation times, and product temperature profiles of production batches that are inconsistent with those observed in stability or clinical batches as significant changes to the process and, therefore, potential sources of concern.

More specifically, the firm should know the thermal behavior of the product, including its freezing point, eutectic point (if one exists), glass transition temperatures, and any other pertinent transition points. There should be a scientific justification for the lyophilization cycle that is based on data that support the cycle parameters of shelf and product temperatures, chamber pressures, and cycle times. And finally, the written manufacturing procedure should specify time, temperature, and pressure limits for each step of the cycle, and should include ramp rates for shelf temperature changes during the cycle.

Leak Rate Testing

Because lengthy cycles stress lyophilization equipment severely, it is not uncommon for mechanical malfunction or failure to occur during a cycle. For example, leakage of several types can occur in a lyophilizer chamber, such as air from the environment, heating/cooling fluid circulating through the shelves, refrigerants from compressors, or oil vapor that migrates from the vacuum pumps back to the drying chamber. Leakage is a serious concern, because it may result in the contamination of the product with microorganisms or chemicals. Therefore, it is important to monitor the leak rate of the system periodically in order to maintain its integrity. The frequency of leak testing should be determined from the data generated during validation of the lyophilizer. A limit for the acceptable pressure rise should be established, and the action to be taken in the event of excessive leakage should be included in the operating document for the equipment.

Mechanical Failures

The corrective actions to be taken whenever events such as mechanical failures happen should be defined. The malfunction should be documented, and the possible effect of the malfunction on the product must be evaluated. It may not be sufficient to merely test extra samples of the product and justify the release of the batch on the basis of the test results. In cases where sterility assurance has been jeopardized or fluid such as refrigerants have leaked into the chamber, it may be necessary to reject the batch, regardless of the test results, because the quality and integrity of the product cannot be guaranteed. FDA inspectors will review preventive maintenance logs, quality assurance alert notices, discrepancy reports, and investigation reports during the initial part of an inspection to identify potential problems and batches that may have been affected by them.

Lyophilization Process Control

Once the drying cycle has been established, it must be shown that the lyophilizer is capable of controlling and recording the essential process parameters. Lyophilization cycle validation has been addressed in other chapters of this book, but it is worth mentioning a few of the issues that the FDA has commented about in inspection reports. Some firms market multiple strengths of the same active ingredient and make various batch sizes of products to accommodate their marketing needs. It is likely that each strength and batch size will have its own cycle parameters. If a company is using the same cycle for multiple strengths, this will be a signal to the FDA to focus their attention on the reports supporting the filed cycle, since it is probable that the company's process development and validation are inadequate.

Sterilization of Lyophilizers

In order to manufacture aseptically, it is preferable that the lyophilizer be sterilized prior to loading the sterile product onto the shelves, although sanitization of older units is still tolerated. Many older lyophilizers cannot withstand the rigors of sterilization-in-place (SIP) by steam, but some are able to be sterilized with ethylene oxide (EtO). In this case, the FDA will want to see evidence that residual EtO and its by-products are removed from the chamber and do not contaminate the product during lyophilization. Other lyophilizers can only be cleaned and sanitized with various chemical agents. In instances where a history of successful sanitization exists, the FDA is not currently insisting that the lyophilizer be replaced with more modern equipment with SIP capability. However, if new equipment is being installed, it should be sterilizable.

The FDA continues to be concerned about several issues regarding the adequacy of procedures used to sterilize lyophilizers. If the unit employs a ram to stopper the vials at the end of drying, a potential breach of aseptic processing exists. As the ram extends into the chamber, nonsterile surfaces of the ram may be exposed to the chamber. It is not likely that the lubricant or hydraulic fluid on the ram can or will be sterilized by the SIP cycle, so it is conceivable that organisms might be blown from the oil into the vials during the vacuum break phase at the end of the lyophilization process. On the other hand, the exposure of the ram occurs at the end of the cycle, when the stoppers are being seated in the vials. Nevertheless, due to the dynamics of the vacuum break (airflow patterns and velocities in the chamber), the FDA remains concerned about the risk of contamination, especially when several batches of the same product are made in one campaign, without cleaning and SIP between cycles. In assessing the risk of product contamination, it may be helpful to monitor the stoppering hardware of the lyophilizer for trends in the level of microbial contamination.

Filter Integrity Testing

Filters are used to sterilize air, nitrogen, or other gases that may be introduced into the drying chamber. It is preferable that the filters be sterilized and integrity tested in place. This avoids the need for aseptic connection to the chamber, but it is somewhat difficult to do. Filters must be wetted to conduct an integrity test. For hydrophobic filters, the wetting agent is generally alcohol. If the filter is tested in place, the wetting fluid will be forced through the filter and into the chamber, where it becomes a potential contaminant for the product during the subsequent lyophilization cycle. However, with appropriate valving and piping, the wetting fluid should be able to be purged from the filter and lines before it enters the chamber, thereby minimizing this concern.

Historically, it has been shown that currently available filters can withstand multiple SIP cycles and maintain their integrity. Nevertheless, if the integrity test is not conducted after SIP, there is no guarantee that the filter has maintained its integrity. Therefore, many companies are using redundant filters, steaming them in place, and then conducting integrity tests after the drying cycle. These companies understand that if both filters fail the integrity test after the lyophilization cycle, the batch will almost certainly be lost due to insufficient sterility assurance. Their position is that it is very unlikely that both filters will fail at the same time, and the risk of losing a batch of product for insufficient assurance of sterility is small. Since the use of redundant filters is obviously not completely foolproof, the debate about how to handle filter integrity testing continues.

Validation of Computerized Control Systems

For units that use microcomputers to control the process, there should be a flowchart or logic diagram that describes the functions of the controller. The controller should be validated to assure that it is capable of consistently running the cycle as defined in the manufacturing directions. The validation program should include normal cycles and aberrant cycles where power failures or mechanical problems occurred to be sure that the controller makes appropriate adjustments to protect the integrity of the product. Basic concerns about the validation of controller software should include software development, program modifications, and system security.

Lyophilization Cycle Validation

Sometimes validation is performed retrospectively by extracting information about the lyophilization cycles from historical manufacturing batch records. Companies have been cited for issuing reports for retrospective validation that contained obsolete, nonspecific, or inappropriate information. In particular, the reports did not contain detailed summaries of critical lyophilization parameters during various freezing and drying phases of the cycles. If information is gathered from batches made in older equipment, it should be kept in mind that the recording and controlling devices may not have been sophisticated enough to generate data that can meet current standards for the validation of lyophilization cycles.

LYOPHILIZER DESIGN AND STERILIZATION

Sterilization and Sterility Assurance

For lyophilizers that cannot tolerate steam sterilization, ethylene oxide sterilization or chemical cleaning and sanitization may be used for controlling bioburden. Unfortunately, sanitizing agents are not able to access piping used to transport nitrogen and air to the chamber, and generally cannot be used to sanitize condenser surfaces, especially if the condenser is optically dense, or configured so that its surfaces cannot be wiped down with the chemical agent. For EtO treatment, the gas must be dispersed evenly throughout the lyophilizer, humidity control is required to ensure effective sterilization, and monitoring for residual EtO and its by-products is necessary to insure that the aeration process at the end of the cycle is adequate.

The most common method of sterilization is steam under pressure. The process is similar to autoclaving, and the problems associated with steam sterilizing a lyophilizer are similar to those encountered in autoclaving. Provision should be made to remove condensate from the chamber, condenser, and associated piping during the SIP cycle to maximize the effectiveness of the process. It is generally accepted that lyophilizers should be sterilized after every cycle, due to the possibility that shelf support rods can become contaminated, and because the manipulations involved in unloading and cleaning the chamber can increase contamination levels. Of course, this is particularly true when the lyophilizer is a double door type, and the door used for unloading opens into a nonsterile room. Due to their concern about contamination from the nonsterile room, the FDA has recommended that the unloading area for a double door lyophilizer should be a cleanroom, with appropriate microbiological controls in place if sterilization is not performed after each load. The doors of all double door units must be properly interlocked to insure that the door on the cleanroom side cannot be opened before the unit has been sterilized.

Many of the problems that have occurred with SIP are the result of poor circulation of steam. Some large lyophilizers collapse the shelves together to facilitate loading and unloading. The shelves must be separated during SIP to allow the penetration of steam into all areas to be sterilized. In at least one instance, the FDA has objected to a company's practice of sterilizing the trays used to transport vials from the filling line to the lyophilizer during SIP of the chamber. The trays impeded steam flow across the shelves and resulted in an ineffective sterilizing process.

Most newer lyophilizers are capable of sterilizing the chamber and the condenser, even if the condenser is external to the chamber. This provides better sterility assurance for the product, especially in the event of a mechanical problem that allows the chamber to be at a lower pressure than the condenser, thereby increasing the probability that contaminants might migrate from the condenser to the product being dried in the chamber. During the validation of the sterilization process, it is common practice to monitor the chamber, condenser, and gas supply lines with calibrated thermocouples. In addition, the sterilization cycle is generally challenged with biological indicator strips (usually *Bacillus stearothermophilus*) to confirm that adequate steam penetration occurs throughout the lyophilizer and to insure the sterility of the chamber, the condenser, and gas supply lines (piping).

One of the more serious problems associated with SIP is that there is frequently some amount of condensate on the floor and shelves of the lyophilizer after sterilization. Some companies drain this water while the chamber is still under positive pressure. While this might be effective and acceptable practice, others have left the drain open and allowed the chamber to come to atmospheric pressure. This practice can allow nonsterile air to enter the chamber from the drain line, and at least in one instance, contamination of the chamber with *Pseudomonas* has resulted. The FDA is alert to this problem, and they will want to see evidence that the system being inspected is not liable to this type of contamination.

Backstreaming

During lyophilization at very low pressures, it is possible for oil vapor to migrate from the vacuum pump to the drying chamber, especially in older units where the condenser is not designed to prevent this from happening. Newer units are equipped with optically dense condensers; that is, condensers with convoluted passageways that inhibit vapor flow through them, thereby enhancing the likelihood that vapors will be trapped in the condenser, rather than escaping to the vacuum pump (water vapor from the product) or back to the drying chamber (water vapor or oil vapor). This "backstreaming" of oil into the drying chamber and into the product must be prevented.

There are essentially two ways to stop backstreaming. The first is to increase the chamber pressure with an inert gas such as nitrogen during drying. This method increases the number of gas molecules flowing toward the vacuum pump. The gas molecules collide with backstreaming oil vapor and physically prevent it from reaching the chamber and product. The second method is to improve the design of the lyophilizer to make the path from the vacuum pump to the drying chamber more tortuous, thereby making it more difficult for oil vapor to reach the chamber.

FINISHED PRODUCT TESTING

There are many aspects to finished product testing for lyophilized products, but the four that are of primary concern in lyophilized products are dose uniformity testing, moisture testing, stability testing, and sterility testing.

Dose Uniformity Testing

The United States Pharmacopeia (USP) includes two forms of dose uniformity testing. Weight variation may be applied to solids that have been prepared from solutions and lyophilized in the final container. But if excipients or other additives are present, weight variation may only be applied if there is a correlation between sample weight and potency results. If potency is determined by assaying the entire contents of the reconstituted vial, the label claim can be confirmed. But without knowing the sample weight, dose uniformity cannot be assessed. Initial and stability testing for potency should be performed on a known weight of sample to be sure that fill weight variation within the batch does not bias potency testing.

Moisture Testing

The main premise underlying the decision to lyophilize a product is that the product is not stable in the presence of water. A primary concern then is the achievement and maintenance of acceptably low moisture levels initially and throughout the shelf life of the product. The basis for the moisture specification at release and on stability will be reviewed by the FDA. The expiration dating and moisture specification should be developed from worst-case data (highest moisture) to ensure adequate stability throughout the product's shelf life.

Stability Testing

The USP points out that compendial standards apply at all times during the life of the product. Therefore, the stability of reconstituted solutions should be conducted on aged samples throughout the shelf life of the product, and particularly at the expiration date interval. Following reconstitution, samples should be held for the maximum time allowed in the product labeling prior to testing. And since the most concentrated reconstituted solutions will generally exhibit the fastest degradation rate, samples of the most concentrated and least concentrated reconstituted solutions should be included in the stability assessment.

Sterility Testing

There is a concern with the solution used to reconstitute the product for sterility testing. Although product labeling may allow reconstitution with bacteriostatic water for injection, sterile water for injection (SWFI) should be used for the sterility test. Many hospitals do not use bacteriostatic water for injection, due to its potential toxicity. Also, bacteriostatic water for injection may kill vegetative organisms that may be present, thereby masking the actual level of contamination in the product. Contaminants detected in the test should be identified and reviewed.

FINISHED PRODUCT INSPECTION

The FDA believes that it is good pharmaceutical practice to perform 100 percent visual inspection of all parenteral products, including sterile lyophilized powders. Among the critical properties of the product are cake volume and cake appearance. One of the major defects to look for is meltback. Meltback occurs when the product changes from the solid state to the liquid state during the lyophilization cycle, and its presence means that sublimation was not complete in that particular vial. The change in physical form of the drug substance (conversion from the crystalline form to the amorphous form, for example) or excess residual moisture in the product associated with meltback may cause decreased product stability, or to look at it another way, increased product degradation.

It should be understood that meltback is a true indicator of product quality, not just a cosmetic defect. It is an indication that the lyophilization cycle was not controlled properly, or that the cycle is not appropriate for the product. With this in mind, the manufacturer should establish acceptance criteria for physical defects such as partial meltback, and develop stability data for products exhibiting partial meltback. Excessive frequency of meltback should trigger a full investigation, including analysis of the drug product for impurities and degradation products, as well as an examination of the cycle and lyophilizer controls. If partial or complete meltback occurs regularly in production batches, the FDA considers the process to be out of control. This is a clear violation of good manufacturing practices and should be addressed with appropriate urgency by the manufacturer.

CONCLUSIONS

This discussion of the FDA perspective on lyophilization is based on guidelines published by the FDA and actual observations made by the FDA during inspections of companies that manufacture lyophilized products. Overall, the FDA recognizes that lyophilization is a complicated technology and that there may be more than one way to meet the goals of a validated lyophilization process. They will, therefore, be somewhat flexible in evaluating a firm's capabilities to manufacture freeze-dried products reproducibly.

However, this position should not be construed to mean that a process does not have to be rigorously characterized, validated, and controlled. On the contrary, the FDA expects that lyophilization cycles will be established on the basis of well-grounded scientific evidence and experimental data and that a written report will be prepared to document the development of the cycle. The cycle should be detailed in written manufacturing procedures and run the same way every time the product is made. It is not acceptable to fine-tune the cycle during production. Operating parameters should be established and validated before commercial-scale production begins.

In summary, cycle development should be conducted and documented prior to introducing the process to production. Appropriate process controls should be in place to ensure that the cycle will run consistently and reproducibly. The lyophilization process, though it may be very complicated, must be rigorously validated and robust enough to guarantee product of consistent quality before commercial lots are distributed for use.

ACKNOWLEDGMENTS

The author would like to thank Mr. Edward H. Trappler of Lyophilization Technology, Inc., for his assistance in preparing this chapter, and Dr. John Levchuk of the FDA for his helpful editorial comments.

6

FREEZE DRYER STERILISATION

Kevin Kinnarney

Bio Products Laboratory
Herts, United Kingdom

The production of pharmaceutical products requires manufacturing in a clean environment or even under totally aseptic conditions. As equipment for use during the manufacturing process will have clearly defined levels of acceptability for use, the freeze dryer must also meet these standards. Amongst these standards is cleanliness or sterility. The freeze dryer should be viewed as another piece of process equipment and treated in the same manner. If a product is filled aseptically, it would be inadvisable to use a freeze dryer that has not been cleaned or sterilised in an acceptable manner. Many companies operate sterilisable freeze dryers, and the current preffered method of sterilisation is steam. There are still many older units in operation that do not have the ability to accept steam sterilisation, and other methods exist to render the equipment suitable for its intended purpose. Whatever type of equipment is in use, or its method of operation and maintenance of cleanliness, GMP guidelines should be followed.

SANITATION/STERILISATION METHODS

Disinfectants

The inner surfaces of freeze dryer chambers are wiped or sprayed with some form of disinfectant solution. This solution must be carefully selected so that it will have no adverse effect on any of the materials of construction during the cleaning period. Equally, any residue left behind must have no effect on either the material of the equipment being cleaned or the product itself. The cleaning of the chamber is not made any easier by the fixtures and fittings inside, which are necessary to the freeze drying process. During design and building of the freeze dryer, the future cleaning and sanitisation of the plant may not have been of the highest priority. The interdistance between shelves, flexible connection hoses, and stoppering systems form areas that are difficult to reach and effectively sanitise, as access is only usually available from the loading door. More modern plants will have considered this need for cleaning and sterilisation, although the same constraints of fixtures and fittings limiting access still exist.

Any type of sanitisation exercise is difficult to perform routinely with consistency, as it is usually carried out manually. Because of the difficulty in ensuring consistency of any sanitisation routine when carried out manually, validation of the efficacy of this action becomes difficult to achieve. Areas that are easy to reach will be effectively treated, possibly limiting the effectiveness to the chamber only. Pipework and attached valves that are difficult to reach may not be effectively treated, if at all. Sterilisation of the gas inlet vent filter will have to be carried out separately and attached back onto the plant before any freeze drying operation can begin.

When disinfection is the main form of reducing contamination, then care must be taken to rotate between different disinfectants to prevent increasing microbial resistance to these solutions. Monitoring of the disinfectants should be carried out to check that they are not themselves contributing to any source contamination.

Gases

Gases used to sterilise freeze dryers include formaldehyde, ethylene oxide, and vapour phase hydrogen peroxide. Formaldehyde has long been a favourite sterilising agent for equipment, but it has many drawbacks, including the difficulty in completely removing trapped residues. Ethylene oxide also suffers from the same disadvantage. The effectiveness of these gases depends on controlling the environment in which they are used and monitoring these conditions. These two gases are reactive and may attack some of the materials present in the freeze dryer, leaving unwanted residues. They also present a problem during removal following the exposure period without careful exhausting, they present a health and safety hazard. It may be necessary to vent and flush the freeze dryer many times to remove all gas residues trapped behind O-rings or other seals. After the gas has been removed and any air flushing completed, any remaining residues should be at an acceptable preestablished limit. Effective microbial kill relies on good contact between the gas and any microbial contamination present; large deposits of spilt product may reduce the penetration of the gas, which could allow microbial growth to flourish. Effective cycles rely on controlled humidity, temperature, and also time—all of which should be carefully monitored. Biological indicators of a suitable type are the only effective method of checking the level of sterilisation efficiency, and it may be necessary to incorporate these in each cycle. Sterilisation of the vent filter may require removal from the plant, separate sterilisation, and reattachment aseptically.

Hydrogen Peroxide Vapour

A sterilisation process with hydrogen peroxide used in its vapour phase. Hydrogen peroxide in this form is more effective in destroying spores than as a liquid. Sterilisation using this method may be carried out at room temperature. The vapour is generated externally and led to the vessel undergoing treatment. Following sterilisation, the gas is decomposed into water and oxygen, leaving no dangerous residues behind. A catalytic converter fitted to the freeze dryer is used to decompose the gas, which is then pumped clear of the system. The normal rotary vacuum pump cannot be used for this purpose, as the water produced on chemical breakdown will contaminate the pump; therefore, a second type of pump is required. The advantages are that this process is carried out at low temperature and low pressure, without any harmful residues left by the gas itself.

Successful sterilisation of the freeze dryer relies on certain conditions being met. All parts of the system undergoing treatment must be the same temperature, as different temperatures affect the exposure time required. Also, there must be no water, or ice, present that can cause condensation of hydrogen peroxide vapour. Freeze dryers, therefore, need some form of drying without the use of the condenser, as this may cause ice to form.

Gas distribution of hydrogen peroxide vapour is achieved by lowering the pressure in the plant to below 10 mbar and then allowing the vapour to enter the plant until a satisfactory pressure has been reached. A hold time follows before the gas is discharged. The system is then pumped clear of all gas, using air flushing if necessary.

This method of sterilisation has other problems to consider. All materials used in the plant must be resistant to the gas and not act as a catalyst. Any rust in the plant causes hydrogen peroxide gas concentration to decrease rapidly; therefore, a thorough check of the materials of construction should be undertaken. The method of determining the efficiency of sterilisation in all areas of the plant may rest solely on the use of biological indicators. The ease with which these can be positioned and retrieved may cause difficulty with monitoring. Temperature distribution across the system must also be checked, as this will determine the time needed for sterilisation. A check for clearance of the vapour before use in freeze drying or any possible remaining residues must be undertaken and the routine cycle adequately validated.

The main advantages of this method are the capital savings on purchasing a freeze dryer that is, in fact, a pressure vessel. The large temperature range covered by a steam sterilisable freeze dryer and the resultant stresses are less if this method of operation is adopted. The need to generate quantities of clean steam and the energy costs in recooling the plant after sterilisation are also eliminated.

Extra equipment is needed to generate hydrogen peroxide vapour and convey it to the unit using this method of sterilisation. Complete drying of the plant internally prior to treatment and ensuring an even temperature are also prerequisites. Effectiveness of the process may only be determined by using biological indicators at present; the result of the sterilisation cycle will not be known immediately.

STEAM

Steam sterilisation is the accepted method of sterilisation, particularly in the pharmaceutical industry. The methods and mechanics of sterilising many different types of equipment are well known and widely practised, and there is a long history of successful operation. All types of vessels, tanks, and processing equipment, including freeze dryers, may be sterilised using steam. Regulatory bodies in both the United States and United Kingdom accept, and may even recommend, this method of sterilisation because of the above reasons. The cost of a new freeze dryer will be substantially higher for a steam sterilisable unit because of the pressure vessel standard required; but this is obviously not a feature that can be added later.

Steam does not present the same problems associated with gases or disinfectants, as there are no harmful residues left following sterilisation, and there are no toxicity and few environmental problems with waste. Additional equipment to render the sterilant harmless is not necessary because natural cooling and condensing of the steam can be allowed to take place. The steaming process itself can assist in the cleaning of the freeze dryer chamber, condenser, and associated components, especially as high quality steam should be used.

As steam sterilisation has been used in many applications the accepted operational criteria and methods of validation have been well tried and tested. Equipment is, therefore, readily available to use for these validation and monitoring purposes.

Design of the Freeze Dryer to Allow Sterilisation

The reason for wanting to sterilise freeze dryers is to provide an acceptable environment for processing an open product. The product to undergo freeze drying is often at the final stage of processing and may be contained in partially stoppered vials or ampoules. In this state, there is a potential for contamination from the surroundings; therefore, every effort should be made to ensure contamination risk is minimal. Freeze drying cycles may be relatively long, and the exposure time of the product inside the plant can be significant.

The inside surfaces of the freeze dryer are themselves sterilised, as opposed to an autoclave that sterilises materials introduced into the chamber. The same characteristics as seen in autoclave design do not extend very far because an autoclave is usually a jacketed vessel consisting of only one single, empty, chamber. A freeze dryer, usually, consists of a chamber connected to a separate condenser which limits access for validation. A freeze dryer has primarily been designed with the freeze drying cycle in mind; the sterilisation cycle plays an important but secondary role. Basically, a compromise between the practical and the ideal exists.

General

The unit should be designed to allow all possible parts of the freeze dryer in contact with the product or the subliming vapour to be sterilised. Any part of the freeze dryer open to the product during the freeze drying phase is a potential source of contamination to the product. Most modern freeze dryers are constructed using high grade stainless steel, wherever possible, which is not affected by steam. Obviously, there are some components used that are not possible to steam sterilise but these must be minimised and any potential risk to the product limited. A major item that cannot be steam sterilised is the rotary vacuum pump, which must be isolated during the sterilisation phase. Careful design of the method of using this pump during freeze drying can reduce the source of potential contamination; alternatively, a sterilisable filter could be fitted before the entrance to the pump.

A pressure vessel capable of withstanding the pressures generated during the sterilisation process is required. Pressure vessel requirements for the chamber also apply to the condenser and any relevant pipework; and this rating will depend on the temperature range specified, but not less than 3.5 bar$_a$ would be recommended.

The high pressures generated during steam sterilisation make the design and locking of the door very important. The door must be of suitable material and strength to withstand the temperature and pressure during this time and the locking mechanism must be able to hold the door closed safely to prevent the escape of steam. Even for a relatively small freeze dryer, the pressure exerted on the door locks during this period will reach several tonnes.

Safety valves must be fitted to the system to prevent the possibility of overpressure. The material of construction of these valves and any internal seals should conform to the standard of the rest of the freeze dryer, which will usually be high grade stainless steel.

Leak Tightness

During the sterilisation process, the components of the freeze dryer will be subject to high temperatures. Any joints in the system will undergo movement and stress resulting from the expansion of pipework, and so on, caused by heat. To minimise any possible leaks at these joints, it is advisable to use welded joints where possible—all of which must conform to pressure vessel standards. They must also be suitably finished inside to meet GMP standards, in that they are finished flush and are crevice free. Automatic welding machines offer better finishes than manual welding. The possibility of any leaks will affect the sterilising cycle and may also have health and safety implications. Leaks may show up on subsequent cooling down of the vessel and may allow particulate matter or microbial contamination to enter the freeze dryer. The previously sterilised freeze dryer may, therefore, suffer a breach of integrity, negating the action of the sterilisation cycle. It is not possible to completely eliminate joints by welding, as some components must remain removable for calibration or validation purposes.

Steam Penetration

It is necessary to ensure complete sterilisation of the unit, and steam must be able to penetrate all parts of the freeze dryer, including pipework and component parts. To enable this to take place, these items should be made with as large a bore as possible and kept as short as possible. There is an optimum ratio of pipe diameter to length for dead legs, and this should be taken into account when designing the plant. (Ideally, this ratio should be 1* the diameter for pipe length.) None of this pipework should be positioned or angled in such a way that it can fill up with condensate during this period, as free draining is necessary to ensure good steam penetration. The position of some pipework may also offer a potential area of air entrapment that may prevent adequate penetration of steam and adversely affect the efficacy of the sterilisation of that region. It is possible to overcome the potential problem of air entrapment by designing the system to eliminate this as much as possible and by negative pulsing during operation.

Condensate Removal

A large volume of condensate is generated during heat up and sterilisation of the freeze dryer, and this must be removed quickly and efficiently to allow the system to reach its operating parameters. To assist in this, a large drain is fitted to the lowest point, or points, in the system. The number of drain pipes and their size will be determined by the size, layout, and type of freeze dryer. Attached to the drain (or drains) should be a suitable steam trap with, perhaps, a bypass line and isolation valve to allow the condensate to escape quickly during the warm-up period.

To assist draining of the condensate, all chamber and condenser floors should slope to drain. All pipework must allow easy draining of the condensate, and the number of dead legs present should be minimised. It may also be advisable, if possible, to angle the shelves to allow the condensate to run off quickly and not form pools.

If a vent filter is integral to the system, this should be included in the sterilisation process, thus eliminating the need for removal for separate sterilisation. Penetration of steam and condensate removal in the filter and housing may be more difficult to achieve due to position and pipework size. These problems should be considered at the design stage and appropriate action taken. It may be possible to reposition the filter housing and attach a separate steam supply and condensate trap to allow successful operation. Care must be taken in the design to prevent the vent filter from being damaged by high differential pressures across the filter media during the sterilisation process. (Filter manufacturers can supply data showing allowed pressure drop across the filter and any other operating constraints.)

System design will ensure that the filter is not subjected to damaging pressures at elevated temperatures. There are two simple methods to overcome this problem. One method is to introduce the steam directly into the plant and allow penetration from the chamber to the filter housing. With this method, pressure is slowly increased in the filter housing and the filter media does not suffer sudden changes. A check must be made on the penetration of the steam through the filter media. If steam is usually introduced into the freeze dryer via the vent filter pipework, then large pressure differentials will exist when the sterilisation cycle begins. At this time, the plant will be under a vacuum, and steam will be entering from the supply line at approximately

1.5 bar$_g$. This is the magnitude of differential that can prove fatal to modern vent filters! By fitting a bypass line around the filter housing, steam may be introduced into the plant via this route or through the filter. Both the filter housing line and the bypass line require isolation valves. The filter may be isolated using the line valve, and steam is allowed to flow via the bypass. When the pressure in the plant reaches its preset level, the bypass line isolation valve closes and the filter line valve opens, allowing steam to penetrate the filter. Subsequent maintenance of pressure in the unit is via the filter. With this method, the filter is protected at warm-up and pressure increase, but then has a period of direct flow sterilisation.

It is usual to have an isolating valve between the outlet from the freeze dryer and any condensate trap. This valve should be positively controlled to open only above atmospheric pressure and will prevent any possibility of condensate being sucked back into the plant during any vacuum phase, which could compromise system integrity.

Components

All components must be able to withstand the pressures and temperatures reached during sterilisation, including vacuum gauges, pressure gauges, and temperature measuring devices. It is not desirable to isolate these components before sterilisation and then reconnect them following completion of the process. Valves should be capable of sterilisation and be hygienic in design, enabling all condensate to drain completely. Depending on the type fitted, these valves may need to be fitted at an angle to ensure adequate draining. The material used for all types of seals, including valve seals, must be of a suitable type and capable of withstanding high and low pressures and temperatures. All other O-rings and any sealing material must be compatible with the system, including internal fittings in components, such as steam safety valves and Pirani gauges.

Suitable validation ports must be fitted to the plant to allow temperature sensors to be inserted for the adequate temperature mapping of the sterilisation process. Lagging should be provided to prevent heat loss and reduce cold spots; this is also a safety protection for personnel. It is inadvisable to lag inside the door, as this may be in a clean room and the lagging will act as a breeding ground for possible contamination. Safety protection may take the form of a double skin to the outside surface to prevent accidental injury.

Valves

There are many different types of valves used on freeze dryers, some dating back before the advent of hygienic designs. The main concern when selecting the type of valve is its suitability for both freeze drying and sterilisation cycles. Valves must be acceptable for both operational constraints and comply with the latest GMP criteria. The material of construction should match that of the plant, and the seal must, as has previously been mentioned, be inert to the product and process. Valves must be capable of operating in the temperature range of at least –80°C to 125°C and a pressure range from 0 to 3 bar$_a$ without any change in efficiency.

Over the years, many types have been used. Commonly used valves included angle seat valves, ball valves, and diaphragm valves. Some of these have inherent problems when sterilised and others have perceived problems. Currently, the preferred choice appears to be diaphragm valves that because of their design, allow easy sterilisation of all parts in contact with the freeze drying environment. The construction of these is relatively simple in that the diaphragm surface is the only moving part exposed to steam. Opening and closing the valve consists only of tightening or loosening the diaphragm against a stainless steel surface. There is no necessity for any gland or face seals and different materials may be used for the diaphragm. They are hygienic in use and, provided they are fitted correctly, allow complete draining of any condensate formed.

Angle seat valves do not offer the same advantages in that there are more sealing sites in the construction. These valves require a gland seal on the operating shaft; the fact that the shaft is withdrawn during sterilisation means it cannot be completely sterilised. If the valve is open during sterilisation, then when it is closed, the unsterile shaft is allowed back into the system. This may not be a problem in some applications if any flow is only from the clean side to the dirty. Again they must be fitted at the correct angle to allow good draining of any condensate formed.

Ball valves are often used on freeze dryers and have proven to be popular for many applications. Whatever position the valve is in, not all the surfaces of the ball can be sterilised at any one time. The whole valve may be heated to a high temperature, but some of the surfaces will not be exposed to steam. The angle at which these valves are fitted is not critical to good condensate drainage.

Validation

The sterilisation cycle must be validated adequately and the results of the cycle must conform to an internationally acceptable exposure to dry saturated steam. Whatever time/temperature relationship is adopted for acceptance of this cycle, it must meet the requirements of any quality control or regulatory authority. Because the design is not primarily for an autoclave it may be necessary to widen the acceptable limits above the sterilisation criteria normally encountered during autoclave steam sterilisation. To successfully validate a freeze dryer's sterilisation cycle the following steps should be considered.

Target of Sterilisation Cycle

The first step is to determine what the sterilisation cycle should be to achieve its target. This is only the first pass and may need to be modified in the light of results encountered during validation. A basic cycle could consist of a vacuum stage to remove air from the system, followed by the introduction of steam. It may be considered necessary to use a series of negative pulses to remove any noncondensable gases from the system. If the rotary vacuum pump is used to draw a vacuum before the admission of steam, a much lower pressure can be achieved in the plant. One pump down will only be required, and pulsing may be omitted, as better removal of noncondensable gases may be achieved at very low pressures.

Temperature Uniformity

The next step is to determine the uniformity of the sterilisation temperatures within the freeze dryer. Temperature probes are located, via any validation ports, throughout the freeze dryer. Locations are chosen that will include all pipework and potential dead legs. Locations such as the vent filter and its pipework, safety valves, Pirani gauge heads, and pressure transducers should be considered. Attention should also be paid to large components that may take time to heat. Included in this category are shelf lifting rods, the door, and flexible hoses. Some examples of potential cold spots to monitor are shown in Figure 6.1. This temperature mapping should be as thorough as possible to ensure that all potential cold spots have been identified, the work may require a number of runs to complete the task. If all tested areas reach the required temperature, then the time period can be adjusted to suit the acceptance criteria. A time is usually set that allows the coldest spot identified to reach the stated sterilisation temperature and hold for the minimum time, although this may mean other areas in the plant have excessive time at, or above, the sterilising temperature.

If there is a problem with a cold spot not reaching temperature, without excessive overkill in the rest of the plant, the reason should be investigated. It may be the result of poor steam penetration or the presence of noncondensable gases. These problems could be overcome by additional negative pressure pulsing before sterilisation begins. Alternatively, a different method of introducing the steam into the system may be considered. Direct injection of the steam into the cold area

Figure 6.1. The areas of the plant that should be considered for monitoring during sterilisation validation. Key: A. Chamber pressure sensor; B. Safety valve; C. Vent filter; D. Chamber vent valve; E. Condenser vent valve; F. Condenser vent valve; G. Vacuum valve line; H. Condenser cooling coils; J. Main valve; K. Condenser drain valve; L. Chamber drain valve; M. Hydraulic ram and seals; N. Door seal.

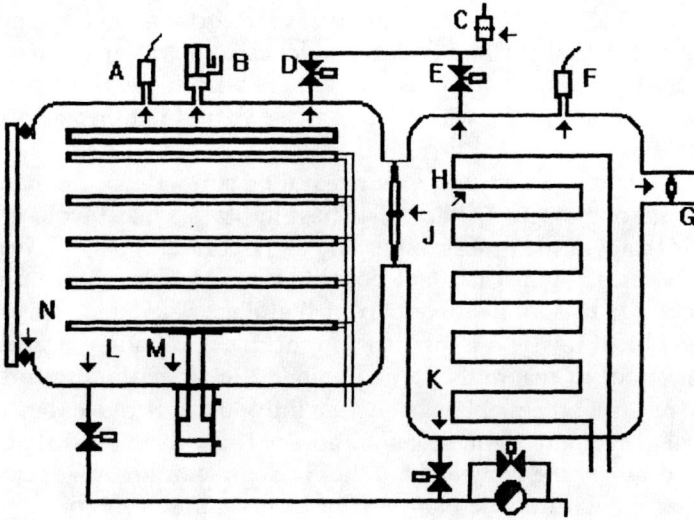

using an additional supply, or an additional steam condensate trap to remove condensate, may be all that is necessary to overcome the problem. The use of extra insulation around gauge heads and so on may also reduce heat loss, resulting in improved temperature stability.

When all the temperature mapping has been completed and the position of the coldest spot has been determined, this may be used to control the sterilisation cycle. In practice, it is usual for the temperature probe positioned in the condensate drain line to control the cycle, as this is often the coldest spot.

Reproducibility

Having determined the position of cold spots in the freeze dryer, and as far as possible eliminated any problem areas, a final temperature mapping exercise may be undertaken. Temperature probes should be positioned in all the known hottest and coldest places within the freeze dryer, and the sterilisation cycle operated following the documented procedure. Providing no unexpected results are generated, this cycle should become the definitive cycle for that particular plant. There may have been modifications from the sterilisation cycle first envisaged when the process began that takes into account subsequent observations.

Recordings should be taken using suitable calibrated data collecting equipment, with a satisfactory scale resolution, throughout the exercise, and a satisfactory number of recording probes should be utilised. Usually, three cycles should be undertaken to show reproducibility. If all the previous studies have been successfully completed, this final part of the validation exercise should not present any problems.

Temperature studies may need to be supported, or enhanced, by the use of biological indicators. These indicators may be placed alongside temperature probes, especially in the coldest spots. They may also be necessary when it is not possible to use a temperature probe, for whatever reason, in some part of the plant. The biological indicator must be of the type recommended for this application. It is also very important to ensure the same number of biological indicators are removed from the plant as have been introduced! Because they are relatively small and light, it is not impossible for them to be flushed into the drain by the movement of the condensate or to some relatively inaccessible part of the plant. Major dismantling of the plant to find a spore strip is not recommended!

The reasons given above should serve as a warning to the casual use of spore strips. It may be better to forego their use if the alternative is the risk of leaving an introduced contamination in the plant. Discussion with the regulatory bodies will clarify this point.

Sterilisation Cycle

General

Having carried out the validation work, there should be sufficient data to formulate the final routine sterilisation cycle. The cold spot in the freeze dryer should now have been positively identified, in most cases, as already mentioned, this will prove to be the condensate drain line. A permanent temperature probe should be fitted at this point (or wherever the coldest spot is in the system). This point should be recorded during operation; in some cases this may be the only point that must be monitored to achieve a satisfactory cycle pass. The control settings can now be fixed to achieve the temperature required for the monitoring probes. (Times and temperatures may be different to those normally encountered in an autoclave.) These settings and the pass criteria for the cycle now become the operational criteria.

Following the sterilisation cycle, there must be no possibility of compromising plant integrity by unsterile air being drawn into the plant, and a positive check on this possibility must be made during validation. Drain valves must be checked to ensure that they only open under positive pressure, unless they are protected by a filter or some other means.

Revalidation

A routine revalidation schedule should be adopted that will test the compliance of the cycle at predetermined retest times. It may be advisable to check that the coldest spot in the plant is still at the same position as on previous tests. Revalidation will normally follow calibration of control system instruments, recorders, and temperature probes and is usually carried out at least annually.

The Sterilisation Cycle

Two examples of sterilisation cycles are shown below.

A Liquid Ring Vacuum Pump. The condenser may be defrosted following the previous freeze drying cycle. It is not absolutely necessary to defrost the condenser, as the steam entering during the sterilisation heat up will melt the ice. Defrosting during unloading of the freeze dryer will save time, and using water is also a savings in cost over that of clean steam.

The liquid ring pump is switched on and the plant pressure allowed to fall to below 100 mbar. When the pressure is low enough, the ring pump is isolated and steam is injected into the plant to bring the system back to atmospheric pressure.

This pulsing of vacuum followed by steam injection may be carried out more than once to ensure all noncondensable gases have been purged from the system. The actual number of times required will have been determined during validation; three times would not be unusual.

Following the final negative pulse with the liquid ring pump, steam is injected to increase the system pressure, and, therefore, temperature, to the sterilisation level. When temperature at the coldest point is reached, the sterilisation time commences. It may be advisable to monitor pressure that will confirm the temperature and both readings should be logged with the system recorder.

Following the time at temperature (and pressure), the steam supply can be isolated. The steam pressure is removed from the system and the plant cooled. Pressure removal may be achieved by various methods.

- The pressure may be reduced by simply allowing natural condensing of the steam in the unit.

- A bypass valve around the condensate trap can be used to vent the steam to drain more quickly, with closing just above atmospheric pressure.

- Operating the condenser cooling will speed up the condensing of the steam. This coupled with the operation of the liquid ring pump will quickly reduce the system pressure. The liquid ring pump is left running to flash off the remaining water whilst the system is hot.

- The liquid ring pump should operate alone until all the free water has been removed and a vacuum remains in the plant.

- Some systems are fitted with cooling jackets to assist in cool down.

Final drying of the system may take place by the operation of the condenser cooling, and any remaining water will be trapped on the coils. Operation of the liquid ring pump for long periods is not recommended. Other than the extra wear and tear on the pump, there is the question of whether the pump and its pipeline offer a risk to the integrity of the system. Liquid ring pumps rely on constant water supply for their effectiveness; consequently, if there is a severe fluctuation in this supply, there is the possible risk of the low pressure not being maintained and suck back into the system occurring.

Without a Liquid Ring Pump. The condenser may be defrosted as previously, although this is not necessary. The condenser cooling is started and the condenser cooled to below -40°C. When the condenser is cool enough, the rotary vacuum pump can be switched on and the total system pressure reduced to below 1 mbar. At this pressure, very little in the way of noncondensable gases remain. The vacuum pump may be switched off and steam injected to increase the pressure and temperature.

When the sterilisation temperature has been reached, as measured by the probe in the coldest spot, then the time sequence begins. Starting the steam injection at such a low pressure in the system may aid steam penetration within the plant.

Following the hold time at temperature, the steam supply is valved off and the pressure removed from the system.

- The pressure may be allowed to decay by natural cooling and condensing of the steam.

- If a bypass valve is fitted around the steam trap, this may be opened to release the pressure to drain, ensuring this valve closes above atmospheric pressure to prevent the possibility of suck back.

- The condenser cooling may be switched on to condense the steam and trap the condensed water on the coils as ice.

Whatever method is used to release the pressure, the next stage is to operate the condenser cooling until the coils have cooled down to below -40°C. When the temperature has been reached, the rotary vacuum pump is switched on and a vacuum drawn on the system. This will draw any water present onto the cooling coils leaving the chamber dry.

Conclusions. Whatever method of steam sterilisation is undertaken, the plant will still be in a fairly hot condition although the chamber should be left completely dry. The plant may have to be left to cool by natural means or there may be a built-in jacket cooling system around the chamber to assist this cooling. Other ways of assisting cooling include continuing with condenser cooling and allowing the plant to reach atmospheric pressure with clean, filtered air. This will assist heat transfer from the walls of the condenser and speed up the cooling of the condenser walls. Likewise, operating the shelf cooling system with the chamber at atmospheric pressure will cool the walls of the chamber. Ensure that the shelf temperature does not cool low enough to start condensing water or to draw water back off the condenser coils.

It is usual for modern freeze dryers to have some form of automatic control for the sterilisation cycle. The use of an automated system will ensure conformity to the validated criteria, a consistency is lacking when operated manually.

Routine Operation

There are different views regarding how often a freeze dryer should be sterilised and in what circumstances. The time taken for a sterilisation cycle followed by cooling down may have a significant impact on any production schedule, as it may take a full working day to complete this phase. The final decision of how often sterilisation is necessary rests with the user, but there are some considerations to be taken into account.

Sterilisation between each product batch dried is, possibly, the ideal scenario, as this acts as a barrier between cycles. It effectively sterilises after the first batch, leaving the plant ready for the next batch. If the first batch fails its quality control stage for whatever reason the second batch is protected because sterilisation of the plant has taken place. When no intermediate sterilisation has taken place, the second batch could be subject to contamination from the first, rendering release for use questionable.

The type of container for the product undergoing processing may have a bearing on sterilisation frequency. It may be argued that "closed" containers, such as vials with partially inserted stoppers, do not offer the same risk of contamination as "open" trays. Where a batch of starting material is divided into multiple loads for drying, and this is carried out subsequently in the same plant, there may be justification in not sterilising between loads. This is certainly acceptable for some types of intermediate product that have further downstream processing.

"Campaign" freeze drying may also be carried out with the freeze dryer only being sterilised when the type of product being processed changes, or after a specific time period. Whatever routine is adopted, a sterilisation routine must be defensible when expertly examined. The routine adopted may require microbiological validation to support the frequency of sterilisation. As with most other sterilised equipment, a "use by" date should be imposed. A typical time period between sterilisation and use may be 10 days; if this period is exceeded, then the plant would require resterilisation, although this is almost impossible to validate. Plant integrity may be compromised, and the need to sterilise between each batch made necessary, if the stoppering system relies on a "nonsterile" ram being introduced into the chamber. As the ram has not been previously sterilised or kept in a clean environment, when it enters the chamber it carries with it some contamination on the metal surfaces. The level of risk to the product undergoing closure may be minimal, but the plant itself has become contaminated from an outside source (i.e., a hydraulic oil system).

Routine Maintenance

During a freeze drying cycle, temperatures in the condenser and the shelves may reach $-80°C$ and the pressure in the system will be 0 bar_a. During sterilisation, the temperature will be in excess of $121°C$ and the pressure up to 2.5 bar_a. The stresses generated by these changes in temperature and pressure are significant. Seals at joints and in valves are particularly affected by this type of stress. Some materials may start to break down under the physical changes taking place, causing later problems with the operation of the plant. A routine maintenance regime should be adopted that will include the inspection and renewal of all critical components that are subject to possible deterioration.

Part of the routine maintenance of the plant will include calibration of critical measuring equipment. It is essential that all temperature sensors and recording instruments are regularly calibrated against a traceable standard.

Steam Quality

The quality of steam used in the sterilisation process should be carefully considered. For many years, the only readily available quality of steam was plant steam, which was normally used for heating and the generation of hot water. Occasionally, filtration of this steam was attempted to render it suitable for pharmaceutical use. The degree of filtration was not necessarily effective, and boiler treatment chemicals could be "carried over" into the plant. The inside of the chamber could thus become contaminated with chemical particulates that could affect the product or plant. It is now normal practice to use clean steam, which usually meets the standard expected of WFI. The steam should also contain only very low levels of noncondensable gases, and must be regularly tested for their presence. As it is important to remove these gases to sterilise the plant, it is undesirable to introduce them with the steam. There are standards for acceptable levels of noncondensable gases and also the dryness fraction of the steam.

If quality is important then there must also be sufficient quantity. If there is an insufficient volume flow of steam, the sterilisation temperature may not be reached or the cycle time may be extended. The steam generation plant and the connecting pipework must be able to cope with the maximum demand of the plant. Attention must also be paid to the materials of construction of the connecting pipework and generation plant; as with the freeze dryer itself, high grade stainless steel should be used. Any gasket or sealing materials should also be made of an acceptable material.

7

LEAK RATE TESTING

Kevin Kinnarney

Bio Products Laboratory
Herts, United Kingdom

Freeze dryers are pieces of equipment that are designed to operate under negative pressure during normal product processing. Pressures that are encountered in the freeze drying process may be in the region between 1 and 0.001 mbar. With atmospheric pressure acting on the outside of the plant, any leaks into the freeze dryer during this time will cause control of the cycle to be compromised. It is impossible to make this type of equipment completely leaktight; therefore, the problem of air leakage into the freeze dryer must be accepted as a process hazard. The degree of leakage will have consequences on the contents of the plant; therefore, the leak rate should be measured, with any likely effect on the final product being assessed.

When new equipment is purchased, a leak rate is usually specified by the manufacturer in conjunction with the customer. In the past, it has not been made clear what areas of the equipment are covered by this leak rate, as some manufacturers have not included all component parts in any specification and have only tested the actual freeze drying chamber. If a high leak rate is found after completion of manufacture, then it is possible for a larger vacuum pumping set to be added to the plant. This approach only addresses the need to keep the chamber at a certain pressure level and ignores any other consequences. The constant movement of air through the leak site to the pumping set may give a vapour "sweeping" effect over the product. This may mean that a different drying regime has taken place over the vials under this vapour path, and the product could show a wider variation in final moisture content, from vial to vial, than expected. The theory of the effect this phenomenon may have on the product may differ from practice and, as a consequence, no real problem may be apparent, as all tested qualities may be within the final product specification.

High leak rates can, therefore, affect the operation of the equipment. High, in this instance, may only be leaks that are perfectly acceptable on other pieces of equipment. Leaks may not only affect the physical operation of the plant, but may also affect the final dryness of the product.

What is of greater concern is the quality and quantity of air being drawn into the freeze dryer and the challenge this creates the product. If leaks occur from the relative dirty air outside the plant to the clean chamber during processing, there is the possibility of product contamination taking place. Most freeze dryers are positioned with the door and surround in the clean room and the remainder in the plant area, including the chamber, condenser, associated pipework, and equipment. It is not normal practice to control the environment of the plant room very strictly, as dust and oil vapours may be generated by the operation of the equipment. There may be air conditioning units and filtration systems but the object is not aimed at providing a clean room. The freeze dryer itself will produce contamination in the plant room from the action of the vacuum pumping system and other components. As only a small portion of the freeze dryer is inside a clean area, we must accept that nearly all contamination entering the internal environment will be from the plant room.

Assuming normal plant room conditions, there will be airborne contamination with the potential hazard of entering the product inside the chamber. This hazard may be in the form of colony forming units that are drawn through the leak site into the freeze drying chamber. It may be possible to reduce this potential by upgrading the status of the plant room to minimise the contamination possibility.

SOURCES OF LEAKS

A standard steam sterilisable freeze dryer is a relatively complicated piece of equipment. It must perform the task of self-sterilisation under pressure and then must freeze dry products under negative pressure at low temperatures. Every piece of equipment added to assist the plant in meeting these criteria adds a potential leak site. Some of the likely areas of leakage are given below.

- The main chamber and condenser will normally be constructed of high grade stainless steel, which have many welds along their seams. There will also be a number of connection stubs penetrating the walls of the main part of the plant. These flanged stubs allow the connection of measuring equipment and items such as safety valves. All of these welds must conform to any associated safety rules, be leaktight, and meet GMP standards.

- Items attached to these flanges or stubs must also be as leaktight as possible over the temperature and pressure range encountered during use. The connecting gasket or seal between the two items must be designed to minimise any possible leakage.

- Lead-throughs for refrigeration pipes or diathermic fluid manifolds should also be welded, if possible. Other types of lead-throughs (e.g., for temperature measuring probes) should also be considered as a possible leak site.

- Door seals are also susceptible to leakage, especially after they have been in use for some time. During use, they may become damaged by broken glass from vials or by a buildup of debris from the unloading/loading operation. Design of the seal and support groove must be considered as it may distort during use and allow leakage across the sealing face.

- Valves should meet all current GMP standards and are usually manufactured from the same grade material as the freeze dryer chamber. Valve seals may deteriorate with time, especially as they are subject to a range of temperatures and pressures, allowing leakage to occur across the sealing face. Drain valves, in particular, may become damaged by debris from the freeze drying cycle being washed down onto the seal during defrosting or sterilising.

- There are also sources of leaks that are not directly from outside to inside the plant. Leaks may occur from internal components, such as product shelves and will offer the possibility of product contamination. Hydraulic stoppering systems attached to the chamber or condenser refrigeration coils are also areas of concern, as they could leak hydraulic oil or refrigerant.

PLANT SPECIFICATION

When a new freeze dryer is purchased, part of the specification should cover the acceptable leak rate of the equipment. This leak rate should encompass all parts of the freeze dryer that the product may be exposed to during the processing cycle. This rate is obtained by testing the clean, dry plant following completion of construction. Leak rates have been improving along with production methods, and users have been calling for improved performance, with GMP guidelines ensuring that users look critically at this area. A generally accepted leak rate would be in the region of 2×10^{-2} mbar litres/second. Some manufacturers may offer leak rates below this figure, and a relatively simple plant should be significantly better. With the size of leak rate mentioned, this still presents a significant challenge to the contained product. This size of leak represents a significant volume of air being drawn into the plant during the process period when under vacuum. If the quality of the air being drawn into the plant is known, then the potential hazard to the product may be estimated, minimising this leak rate will reduce any potential contamination. Once the leak rate has been specified, there should be no significant change for the worse during the life of the plant.

LEAK TYPES

There are two types of leaks that may affect the freeze dryer. The first type, which was mentioned earlier, is the real leakage from outside the plant to the inner chamber. It must be emphasised that this type of leak presents a real hazard to the control system and to the integrity of the plant. This type of leak is called a "real" leak.

The second type of leak that can be observed may not be a "real" leak. The pressure rise that may be observed by the pressure measuring equipment is an increase caused by outgassing of materials within the freeze dryer. When pressure rise measurements are being made, it is essential that they are made in a clean, dry, freeze dryer. Moisture remaining from cleaning, or other cleaning solvent residues, will exert a vapour pressure, especially under vacuum, that causes large pressure rises in the plant. This could then be mistaken for a leak.

The use of poorly suited materials for seals that could outgas under vacuum will also show pressure rise in the chamber when tested. Similarly, seal and seal housing design should prevent trapped volumes of air from being gradually drawn back into the system, causing false test results. All of these problems that can spoil the pressure test readings, but are not "real" leaks, are collectively grouped together under the title "virtual" leaks.

"Real" leaks and "virtual" leaks show different features when under pressure rise tests. "Real" leaks will show a linear pressure rise during testing when the differential pressure between the chamber and the outside remains roughly constant. If a graph is plotted of pressure rise against time, the pressure rise should be linear.

"Virtual" leaks usually show a rapid pressure rise that quickly tails off and stabilises. As the contaminant in the system vaporises, this will be observed as a rapid pressure rise, when it has vaporised, the pressure rise will cease. These types of leaks may not offer the same risk of contamination from air containing bacteria being drawn into the system, but there is still a risk of contamination from the unwanted vapours.

There is the possibility that both types of leaks may be present at the same time in a system. Leak rates should only be calculated for "real" leaks, any possible contamination causing "virtual" leaks should have been removed. The simplest test to use is the "leak-up rate" test.

TESTING THE "LEAK–UP RATE"

It is necessary to test the freeze dryer from time to time to ascertain whether the leak rate has changed. This testing may be carried out according to the following eight steps. It is important that all parts of the freeze dryer open to the product are included in the test, as far as possible.

1. The freeze dryer should be clean and empty. All previous product should have been completely removed, and the condenser defrosted and thoroughly drained.

2. The condenser cooling should be switched on and allowed to cool to a relatively low temperature. When the condenser is cold, then the vacuum pumping system may be started.

3. Evacuation of the system should continue until stabilisation has been achieved. This may be overnight so as to ensure the system has been pumped clear of contaminants, such as water vapour from condenser defrosting. The temperature reached by the condenser will have a bearing on how low a pressure can be achieved in the chamber.

4. It may assist in any outgassing from seals and so on to heat the product shelves, however in all cases, product shelves should be kept at a relatively uniform temperature.

5. When a stable pressure has been achieved, the test can begin. This pressure could be the ultimate achievable or some

predetermined level, but should be low enough to make the rise relatively easy to measure.

6. The vacuum system is isolated from the freeze dryer by the pumping line valve and may, if desired, be switched off. The condenser cooling and the shelf thermoregulation systems must be left running.

7. The system pressure is now measured using the plant pressure sensors that should be calibrated against an acceptable, traceable source. The system is left in this state for a set time period. This may be several hours when initial testing of the equipment is carried out, but may be shortened with experience.

8. During the test period, readings should be taken at regular intervals and/or captured on a chart recorder or data logger. When the test period has elapsed, the readings may be plotted on a graph of pressure rise against time.

If the resultant graph shows a linear rise of pressure against time, then a "real" leak is present (see Figure 7.1). If the rise shows a rapid increase in pressure and then a levelling out, there is a "virtual" leak present (see Figure 7.2). Usually, with a "virtual" leak, a combination

Figure 7.1. "Real" leaks.

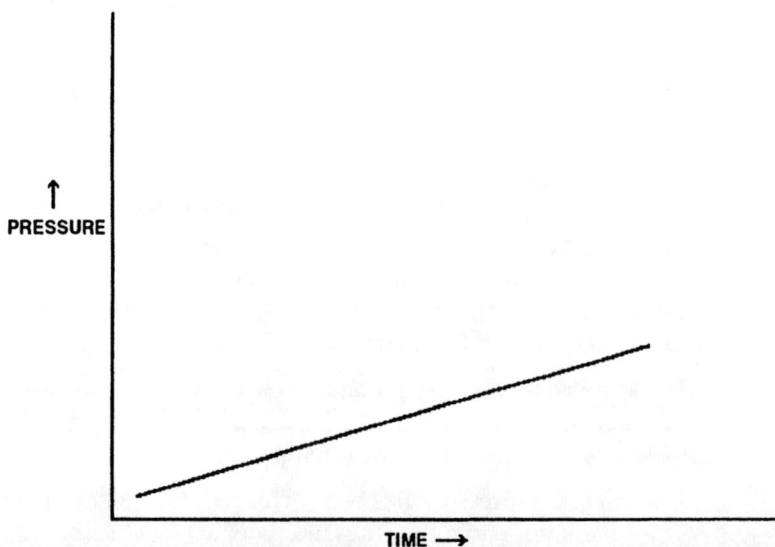

Figure 7.2. "Virtual" leaks.

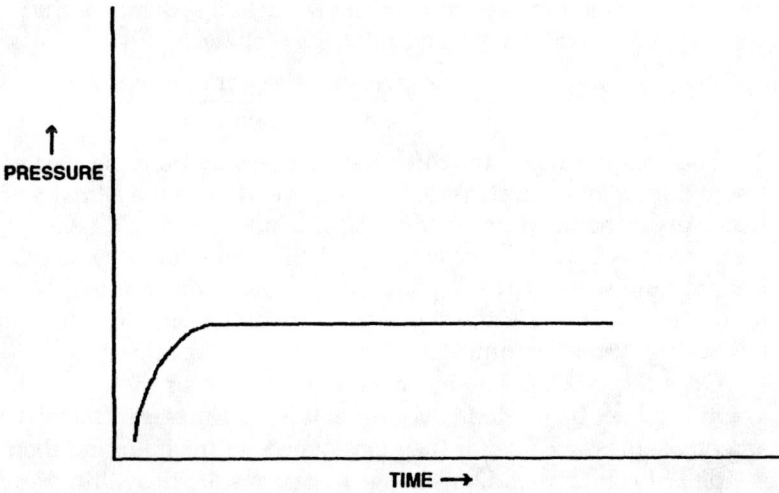

of the two above will be seen, as it is almost impossible to have a plant completely free of "real" leaks (see Figure 7.3).

If "virtual" leaks are present, these must be eliminated before a proper leak test can be completed. This may be achieved by pumping

Figure 7.3. "Real" and "Virtual" leaks.

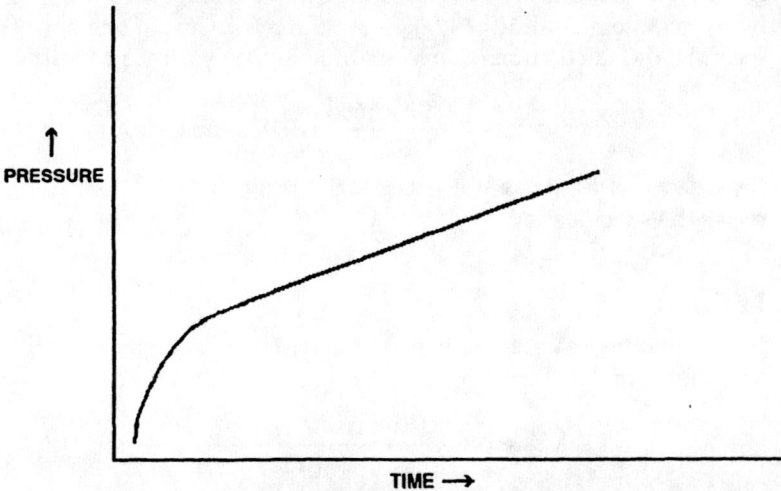

the system for a longer period or rechecking the chamber for contamination. It is only the straight line portion of the graph that will provide the information needed to assess the actual leak rate of the plant.

The leak-up rate may be calculated as follows:

$$\text{Leak-up rate} = \frac{\text{pressure rise per unit time}}{\text{vessel volume}}$$

The pressure rise is the difference in pressure from the start of the test to the end of the test. Vessel volume should include all parts of the freeze dryer included in the test, and this volume should be available from the manufacturer. The leak-up rate is related to the system under test only and will vary from plant to plant based on volume. The leak-up rate will decrease as the vessel size increases, therefore, an accurate measuring system becomes more crucial to successful testing.

Once the leak-up rate has been determined for the plant, then a graph need not be plotted every time. It is far simpler to calculate the acceptable pressure rise for the plant over, say, one hour and then test the plant for this period, ensuring the test results fit within these set limits.

The figures supplied by the manufacturer may be used to set the initial level acceptable for this test. From the acceptable leak rate for the plant, and knowing both the volume and test time, a calculation of the leak-up rate is possible. Routine leak testing during production operations are rendered simple when the pressure rise per hour for the vessel is known.

$$\text{Pressure rise in system} = \frac{\text{leak rate} \times \text{time}}{\text{volume}}$$

A common acceptable leak rate is 0.02 mbar litres/second. Using this figure, a system volume of 1,000 litres and a test time of one hour (3600 seconds) the calculation of pressure rise in the system is as follows:

$$\text{Pressure rise} = \frac{0.02 \times 3600}{1000} = 0.072 \text{ mbar/hour}$$

Provided this figure is not exceeded during the test, then the plant meets the specification.

Leak Rate

If required the leak rate may also be calculated. This can then be used to compare the performance to the original specification.

$$\text{Leak rate} = \frac{\text{pressure rise} \times \text{system volume}}{\text{time}}$$

Using the figure from the previous calculation,

$$\text{Leak rate} = \frac{0.072 \times 1000}{3600} = 0.02 \text{ mbar litres/second}$$

ROUTINE OPERATION AND TESTING

The nature of freeze dryers is such that a fairly large amount of particulate matter is generated. There is also the possibility of contamination from broken containers used to contain the product undergoing processing. These materials may find their way into valves, causing sealing on closure to be affected. The sterilisation process, when carried out using steam, causes expansion and contraction of the materials of construction, which may cause leaks to appear. The material used for the valve seats and sealing may also break down when subject to the range of temperatures and pressures seen during freeze dryer utilisation. Planned, preventive maintenance is recommended to reduce downtime likely to be caused by the above reasons. Poor maintenance is the cause of many leak problems.

Following any maintenance work or any dismantling of the plant, for whatever reason, a leak test ought to be carried out to ensure satisfactory repair. Sterilisation and recooling are the times when leaks are most likely to appear. It is recommended that a leak rate test be performed following this phase, before the plant is used for drying a batch. Leak rate testing is only meaningful if the instruments used are satisfactory for the purpose and calibrated against a traceable source.

LEAK DETECTION

If a leak is found on testing, the next problem is to identify the area and repair it. There are many traditional leak detecting methods that owe a lot to art rather than science, but are, nonetheless, fairly effective. This includes operator experience as to where the leak is likely to be. Substitution of components and isolation of areas of the plant will eventually result in the leak being identified, but this is extremely time-consuming to carry out. Using the main valve, the chamber may be isolated from the condenser and tested separately. Blanking pieces may be attached to component ports to eliminate these from the test.

Solvents, such as acetone or alcohols, have also been used to locate leak sites. With the plant system under vacuum, the solvent is sprayed carefully around any suspected leak and the pressure measuring system observed. As the solvent vapour should diffuse more quickly through any leak site, the pressure inside the system will also increase at a higher rate, indicating the presence of a leak. This method of leak detection requires care when handling solvents and some patience during searching. Time must be allowed for the vapour to clear from around the plant when moving from one test point to another, as the solvent vapour will rapidly diffuse to other areas.

Modern methods rely on specially made leak detectors. There are many different types on the market that are acceptable for leak detection on all manner of equipment, including freeze dryers. These detectors are attached to the plant, and a vacuum is drawn on the system for normal leak testing. The leak detector, a form of mass spectrometer, is already set to indicate the presence of the search gas. The search gas, which in most cases is helium, is gently sprayed around the area under suspicion. Indication of the appearance of the gas at the detector shows that the search gas has entered the system. If the plant in general is to be tested, it is usual to start at the top and gradually work down the plant. This is to ensure that the helium, which is lighter than air, can disperse away over areas that have already been tested and not give a false leak indication. Using helium leak detection equipment, a complete freeze dryer may be tested, repaired, and retested in a relatively short time.

CONCLUSIONS

The acceptable leak rate for a freeze dryer, at present, will not guarantee that contamination cannot be drawn into the plant through these leak sites. To ensure contamination-free operation, leak rates must be reduced substantially. The balance between the ideal and the practical must be accepted, but that does not mean that no standard should be applied. Reducing leak rates to a manageable level will reduce the potential exposure to contaminants being drawn into the plant from external surroundings. Even with these low levels of leaks, the amount of air drawn into the system is approximately 1 litre every 14 hours, resulting in over 5 litres of potentially contaminated air entering the system during a 3 day freeze drying cycle. Consideration should be given to minimise potential leak sites when purchasing new plant. The quality of the conditions in which the plant is installed and maintained must also taken into account.

Although the leak rate acceptable does not stop potential contamination, it is unlikely that all of the leak is at one site alone, the leak rate is a combination of many smaller leaks, all of which could be too small to allow the entry of bacteria. It should be assumed that the worst case could exist and that contamination is entering the plant, thereby exposing the product to risk. The sweeping action of vapour during freeze drying may well entrain anything entering the plant and trap it on the condenser coils. There does not appear to be a universal outbreak of product contamination from leaks such as those described; therefore, the possibility of product compromise remains very low.

As the leak rate into the plant is fairly fixed by the acceptable standards achievable the only variable is exposure time. It is recommended that freeze drying cycles should not be longer than necessary, thus reducing the risk even further.

8

INLET FILTER INTEGRITY TESTING

Peter Cameron

Tanvec Limited
Elstead, Surrey, United Kingdom

This chapter deals with the integrity testing of the freeze dryer inlet filter and examines the advantages and disadvantages of the various options. Although the methods are outlined, the exact details of each test will depend on individual installations, therefore, consultation with filter manufacturers is considered desirable.

At the end of the freeze drying cycle, it is necessary to break the vacuum within the chamber by the introduction of a gas, either completely or, more often in the case of part-stoppered vials, partially. On many of today's freeze dryers, the injection of gas is also carried out to adjust the level of vacuum within the chamber. This is usually an inert gas, such as nitrogen, and considering the exposed nature of the product at this point, the introduction of this gas must not adversely affect the quality of the dried product. It is, therefore, imperative in sterile processing that the gas be free of microbiological and particulate contamination as well as chemical. This is achieved in the modern freeze drying plant by the installation of a sterilising grade filter immediately before the chamber, in addition to supplying chemically pure gas with a low bioburden.

Due to the critical nature of this filter, it is important that its sterilising efficiency is routinely assured for each cycle of the dryer. This is achieved by the validation work carried out by the filter manufacturer and the routine integrity testing of individual filter elements, as well as by ensuring that the correct filter has been specified and installed correctly.

Up until the mid 1980s, regulatory concerns regarding freeze dryers were centred around sterilisation and stoppering methods. Steam sterilisable plants were only just breaking into the market, and there were many older freeze dryers in use in critical areas where bladder-operated stoppering mechanisms were still employed. Since that time attention has been turning on the use of the inlet filter and, in particular, the testing of its integrity. Most users of freeze dryers did not routinely test their filters, and the few that did invariably removed the filter from its installation in order to carry out the test. However, reacting to market needs, filter manufacturers developed in-line testing systems meeting, where possible, the requirements and restrictions of freeze drying systems. There has, therefore, been a lot of activity in recent years, resulting in more and more production departments integrity testing their freeze dryer inlet filters in situ.

FILTER TYPES

Any sterilising grade filter that has been shown to meet the requirements of regulatory bodies can be used as the inlet protection for the exposed product. However, in modern steam sterilisable plants a hydrophobic, polyvinylidene fluoride (PVDF), or polytetrafluoroethene (PTFE) filter membrane is normally employed. The membrane, typically rated at 0.2 μm nominal pore size, is usually manufactured as a pleated cylinder encased in a polypropylene support mesh and sealed with solid end caps.

The assurance that the filter is fit for use starts with the work carried out by the filter manufacturer in validating the design and production of the filter. The comprehensive studies would include biosafety tests (analysis of eluates, cytotoxicity, pyrogens, etc.), stability and performance tests, as well as retention tests (bacterial challenge testing, particle counting and throughput determinations). It is important that the relevant documentation, available from the filter manufacturer is included in the freeze dryer's validation protocol.

The individual filter cartridges to be utilised in the freeze dryer should also have certificates of conformity relating to them. These will cover some of the areas examined in the filter's validation protocol that are carried out on every batch of filters manufactured, such as toxicity, extractables, bacterial retention, pyrogens and some aspects of performance. Also on the certificate should be the assurance that the individual filter cartridge was successfully integrity tested prior to packaging.

Being hydrophobic, these cartridges can only function efficiently if the membranes are dry; even very small amounts of moisture can dramatically reduce the flow through the filter. So it is imperative that all gases to be filtered are sensibly dry and that after steam sterilisation all residual water is removed from the filter and associated pipework.

FILTER INSTALLATION

The filter cartridge is housed in a stainless steel housing, designed to withstand the pressures encountered during a typical steam sterilising cycle. The housing is located between the freeze drying chamber and the air inlet steam and gas supplies. Some plants, particularly more modern dryers, have valved pipework around the housing to act as a steam bypass during the build up of pressure during the initial stages of sterilisation.

Most filter cartridges are not rated by the filter manufacturer to withstand high pressure differentials at the elevated temperatures associated with these first stages of sterilisation. Therefore, it is important that the sterilisation process be carried out in such a way that the filter element does not encounter a pressure drop in excess of that quoted by the filter manufacturer for high temperatures. This is to minimise the stress experienced by the membrane, reducing the risk of integrity failure or filter collapse.

In order to carry out in situ integrity testing, the pipework layout must be specified when purchasing a new plant or modified in existing dryers to accommodate the testing. It is recommended that all pipework be of welded construction, although the joints on either side of the filter housing are usually kept as sanitary connections to enable the housing to be removed. The pipework should be designed to assist in the draining of test liquids used in the integrity testing and of the condensate formed during the sterilisation process.

The inlet filter is often located on the top of the freeze dryer chamber, subsequently creating logistical problems for the manual operation of valves or the connection of equipment associated with integrity testing. This can be overcome by moving the filter housing and associated pipework to a more easily accessible location or by installing an automated system for integrity testing.

If pipework that is sterilised forms part of the modifications, then consideration must be given to revalidating the sterilisation cycle. This is particularly the case if any dead legs have been introduced to the system that would present an increased challenge to sterilisation.

TESTING FREQUENCY

It is the expectation of the regulatory authorities that all critical filters be integrity tested. They do not, however, stipulate how often testing should be carried out, leaving the decision on testing frequency to the manufacturing operation. The risks involved are, of course, obvious: If a filter fails an integrity test, then all batches of product processed since the last successful test must be suspect and risk rejection. It follows that due to the high value of most freeze-dried products the tendency is for integrity testing of the filters to be carried out at least once during the sequence of sterilisation, leak rate testing and freeze drying.

As the most stressful conditions that the filter element experiences is during steam sterilisation, it is often the desire of production departments that the integrity of the filter be assured before risking the drying of a particularly high value batch, as well as immediately afterward. This approach not only requires that the filter be tested in-line, but that the integrity of the pipework and equipment downstream of the filter not be compromised. Although methods now exist to satisfy this demand, it does require a more stringent evaluation of the process and more attention given to the practical aspects of actually carrying out the test.

As has been mentioned, there are no official guidelines for the frequency of testing, but it is not difficult to imagine that within the foreseeable future testing at least once per cycle will become the expected norm.

TEST EVALUATION

To be able to decide which integrity test to adopt, it is important to evaluate the requirements and constraints that will be put on the system. These criteria must be discussed with the filter manufacturer, together with the specification of the filter to be adopted. It is important to realise that not all tests are appropriate for all filter types. In the light of current trends toward in situ testing after steam sterilisation, this chapter will discuss the available tests with this in mind, although the points made can be easily adapted to presterilisation or off-line testing.

For a test to be suitable, it should meet the following criteria.

Reproducible

It is obviously an important element of any test of this nature that it will reliably give the same results each time the same test conditions are employed. Any differences in results should be accounted for by errors inherent in the system.

Validation

The test must have been shown to be capable of distinguishing between an integral and nonintegral filter. The tests covered here have all been the subject of such validation studies by filter manufacturers. The basis of this work is a correlation between a bacterial challenge test (virus and phage challenge studies are sometimes carried out) and the test itself. Differing criteria are used by the different companies, but all use as a minimum the limits stipulated by the United States Food and Drug Administration (FDA) based on the Health Industries Manufacturer's Association (HIMA) challenge test. This defines a sterilising grade filter as one that gives a sterile filtrate when challenged with 1×10^7 *Pseudomonas diminuta* (grown under specified conditions) per square centimetre of filter membrane. The term *integral* when applied to a filter in this text is meant to mean one whose sterilising efficiency meets this criteria.

The studies usually determine the integrity test values of a number of filters, covering a wide range of results. The filters are then challenged with a bacterial suspension and the filtrate monitored. The results are then analysed to determine the correlation and the particular value that signifies the lower limit for meeting the sterilisation criteria set. Although many filters are tested, it is often the case that scientists have great difficulty in obtaining filters whose integrity test values are close to the limit between integral and nonintegral filters.

Safe and Practical Limits

The limits set for a particular filter type when carrying out a specified test must have a sufficient safety margin with respect to the data derived from challenge testing, to ensure that any filter with a value above the limit is integral. It is also important that the limit is not so conservatively set that a significant proportion of integral filters fail.

Regulatory Approval

The test must be acceptable to the regulatory authorities. It is rarely the case that any of the regulating bodies would specify or recommend a test or even give written approval of a test, but it is obviously important to pharmaceutical producers that their chosen method of assuring a filter's sterilising efficiency is accepted by regulatory inspectors. This can only really be achieved by producing comprehensive validation protocols and documentation to support the route taken. Of course, it is always comforting to know that similar methods are being used by companies with regulatory approval.

Nondestructive or Contaminating

The test must not adversely affect the filter or the associated pipework. Rendering areas of the filter hydrophilic will reduce the filtering efficiency of the filter, and contaminating the element or pipework will put the product at risk.

Dryness

The filter should be dry after the completion of the test. With any vent or vacuum break filters, especially freeze dryer inlet filters, it is important that they are sensibly dry before use. The level of dryness required is very difficult with which to be precise, but it is important to prevent not only the reduction of gas flow through the membrane but also the risk of water freezing within the element (when the filter is exposed to a high vacuum at the beginning of air replacement) and distorting the pore structure. During the vacuum break the gas entering the chamber is also likely to carry any excess water from the filter to the dried, exposed product.

Safety

Any safety issues must be addressed and controlled with regard to safe working practices.

Practicality

When adding another step to the already long process of freeze drying, especially one that does not directly add value to a product, it is important that it can be carried out quickly, efficiently and easily. As has been mentioned, certain modifications can be done to facilitate tests operation. Included in this would be automation of valve sequencing coupled with the use of an automatic integrity tester. However, this approach requires considerable investment of resources at the beginning of the project, not only of money but also in terms of design and validation.

In Situ Testing

Although many firms do still test their filters off-line, there is still the risk of leaks being created on reinstallation. This is especially true at the connections where seals are likely to be a weak point on pipework that is regularly steam sterilised.

Poststerilisation

To assure the filter's integrity following the stresses experienced during steam sterilisation before committing a batch of product, any manipulations downstream of the filter must be very critically assessed and controlled. It is imperative that the integrity of the freeze dryer is not compromised between sterilisation and the completion of freeze drying.

AVAILABLE TESTS

The tests that are discussed in this chapter are not necessarily supported by all filter manufacturers. A large amount of work has been carried out recently by filter manufacturers, leading to an acceptance of a broader range of tests. Certainly, the leading suppliers will look at individual applications closely and take into consideration customers' testing requirements.

Two of the tests—the diffusive flow and bubble point tests—are well established and are based on the testing of hydrophilic filters requiring the wetting out of the element prior to testing. The remaining two—the water-based integrity test and the aerosol challenge test—are both more recent in terms of being refined for practical use.

The Diffusive Flow Test

Integrity testing of hydrophobic filters by diffusive flow is carried out in a similar way to the testing of hydrophilic product filters, except that the element is wetted out with a standard test solution as opposed to the product. It is always advisable to consult with the filter's manufacturer for advice on procedural details, particularly suggested test fluids, and diffusive flow test parameters and limits. The test solutions are typically 60 or 70 percent isopropyl alcohol or 75 percent tertiary butyl alcohol. The test parameters include the temperature at which the test is to be carried out, which must, as in all integrity tests, remain stable during the measuring phases; stabilisation and test times—with modern automatic integrity testers these times are often optimised during testing; and test pressure.

Manufacturers will be able to provide the maximum diffusion value that, under the conditions of the test, will assure the integrity of the filter as related to their validation work with bacterial challenge testing. This limit will be dependant on the test gas used, often nitrogen or compressed air, which must be specified.

A common version of the diffusion test is the pressure decay test, which relies on monitoring pressure changes upstream of the filter and converts these changes to gas flow. In order to carry out this conversion, it is necessary to know the upstream volume of the filter test system. This can often be measured by the automatic integrity tester.

Method for In Situ Testing, Poststerilisation (Figure 8.1)

1. Autoclave the test solution receiving vessel setup.

2. Aseptically connect the vessel to the pipework downstream of the filter.

3. Steam sterilise the freeze dryer and filter.

4. After cooling, connect the test solution supply vessel to the pipework upstream of the filter.

5. Flush the filter with test solution, ensuring that it is bled of air.

6. After all the solution has passed through the filter, connect the integrity tester to the upstream side and commence testing.

7. The upstream side of the filter is pressurised with the test gas up to the test pressure and then the stabilisation time

Figure 8.1. Layout for diffusive flow and bubble point test.

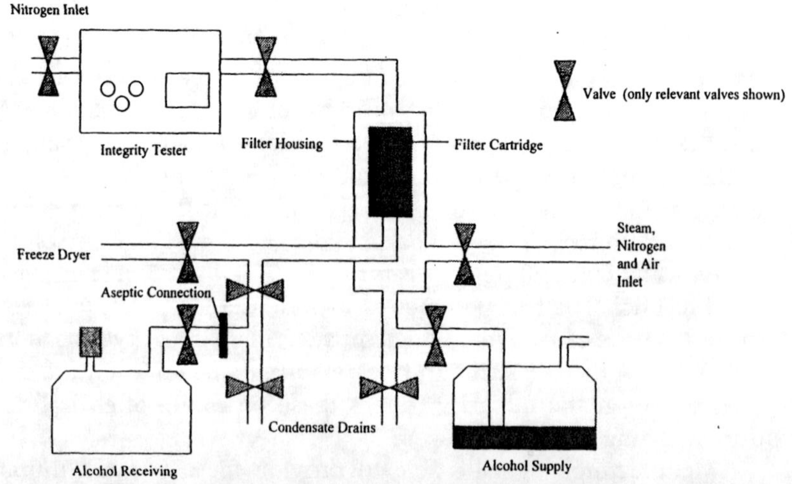

commences, with the pressure maintained at the test value. This allows for the compression of the element under pressure. Any gross pressure drops during this time will indicate a failure, and the test will normally be aborted if an automatic integrity tester is used.

8. After the stabilisation time has elapsed, the test time starts and the rate of diffusive flow is measured over the specified time. This can be either indirectly by measuring the drop in pressure and calculating the flow related to the measured upstream volume, or by directly measuring the amount of gas flow (by the use of sensitive flowmeters) at the maintained test pressure.

9. After venting the system, the filter and pipework must be fully purged of test solution and thoroughly dried. This is usually carried out by flushing nitrogen or compressed air across the filter. The regime often cited by filter manufacturers is to flush the filter with gas for 10–20 minutes. This may be adequate for other, less critical, vent filters, but this has not been found to leave the membrane dry enough for freeze drying purposes. A drying time of 2 hours has been found to be more appropriate in this case. This extra time may become excessive for some operations on tight turnaround times, but the drying efficiency can be enhanced by other means. Allowing the gas to pass over the filter as well as through it helps to dry the membrane, however, to really reduce drying times, the application of heat either in the form of heated gas or by directly heating the filter housing has been found to be effective.

There are slight variations to the above method and it is important to look at each installation separately, taking into account the filter manufacturer's recommendations.

Comparison With Desirable Criteria

- **Reproducible** The test has a long history in the industry and this, together with studies carried out by both filter manufacturers and pharmaceutical companies, has shown the test to produce results that are consistent and reliable.

- **Validation** The test has been part of the validation programmes of most major manufacturers for their filter membranes. These studies will have included correlation with the bacterial challenge test, producing limits and test parameters for the filters.

- **Safe and practical limits** Validation work has produced limits that ensure that only filters with sterilising efficiencies well above that of the HIMA standard will pass the test. The quality of filter manufacturing processes produces membranes with efficiencies well above that represented by the limit, ensuring very few filters are caught in the border zone.

- **Regulatory approval** The test has been used widely for many years by pharmaceutical companies across the world and has been shown to be acceptable to regulating authorities.

- **Nondestructive or contaminating** As long as the test fluid is completely removed from the filter and pipework, and the membrane is dried sufficiently, then the filter system is not adversely affected by the test.

- **Dryness** As has already been discussed, the drying phase of the test must be extended or enhanced in order to produce a sufficiently dried filter.

- **Safety** Apart from normal safety precautions associated with using instrumentation and pressurised gas lines, the only extra measures required are those for handling flammable liquids.

- **Practicality** The time needed to carry out the test is significant and may well encroach on valuable processing time, though this can be kept to a minimum by careful design and planning. The test does require the operation of several valves in a specified sequence and would benefit greatly from automation.

- **In situ testing** The test can be carried out in situ but it does require a valved inlet upstream of the filter and a valved outlet downstream. Therefore, unless the test was accounted for in the original specification of the dryer, then the pipework would require modification.

- **Poststerilisation** The test can be carried out after the plant and the filter have been sterilised, but does require the sterilisation of the collection vessel and its aseptic connection downstream of the filter. Therefore, very tight controls must be put in place to ensure that the integrity of the freeze dryer is not affected, particularly that the aseptic connection is likely to be made in what is commonly an engineering plant room.

Bubble Point Test

The bubble point test, like the diffusive flow test, has been used for testing the integrity of filters for many years. Again, it is based on a membrane that has been wetted out in order to carry out the test. Rather than measure the rate at which gas diffuses through the test fluid held within the pores, it measures the pressure at which the liquid is forced out of the pores, usually termed the bubble point. Filter manufacturers must be consulted regarding the test conditions, appropriate test fluids, exact methodology and, of course, the minimum bubble point applicable to the specified filter.

Method for In Situ Testing, Poststerilisation (Figure 8.1)

1. The filter is flushed through with test fluid as in steps 1–6 of the diffusive flow test method.

2. The test proceeds by slowly increasing the pressure to a predetermined point, well below the minimum bubble point. This pressure is then held for a time to allow the cartridge and conditions to stabilise.

3. The pressure is then slowly increased in small incremental steps and held for the drop in pressure to be measured. The pressure at which there is a large increase in the rate of pressure decay is the bubble point.

4. The test fluid must be completely flushed from the filter and pipework and the whole system dried as in step 9 of the diffusive flow test method.

Comparison With Desirable Criteria

The comments under this section of the diffusive flow test also relate to the bubble point test.

Water-Based Integrity Test

The water-based integrity test was developed several years ago, but has only recently been promoted as a practical, viable test with validated data available for the testing of hydrophobic filters. It was developed to address the problems associated with the alcohol diffusive flow test of downstream manipulations, the need to hydrophilise the filter in order to test it and the use of alcohol in sensitive systems (notably freeze dryers).

Although not all major filter manufacturers support the test in terms of recommending it to assure sterilising efficiency, there is considerable interest in the test and studies are being continued with a view to accepting the test for a wider range of applications.

Method for In Situ Testing, Poststerilisation (Figure 8.2)

1. After steam sterilisation of the freeze dryer and the filter, the upstream side of the filter housing is filled with water to cover the filter element completely.

2. The integrity tester is then connected to the top of the housing. There must be a certain volume of gas between the water and the tester to optimise the sensitivity of the measurements. This is often provided by a standard volume reservoir, as it is imperative that during the test the water level does not drop below the top of the filter cartridge.

3. A constant pressure, below that of the water breakthrough point, is then applied to the system. After a stabilisation time, the rate of water flow is measured. This is usually measured either by pressure decay over time or by gas flow; in either case, it is necessary to convert the readings to water flow.

Although there was some controversy over the mechanism of the water flow observed (bearing in mind that the filter membrane is hydrophobic and impermeable to water at the pressures applied in the test and does not, therefore, become wetted out during the test), it is generally accepted that at pressures below the water breakthrough point, water vapour will "diffuse" through the membrane's pores and condense on

Figure 8.2. Layout for water-based integrity test.

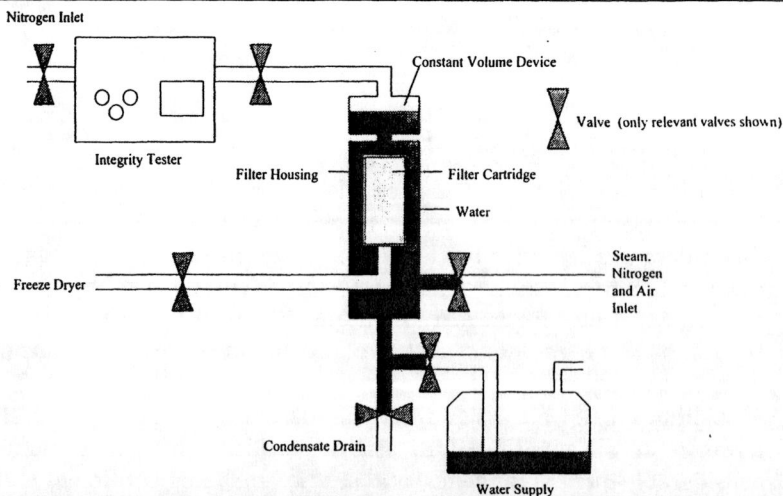

the downstream side. The rate of vapour flow will, therefore, be related to the porosity of the membrane.

4. . After the completion of the test, the pressure is released and any water that may have intruded into the membrane is forced back onto the upstream side. The water is then drained from the housing and associated pipework.

5. Although the membrane is free of water, there will be significant quantities held in the support meshes and structures of the cartridge, as well as numerous droplets within the housing and pipework. It is, therefore, necessary to carry out a drying phase. For freeze drying systems, this must be extended beyond the minimal drying recommended for general vent filters, as with the diffusive flow test.

Comparison With Desirable Criteria

- **Reproducible** Although an early study questioned the reproducibility of the water-based integrity test, all other studies carried out by both filter manufacturers and pharmaceutical companies have shown a consistency that matches other tests. There are indications that the test is more sensitive to temperature changes during testing, and this condition may require tighter controls than in the other integrity tests.

- **Validation** Correlation to bacterial challenge tests have been carried out for some of the commonly used filters and, at the time of writing, testing of an increased range is being undertaken. There is an almost universal approach now amongst the major filter manufacturers to correlate the water-based integrity test against the bacterial challenge test for all new hydrophobic filter cartridges.

- **Safe and practical limits** For filters that have data available from validation studies, the limits appear to have a reasonable safety margin to ensure integrity whilst not being too extreme to fail most integral filters.

- **Regulatory approval** The test is being used in the United States and by some companies in Europe that have had regulatory inspections. It would therefore, appear that the regulatory authorities have no great concerns over the test.

- **Nondestructive or contaminating** The test has no adverse affect on the filter system, save for the need to remove the excess residual water by drying.

- **Dryness** As has been mentioned, this test, like the diffusive flow and bubble point tests, requires an enhanced drying phase.

- **Safety** Safety issues are less pronounced than with other tests because no flammable liquid is used.

- **Practicality** The test does present a significant time penalty, but this can be minimised by enhancing the drying phase. There are less valves to operate than in the bubble point and diffusive flow tests, but there would still be value in automating the test procedure.

- **In situ testing** The test lends itself well to in situ testing and only requires a valved inlet upstream of the filter.

- **Poststerilisation** There is little risk of compromising the integrity of the freeze dryer after sterilisation, as the only manipulations required are upstream of the filter. Thus it is therefore very suitable for poststerilisation testing.

Aerosol Challenge Integrity Test

One filter manufacturer has recently developed a test based on the dioctylphthalate (DOP) smoke testing of high efficiency particulate air (HEPA) filters used in air conditioning systems of cleanrooms to verify the integrity of hydrophobic gas filters. The major change to the DOP test has been to increase the sensitivity of the system and to scale down the equipment in order to deal with the smaller volumes of the filter systems and the smaller surface area of the elements. The test also differs, in-line with common current practice in HEPA filter testing, in that a white mineral oil is used in place of DOP.

The principle of the test is to challenge a membrane with a large number of aerosol particles of a controlled size, and then measure the concentration of particles, using a photometer, upstream and downstream of the filter and calculate the percentage penetration. The concentration found downstream of an integral filter would normally be zero. The range of particle sizes generated are said to be the most searching in terms of filter penetration and are relative to the worst micro-organism challenge. Particles are generated by applying a pressure to a Laskin type nozzle that is immersed in the challenge fluid.

Method for In Situ Testing, Poststerilisation (Figure 8.3)

1. After sterilising the freeze dryer and the filter, the integrity tester is attached to the upstream and downstream

Figure 8.3. Layout for aerosol challenge test.

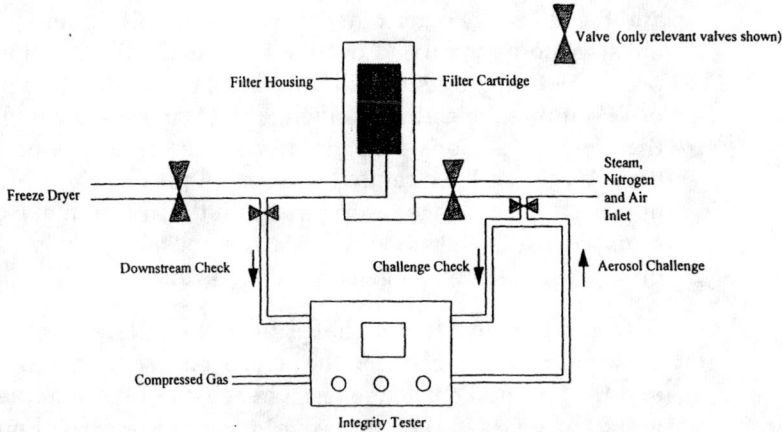

connections. Once the test is started, the unit will pressurise the filter system, helping to maintain its integrity.

2.   The integrity tester then goes through its test procedure, challenging the upstream side of the element with the specified concentration of particles (dependant on filter size and type). Upstream side air is then sampled and measured by a photometer.

3.   The pressure differential across the filter is controlled and the downstream air sampled and its concentration measured.

Comparison With Desirable Criteria

• **Reproducible** Being only recently promoted, there have been few studies carried out by the pharmaceutical industry. The only data readily available come from the one filter manufacturer that has developed the test. The reports released so far show encouraging consistency, but the level of reliability sort by most pharmaceutical concerns would require further studies.

• **Validation** Microorganism challenge testing has been carried out using the smaller bacteriophage as well as the spores and cells of bacteria, including *Pseudomonas diminuta*. However, the tests were carried out using aerosolised organisms instead of cell suspensions described in the HIMA test. That is, hydrophobic filter membranes were challenged in the dry state as they would be in service, rather than being wetted out first and the efficiency determined during liquid filtration. The scientists who have carried out the work maintain that this approach not only tests the filter in the state in which it will be used but that the aerosol challenge test is more searching and therefore is a more exacting test of the filter's efficiency, though this has been refuted by some. Adopting this different approach to challenge testing makes it difficult to make comparisons with other integrity test methods, especially as the only prescribed challenge test is the HIMA one.

- **Safe and practical limits** The results of the studies carried out show a correlation between the aerosol challenge integrity test and the bacterial challenge test. Greater confidence in the test would be given if more intensive studies were carried out, as there appears to be no results for filters that had test results around the pass limit, though it is notoriously difficult to identify such filters.

- **Regulatory approval** The regulatory authorities' view on this test is currently unknown because very few pharmaceutical companies are using the test, particularly for critical applications such as freeze dryer inlet protection.

- **Nondestructive or contaminating** By challenging the membrane with an aerosol of Ondina oil, the element is contaminated with the test fluid, even with integral filters, a risk of penetration to the downstream side is possible. Of course, even though the number of particles is huge (about 10^{12}), the quantities of fluid involved are very small (about 200 µg per 10-inch cartridge), and the amount found downstream would be virtually immeasurable. However, it is difficult to assuage the misgivings from a GMP point of view. It is reported that the contamination would be completely removed from the filter system during steaming. So if the test is performed prior to sterilisation, then the concerns expressed would appear to be less critical.

- **Dryness** The dryness of the filter is not affected by the test and therefore, no drying stage needed.

- **Safety** There are no extra safety precautions associated with this test.

- **Practicality** One of the main advantages with this test is the ease and speed with which it can be carried out. It is simply a case of making a few connections and then initiating the test. The whole procedure can be finished in just a few of minutes.

- **In situ testing** The test can be carried out in-line.

- **Poststerilisation** The test can be carried out after sterilisation if the concerns mentioned about contamination are adequately addressed. The other drawback to the test is the use of quick fit connectors, which may make it difficult to assure the integrity of the freeze dryer and pipework and make it difficult to validate during sterilisation. Changing these couplings for T pieces and hygienic valves may be an appropriate solution, but will require a critical look at the sterilisation process.

SUMMARY

The increased requirement and desire of pharmaceutical companies to integrity test freeze dryer inlet filters in situ over the last decade has been followed by the activities of the major filter manufacturers to support such testings. A great deal of development work to define suitable tests has been undertaken, and the subsequent validation work with respect to individual filters is ever ongoing. Not only are the regulatory authorities now insisting on routine testing but they are fully supportive of the trend to in situ test. Audited companies should not be surprised to find this as the expected norm in the near future.

When choosing a test, it is important, as has been stated, that filter companies are consulted in the decision process. The optimum filter choice of one supplier may not have the validation documentation to support every test, which must be brought into the equation.

The critical nature of the testing and the sensitivity of the tests really dictate the use of an automatic integrity tester. There are many instruments on the market now; however, for tests that require the measurement of flow, there are two main types available. The first measures flow indirectly by monitoring the pressure drop experienced in the gas space upstream of the filter membrane during the test phase. This makes the instrument relatively simple and easy to calibrate, but it requires the measurement of the volume upstream of the filter and is very sensitive to fluctuations in temperature during the measurement phase. Invariably, the accuracy of the test measurement and subsequent flow calculation will be affected by both the change in volume during testing, due to pleat compaction and decompression, and the drop in pressure from the test pressure.

The second type of automatic integrity test instrument is equipped with highly accurate flowmeters and measures the amount of flow directly. As the measurement is carried out at constant pressure and is independent of headspace volume, the errors involved in calculating the integrity test value are potentially much smaller than with the first type.

Diffusive Flow Test

The diffusive flow test has the most history within the pharmaceutical industry and is, therefore, more comprehensively understood. The test is supported by validation documentation for virtually every filter available, with well-defined and secure test limits and parameters. Its acceptability to the regulatory authorities is well known, but some concerns have been expressed about its use in situ and particularly post sterilisation, due to the need to perform downstream manipulations.

The use of alcohol is often cited as one of its major drawbacks. Although the safety aspects can be easily addressed, assuring that the filter and associated pipework are completely clear of contamination after testing is relatively difficult. Practically, the test suffers from a rather complex valve arrangement and really requires the complete automation of the system in order to maintain a high level of test security. If the freeze dryer is to be modified to accommodate testing, then the requirements for the diffusive flow test (along with the bubble point test) are the most extensive.

Bubble Point Test

The comments above for the diffusive flow test relate also to the bubble point test, although it is less often specified for the larger filters found on some freeze dryers.

Water-Based Integrity Test

Although the amount of experimental data for the water-based integrity test has only more recently been significant, current documentation is now based on truly comprehensive studies. The test is more sensitive to environmental conditions, such as temperature fluctuations and, of course, the surface tension of the water, and will fail if any contamination is present on the filter surface. Due to lower test pressures and subsequent flow with PVDF membrane filters due to the lower water breakthrough point compared with PTFE filters, the safety margins associated with the test limit will be less, necessitating the need for a very sensitive test instrument.

Its main benefit, however, is the ability to carry out the test without the need for any downstream manipulations, which makes it eminently suitable for in situ and poststerilisation testing. A simple valve system means that less modifications are required, though automation would still offer distinct advantages.

Aerosol Challenge Test

The limited amount of studies carried out on this test makes it too soon to evaluate—its reliability and reproducibility not have not been fully tested. Questions have been raised regarding the veracity of validation studies using aerosol challenges of bacteria, but there are certainly arguments for it. The problem of contamination is one that many in the pharmaceutical industry find hard to reconcile. If poststerilisation testing is not required, then the steaming cycle after testing may well prove effective in removing both the residual contamination and the associated concerns. Whereas with other tests, measurements are carried out of the dynamic activity of fluid or gas within the membrane, which is then related to porosity or pore size. The aerosol challenge integrity test is a measure of filterability and, as such, more accurately reflects the operation of the filter. However, it does, of course, therefore leave contamination behind.

By far, the biggest advantage in using this test is the speed and ease with which it can be performed. There is very little required in the way of additional equipment, and there are no flushing or stabilisation stages to take up time and resources.

REFERENCES

Dominick Hunter Limited. Validation documentation and technical reports.

Food and Drug Administration. 1993. *Guide to inspections of lyophilization of parenterals.* Rockville, MD: Food and Drug Administration.

MacDonald, W. D., C. A. Pelletier, and D. L. Gasper. 1989. Practical methods of the microbial validation of sterilizing grade filters used in aseptic processing. *Journal of Parenteral Science and Technology.* 43 (6).

Millipore Corporation. Validation documentation and technical reports.

Mouwen, H. C., and T. H. Meltzer. 1993. Sterilizing filter: Pore size distribution and the $1 \times 10^7/cm^2$ challenge. *Pharmaceutical Technology International* (September).

Pall Europe Limited. Validation documentation and technical reports.

Parenteral Society. Technical Monograph No. 8: *Integrity testing of freeze dryer inlet filters.* London: Parenteral Society, Freeze Drying Technical Group.

Sartorius Limited. Validation documentation and technical reports.

Wickert, K. 1990. Vacuum break filter testing. *Manufacturing Chemist* (September).

9

FREEZE DRYER VALIDATION

Peter Monger

Pharmaceutical Consultant
Dunnington, York, United Kingdom

WHAT IS VALIDATION AND WHY IS IT NECESSARY?

The concept of validation is now well established within the pharmaceutical industry, and it is understood that there is a need to validate processes, equipment, and systems to ensure that they consistently achieve what is required of them.

Two of the most commonly quoted definitions of validation are as follows:

1. Establishing documented evidence which provides a high degree of assurance that a specific process will consistently produce a product meeting its predetermined specifications and quality attributes (FDA).

2. The action of proving, in accordance with the principles of Good Manufacturing Practice, that any procedure, process, equipment, material, activity or system actually leads to the expected results (EC GMP Guide).

These definitions encapsulate what is meant by validation; that is, to prove that a process does what it is supposed to do, consistently and repeatably, in order to ensure that the products manufactured reliably meet their required quality standards.

There is a clear analogy to the concepts of *quality assurance* and *quality control;* validation is all about quality assurance. As such, it should be regarded as a continuous process—not something to be done once and forgotten—but an integral part of the systems and procedures used in the manufacture of medicinal products.

In fact, the concept of validation is simply formalisation of what many well-organised companies used to do under headings such as installation, commissioning, acceptance testing, on so on.

THE VALIDATION PROCESS

Validation is a document-driven process. Indeed, the FDA's definition of validation makes it very clear that documentation is an essential part of the validation process.

The purposes of the documentation are as follows:

- To define the scope of the validation exercise and the process or equipment to be validated.

- To describe the validation experiment.

- To specify the acceptance criteria to be applied.

- To record the results of the exercise.

- To identify whether or not the acceptance criteria were met.

This is normally achieved by the use of three main documents:

- The Validation Master Plan (VMP)

- The Validation Protocol

- Validation Reports

This approach is widespread within the industry, and has recently been adopted by the PIC (Pharmaceutical Inspection Convention) in their "Validation Guidelines", which are likely to become an Annex to the EC GMP Guide in time.

Validation Master Plan

The VMP should, as its name suggests, provide the overall framework for the validation exercise to be performed. It will typically cover the following:

- Scope: What is to be validated. In particular, care should be taken to define the boundaries of any system, process, or item of equipment, especially where it interrelates with another.

- The objectives of the validation exercise.

- A description of the overall approach to be taken to the validation activity and the rationale for it.

- The schedule or programme for validation work to be carried out.

- The person(s) responsible both for directing the validation programme and for carrying it out.

- Reference to validation protocols that will provide detail of each validation exercise and validation reports that are to be prepared to provide appropriate conclusions.

Validation Protocol

A validation protocol must be prepared before a validation exercise can be performed. It should provide the following:

- The details of the validation experiment to be undertaken

- A clear statement of the acceptance criteria to be applied

- Provision for the collection of data and a record of the people carrying out the work

- Conclusions as to whether the acceptance criteria were met

Validation Reports

A validation report will normally be required to consolidate the results of the various individual validation exercises performed and defined by separate validation protocols. The report should identify whether the overall objectives identified in the VMP have been met.

THE VALIDATION LIFE CYCLE

Although validation terminology may be new, the concepts are not. The "life cycle" approach may be more clearly exemplified by the use of typical validation terminology and processes (Figure 9.1).

Figure 9.1. Validation can be seen as integral to each step in the life cycle.

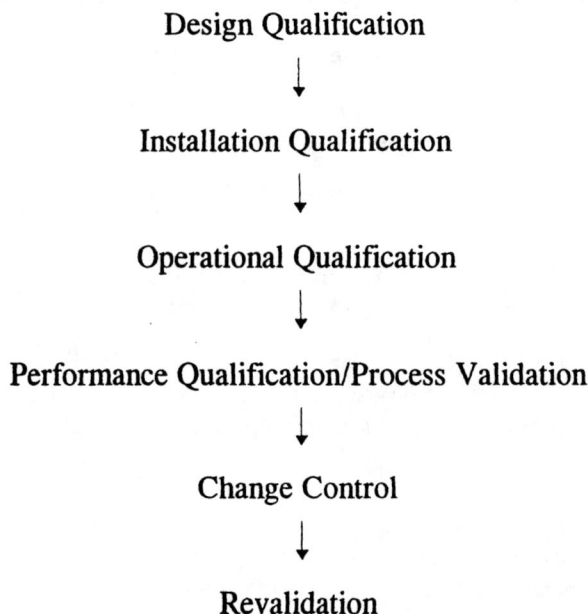

Design Qualification

↓

Installation Qualification

↓

Operational Qualification

↓

Performance Qualification/Process Validation

↓

Change Control

↓

Revalidation

Design Qualification

Design Qualification is the process by which it is assured that an item of equipment, a system, or a procedure has been designed so that it will perform the tasks required and will comply with standards of GMP, safety, and any other relevant considerations. For an item of equipment such as a freeze dryer, this should start with a User Requirement Specification (URS). This is a high level document that identifies what the equipment is to do. It should identify, for instance,

- Product throughput

- Operating constraints (such as shift working patterns, available services and infrastructure limitations)

- Product characteristics (thermal stability, inert gas requirements).

- Essential equipment design features (e.g., sterilisability; cleanability [CIP or manual], loading systems, stoppering mechanism characteristics, filter integrity testing)

- Process requirements, if these are already known (e.g., vacuum/temperature requirements)

- Control system requirements (manual or automated)

- Materials of construction (compatibility requirements, refrigerant considerations)

- Design for validation (e.g., access for temperature probes, absence of dead legs)

- Safety considerations, standards applicable and alarms required

It would normally be expected that the URS would be written by the equipment user, and it forms the basis for a Functional Specification (FS). If the URS identifies what is required, the FS can be seen as showing how this is to be achieved. Thus,

- Throughput requirements can be translated into numbers of batches/batch sizes on the basis of product volumes, cycle times, sterilisation/cleaning requirements, and so on.

- Operating characteristics must similarly be specified to achieve the same product throughput (e.g., heat up/cool down rates, condenser capacity, defrost method/time, loading/unloading system, time to vacuum, leak rate).

- Materials of construction may be specified on the basis of compatibilities. Refrigerant(s) can be identified to provide appropriate temperature and meet other requirements, such as environmental policy.

- Control systems and alarm points can be specified on the basis of product requirements and characteristics.

As for the URS, the FS should normally be developed by the user, although there is often considerable input from equipment suppliers. Together, the URS and FS will form the basis for an invitation to tender and/or a purchase order for the equipment. It is at this stage that detailed consultation is required with equipment suppliers, and it is they who will be primarily responsible for developing the URS and FS into a Design Specification (DS).

It is the DS that translates the requirements identified in the URS and FS into hardware specifications, including but not limited to the following:

- Chamber size/shelf area

- Condenser capacity

- Heat up/cool down rates
- Vacuum pump rates/ultimate vacuum, leak rate
- Refrigerant
- Shelf temperature capabilities and uniformity
- Materials of construction, finishes, dead legs, valves, and gauges
- Stoppering mechanism and capabilities
- Validation access arrangements
- Sterilisation process/cycle times
- Arrangements for air/condensate removal (for steam sterilisation)
- Cleaning system
- Loading mechanism
- Control system: hardware, software, alarms

It can be readily seen that this design exercise is a complex process, and one where the consequences of an error can be highly significant, possibly leading to the purchase of equipment that will not meet the URS or that is deficient in GMP. It is for this reason that these activities should be subjected to formal validation (i.e., Design Qualification [DQ]).

In its simplest form, DQ can be carried out by reversing the original process—by taking the design specification and ensuring that it meets the requirements of the URS, the FS, and GMP. This is best carried out by a multidisciplinary group, since it is unlikely that one person will have the necessary expertise in engineering, process development, production, QA, and regulatory affairs. As with all validation tasks, the DQ process should be carried out formally and should be documented. A checklist approach is often helpful in ensuring that all relevant issues are raised.

Of course, any discrepancies must be identified and resolved before the process can be considered to have been satisfactorily completed, and allow progress to the next stage.

A relationship exists between the elements of the DQ process and the activities that follow in a typical validation programme (Figure 9.2). Installation Qualification (IQ) is the process by which it is established that the equipment has been constructed and installed in accordance with its design specification. Operational Qualification (OQ) is the verification that equipment operates essentially as described by the

Figure 9.2. How the DQ process interrelates with validation.

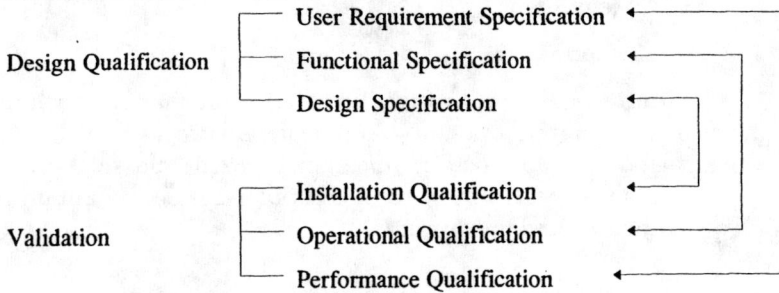

Design Qualification	User Requirement Specification
	Functional Specification
	Design Specification
Validation	Installation Qualification
	Operational Qualification
	Performance Qualification

FS. Performance Qualification (PQ) is the verification that the equipment meets the requirements identified in the URS and is able to perform the processes satisfactorily in order to deliver product of the required quality within the specified processing times.

Installation Qualification

In practice, for complex equipment such as a freeze dryer, some of the IQ testing may be carried out by the equipment supplier, at his premises, under the title of Factory Acceptance Testing (FAT) or Pre-delivery Inspection (PDI). However, it must be emphasised that final IQ and OQ must be carried out after site installation, since it is only then that many potential problems may be detected , for example,

- Improperly sloped drain lines
- Inadequate utility supplies or improperly connected utilities
- Inappropriate siting or access arrangements

Installation Qualification is normally limited to observations and checks that can be made without operating the equipment, (except for motors that should be checked for direction of rotation). The process should be controlled and documented by a protocol and would typically include checks of the following:

- Materials of construction (normally by certification rather than physical testing)
- Correct installation and configuration of major components such as pumps, compressors, shelves, stoppering system, CIP system, loading system, and other fittings, such as valves and gauges

- Correct installation of utilities, drains, and so on (particularly sloping of drain lines, orientation of steam traps, absence of dead legs, etc.)

- Verification of "as-built" drawings

- Confirmation of availability of documentation, including manufacturers operating and maintenance manuals; recommended spares list; certification of welds, passivation, and pressure vessel testing; and computer system definition and software version control

Operational Qualification

On successful completion of the IQ process, OQ can begin. As a prerequisite, however, critical devices must be identified and calibrated so that data from them can be utilised. In a freeze dryer, these would specifically include temperature and pressure/vacuum measuring devices that should be calibrated across their working ranges.

The OQ process typically consists of two phases:

1. System checks

2. Performance checks

System Checks

System checks should verify the correct operation of systems.

- Alarms

  - *Shelf and condenser temperature:* response when the temperature varies from the set point and at the safety cut out temperature.

  - *Vacuum:* response when the required vacuum is not achieved within the specified time or if limits are exceeded during the drying cycle.

  - *Service or compressor failures:* action taken or alarms indicated.

  - *Sterilisation set point failure:* alarms if the temperature is not achieved within the preset time or if it drops during the sterilisation phase.

  - *Pump failure:* response if shelf coolant pump fails.

- Vacuum break system: Operation to required pressure.

- Stoppering system: Smooth operation with stoppers correctly positioned. Funcationality of shelf interdistance adjustment should also be verified where this option is possible.

- Clean-in-place (CIP) system: Where CIP is fitted, its correction functioning should be verified. For multiproduct use equipment, the effectiveness of the cleaning process will require validation.

- Filter integrity testing: Satisfactory operation of in situ system and correct valve sequencing.

- Loading system: Satisfactory operation. This is likely to be a major concern if an automated system is installed.

- Temperature controls: The set point control for shelf temperature should be evaluated for funtionality. At the same time, the performance can be evaluated by measurement of initial overshoot and control accuracy across the range of temperatures for a typical freeze drying cycle using both manual and automatic cycles.

- Cycle sequencing and control systems: Modern freeze dryers are typically controlled by computerised systems and these should be given particular attention to ensure that they are developed and used with appropriate systems and controls. There is a range of opinion as to what is required to validate a computerised control system. What is generally agreed on, however, is the need to adopt a "life cycle" approach, which includes the following major elements:

  - Development of software under a controlled quality system

  - Simulation and functional testing

  - Rigorous change control

  It is as a part of the change control system that software source code is likely to be most valuable. It is not generally productive to attempt to perform a line by line review of source code, although some auditing is desirable. When these elements are in place, then a "black box" approach can be adopted for the OQ phase, which is simply the verification of inputs and outputs and the proper functioning of systems and controls.

Performance Checks
Certain performance checks are also typically performed as part of the OQ activity.

Shelf Cooling and Heating Rates
- The time taken to achieve a pre-set temperature should be measured with temperatures expected to be used for actual cycles used to derive acceptance criteria.

- Determine the ultimate (low) temperature obtainable and correct functioning of the shelf high temperature safety cut out and alarm.

The temperature set point control would not normally be used during these tests, since this would modulate the heating/cooling function around the set point and, therefore, affect the heating/cooling times. Rather, the temperature control is set to the maximum or minimum values possible.

Shelf temperature mapping should be performed at atmospheric pressure at a range of temperatures covering both the heating and the cooling phases of a typical freeze drying cycle. The temperature of each shelf should be measured in order to detect possible restrictions in the flow of thermal fluid.

- Temperature should also be checked across individual shelves to demonstrate uniformity.

- It is essential to have good contact between the shelf and the temperature probe. Probes should be calibrated before and after the test.

- The test specifications should address inter and intrashelf variation and time stability.

Vacuum Pump Performance
- The time taken to achieve a desired vacuum level should be specified and measured with each pump being tested separately when more than one is installed.

- The ultimate vacuum achievable should also be compared to the value specified.

Both of these tests should be performed with the condenser cold and the chamber and condenser dry. This can be achieved by pulling a vacuum in the system for several hours with the shelves at ambient temperature.

The correct functioning of the vacuum control system should also be evaluated. This would normally be first carried out on an empty chamber while running a cycle under automated control; final evaluation would then take place during a placebo or product cycle.

Leak Rate. The leak rate test is normally performed on a routine basis to verify the satisfactory operating status of the equipment and the condition of parts subject to wear or damage, such as seals and diaphragms. Nonetheless, it is important to establish a baseline performance for leak rate achievable with the equipment as installed.

The test is performed by measuring the pressure rise with time (typically one hour) after allowing sufficient time for outgassing to distinguish between "real" and "virtual" leaks. Typically, this is achieved by pulling a vacuum with the shelves at elevated temperature and the condenser cold. The vacuum pump can then be isolated from the system and the pressure rise monitored.

"Virtual" leaks can be caused by moisture evaporation or outgassing from seals/gaskets, and so on. They can normally be distinguished from "real" leaks by evaluation of the pressure curves (Figure 9.3).

Figure 9.3. Pressure curves for the determination of leaks.

A. Virtual Leak

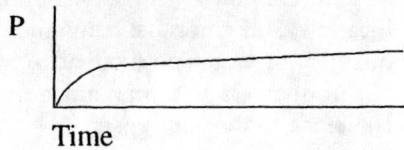

B. Real Leak

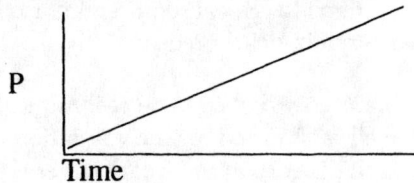

C. Real & Virtual Leak

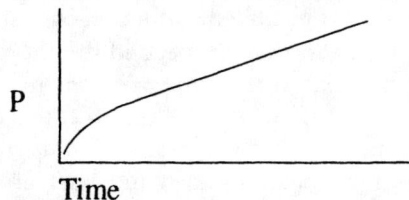

A leak rate of 2×10^{-2} mbar litres/sec is typically achievable in freeze dryer chambers in good condition. This represents a leakage into the chamber of the order of 2 litres per 24 hours, and thus would be regarded as presenting a minimal risk to product integrity, even if the air entering the chamber is heavily contaminated. In practice, the most likely site of leakage is the chamber door seal, and air leaking in through this route will be from the clean room and, therefore, will be substantially free of contamination (although this may not be the case with double door designs). The leak rate test is normally carried out after sterilisation in order to evaluate the effect of elevated temperatures on seals, and so on.

Condenser Performance. The time taken to achieve the lowest temperature and the temperature obtained should be compared to specification values. This test should be performed with and without vacuum to simulate normal operating conditions.

The defrost system(s) should be evaluated to ensure that all ice is removed during the defrost cycle. A visual check is normally sufficient. Where more than one defrost system can be used, then each should be evaluated.

The condenser capacity should also be evaluated against the specification. This can most conveniently be performed by freeze drying a quantity of water equivalent to at least the maximum product load, but in open trays to maximise the rate of sublimation and, thus, the challenge to the condenser.

Sterilisation Performance. Satisfactory operation of the sterilisation system is a critical requirement for freeze drying, and validation of this system is clearly required.

Steam Sterilisation. The techniques required are similar to those now well established for the validation of autoclaves, except that there is no load other than the freeze dryer chamber itself.

Temperature mapping should be carried out to determine the hot and cold spots. Temperature variation is likely to be significantly greater than for an autoclave since the chamber is not normally jacketed or insulated. Although cold spots may be improved by the use of insulation, care is needed in introducing potentially particle shedding materials into clean environments.

A sufficient number of temperature probes should be used to provide a full picture of the temperature range throughout the freeze dryer, including the condenser, associated pipework, and the vacuum break filter. Any cold spots identified should be probed during subsequent heat penetration/reproducibility studies. It is accepted practice to demonstrate satisfactory achievement of sterilising conditions in three consecutive runs.

It is normal practice to use an overkill approach which would require a temperature above 121°C for at least 15 minutes, although a "safety margin" above these conditions is often added to allow for possible temperature variation or control errors.

Satisfactory sterilisation under these conditions requires the presence of saturated steam at phase boundary conditions. To achieve this, it is essential to ensure adequate removal of both air and condensate. Air removal can normally be readily achieved by use of the freeze dryer's own vacuum system followed by steam injection, possibly in a pulsed mode. Removal of the high volumes of condensate formed from the high thermal mass of the often cold equipment can be much more of a problem. (This condensate can provide an effective CIP system for the freeze dryer). Care must be taken during installation to ensure that the chamber and pipework are adequately sloped to drain. Probes should be placed during the temperature mapping exercise in any low points and other areas where there is risk of condensate buildup, so that any such buildup can be detected.

The use of biological indicators (BIs) in the validation and monitoring of steam sterilisation cycles is a somewhat contentious issue. It is normally accepted in Europe that where there is not an unusual risk of inadequate air or condensate removal, then validation of steam sterilisation can be performed on the basis of time and temperature measurements alone. This, of course, implies that it is possible to place temperature probes in all relevant positions. If this is not possible, then the use of BIs may be necessary, although placement of these is also likely to be difficult.

In contrast, the practice in North America is for the wider use of BIs as a routine adjunct to thermal validation studies, in this case, less attention is paid to air removal.

Where BIs are required, a number of issues must be addressed:

- Spore strips (not suspensions) should be used, since the purpose is to show the presence of saturated steam in the freeze dryer, not inside the BI ampoule.

- BIs with a population >10^6 of resistant spores (D value > 1.0) are required. (*Bacillus stearothermophilus* A.T.C.C. 7953 is suitable for steam sterilisation). The population should be verified by the user. D value certification by the supplier is normally acceptable.

- The storage, handling, and incubation of BIs should closely follow the recommendations of the manufacturer since the

D value may be affected by inadequate control of these parameters.

Gas Sterilisation. Where a gas sterilisation process is used then its validation can be achieved by demonstrating the satisfactory kill of appropriate BIs. Although systems exist for the measurement of gas concentration during sterilisation, these data have generally been regarded as useful only in the routine monitoring of cycles, not as constituting an appropriate validation.

The comments noted earlier concerning the handling and placement of BIs still apply. The choice of indicator organism is important and may vary depending on the sterilant used. For ethylene oxide sterilisation, the indicator organism showing the highest resistance is *Bacillus subtilis* var. *niger*. This organism may also be used with gaseous hydrogen peroxide systems, although some workers claim that *Bacillus stearothermophilis* is actually more resistant to this method of sterilisation.

Surface Sanitation. By its nature, this process is not readily controllable and, therefore, cannot truly be "validated". There are obvious variables involved, such as,

- Manual cleaning processes
- The choice of sanitising agents
- Dilution requirements

Other, more subtle changes may occur that are less amenable to control, such as

- Changes in natural flora
- Conditions and cleanliness of the equipment

Therefore, it is normal practice to place a greater emphasis on periodic surface monitoring when this method of sanitation is used, rather than on a "once off" validation exercise. In particular, the deliberate contamination of surfaces with organisms in order to demonstrate the effectiveness of the sanitisation process would be regarded as undesirable and introduces unnecessary risks, since such practices cannot be controlled in the same way as the use of discrete BIs can with gas or steam sterilisation processes.

Freeze Drying Functionality. It is good practice to freeze dry a placebo product when all other stages of the IQ/OQ process have been satisfactorily completed and before committing product to Performance

Qualification (PQ) studies. This may be carried out either in open trays or vials/ampoules as for actual product. The depth of fill should mimic actual product parameters. Of course, stoppering performance can only be evaluated if vials are used.

The cycle sequence should follow as closely as possible the expected product cycle, although times and temperatures for each stage may very. These stages should be carefully monitored for correct system functioning.

The activities of IQ and OQ provide the opportunity for the user to learn a great deal about the freeze drying equipment and its operation. Therefore it is most appropriate to use this information to develop Standard Operating Procedures (SOPs) that should form the basis of PQ and routine operation of the equipment.

Performance Qualification

Performance qualification consists of the verification of two essential elements:

1. The product can be produced reliably and reproducibly.

2. The product can be manufactured in such a way as to maintain its sterility.

These objectives can be met by performing

-   Process validation runs

-   Media simulation studies

Process Validation

The purpose of carrying out process validation trials is to ensure that the equipment will reliably and reproducibly produce materials as established by the URS.

These tests are normally carried out in a concurrent fashion on production lots of materials so that all products and freeze drying cycles are covered. An essential aspect of the testing is the establishment of reproducibility, hence more than one run is necessary, and it is again normally accepted that three consecutive successful runs are adequate.

The tests should be performed essentially as normal production runs, but with the careful control of process parameters and the rigorous evaluation of product quality.

-   It is desirable to run the cycle as closely as possible to the process limits consistent with adequate control. It is not appropriate at this time to investigate the "limits of failure" of the process. Rather the objective should be to provide evidence to support the choice of process control limits. Similarly it is not normally considered necessary to evaluate all of the possible combinations of control parameter ranges (temperature, pressure, etc.), although consideration should be given to determining the validation cycle conditions based on possible interactions or synergistic effects. Thus, typically in three process validation runs, the cycle may be run at "low" values of temperature, pressure, time and so on, at nominal values, and at "high" settings.

- Product should be carefully evaluated after each run. A sampling schedule should be developed to cover product from all areas within the chamber, for example, the corners and centre from each shelf. The conformance of the product against specification should be established for at least the following:

    - Cake structure, height
    - Colour, uniformity
    - Dissolution characteristics
    - Moisture/solvent content
    - Assay, pH, and other chemical characteristics
    - Stability

Media Simulation

The purpose of media simulation is to demonstrate that the whole process is capable of reliably producing sterile products from aseptic manufacturing techniques. To do this, it is necessary to simulate or mimic the entire process. Thus, the use of the terms *media fill* or *broth fill* is not accurate and is disfavoured.

Unfortunately, there is very little actual guidance provided in the EC GMP Guide concerning media simulations. Paragraph 38 of Annex 1 requires that

Aseptic processes or significant modifications should be validated by using a sterile nutrient medium for simulating the process to be performed. That validation should be repeated at defined intervals.

No guidance is provided on how to perform the media simulation, on the number of containers to fill, or on suitable acceptance criteria. Historically, acceptance criteria have evolved steadily, typically as the industry has found it is able to achieve higher standards.

Early limits were proposed by the World Health Organisation (WHO); not more than 1 percent contaminated from a fill of 500 units (1966) and subsequently not more than 0.3 percent contaminated (1973).

The U.S. Parenteral Drug Association (1980) proposed that "manufacturers should strive for a contamination level of less than 0.1 percent" and most recently (1993) the Patenteral Society (UK) suggested that this should be refined so that 0.1 percent contamination could be assured with at least 95 percent confidence. This approach has also been taken by the International Organisation for Standardisation working party TC 198 in the draft international standard on "Aseptic Processing of Healthcare Products". In practice, this means that zero positives can be accepted from approximately 3000 units filled for most batch sizes. Table 9.1 shows the numbers of units that must be filled and the maximum number of positives acceptable to provide 95 percent confidence that the population as a whole is less than 0.1 percent (or 0.01 percent) contaminated. It can be readily seen that the number of units to be filled is large if any positives at all are to be accepted.

None of these limits has been officially endorsed by the regulatory authorities. The UK Medicines Control Agency (MCA) did, however, participate in the development of the Parenteral Society monograph and the draft international standard and could, therefore, be reasonably expected to accept their requirements.

Table 9.1. Media Simulation

Maximum Acceptable Batch Rejects	Batch Contamination Level Will Not Exceed (95% Confidence)	Media Units Required for Given Batch Size					
		5,000	10,000	20,000	50,000	100,000	Infinity
0	0.1%	2,469	2,668	2,808	2,912	2,951	2,995
1	0.1%	3,676	4,047	4,339	4,575	4,670	4,747
2	0.1%	4,684	5,207	5,670	6,044	6,207	6,294
0	0.01%				24,698	26,686	29,944
1	0.01%				46,093	47,047	47,407
2	0.01%					62,911	62,911

It has long been an MCA expectation that media simulations would be performed every three months on each filling line for each shift. This contrasts with the United States where it is generally accepted that up to six months can be allowed between media fills. This is the interval required by the draft international standard. The Parenteral Society monograph, however, suggests twice per year per line for each shift or three times per year per line for single shift operations, so there is no clear consensus on this issue.

There is general agreement, however, that all aseptic processing steps should be simulated. In particular, this must include permitted interventions. For instance, if it is company policy to allow needle changes to be performed during filling, then this should take place during the media simulation exercise. Personnel present should be the maximum number normally permitted.

Sterilisation of the lyophiliser should follow normal practice, and if this does not require sterilisation between each run the media simulation should be performed immediately before sterilisation is due in order to simulate worst-case conditions.

It may be necessary to "split" some processes, for instance, bulk manufacture and holding from filling and freeze drying, to ensure that each step is included in the media simulation. This practice is acceptable.

Media simulation of a freeze drying process is necessarily complex. It is likely to include the following steps:

- Media compounding, using procedures and materials to follow as closely as possible normal operating practices, but omitting, for example, heating and cooling processes, except as necessary to dissolve nutrient materials.

- Sterilisation of the growth medium, again by filtration. This is often a difficult step, since some media will readily block filters. (It is understood that a new low particulate material is being introduced by at least one media supplier).

- Filling.

- Stopper insertion.

- Loading of the freeze dryer using the normal method.

- Simulation of the freeze drying cycle. There is some variation of opinion as to how this should be done. Typical practice is to pull a partial vacuum (500 mbar is typical; too low a pressure may cause the media to boil). Pressure is then vented back to atmospheric via the normal gas inlet system and two more vacuum pulses are pulled. This process simulates the effects of turbulence from air removal and entry and may be regarded as somewhat of a "worst-case" approach.

Some practitioners then recommend holding the media for the normal cycle time. There would appear to be little value in this approach, however, since the media cannot be held under the normal high vacuum and potential air leakage into the chamber will not be reproduced. Therefore, it is regarded as more reasonable to complete the stoppering process after the final vacuum pulse cycle and then remove the filled units for incubation and evaluation.

- Incubation should follow normally accepted practice for the growth medium used. Efforts should be made to ensure that the media is in contact with the closure system (e.g., by periodic shaking).

- Evaluation of the results should be against the criteria presented in Table 9.1. There is no statistical justification for adding together results from more than one media simulation exercise. Each is a discrete operation and must be considered as such.

- It is essential to include positive controls in any media simulation exercise. These should be designed to ensure that low level contamination will be detected, typically by inoculation with 10–100 organisms of appropriate species.

- In the event that positive unit(s) may be found following a media simulation, an investigation in to their cause will be necessary. To facilitate this, it is essential that environmental and personnel monitoring is performed during the exercise. Any isolates should either be identified or retained for comparison with contaminates found in the media.

- Some product types may require variations in the general techniques of media simulation. For instance, for open (tray-dried) products, the use of settling plates may be convenient. For dual chamber vials, the intermediate stopper must be activated so that all parts of the system are challenged. The principle should always be to challenge the system with "worst-case" conditions, following actual production procedures and practices as much as possible.

Revalidation and Change Control

The life cycle approach to validation has been stressed throughout this chapter. In this context it is necessary to maintain a system of change control and to perform revalidation as appropriate to ensure that the equipment and process remains in a state of validated control.

Change Control

The absence of effective change control will lead to failures in system performance. failures that occur in this way are among the most frequently raised observations made during regulatory inspections.

Where critical processing equipment, such as a freeze dryer, is involved, change control assumes great importance. The elements of an effective change control programme include the following:

- Documented system definition, to allow a baseline to be established and judgements to be made on the magnitude and significance of proposed changes. Documentation should include

  - System description and specifications

  - As-built drawings and Pipework and Instrumentation Diagrams

  - Hardware and software configuration for control systems

  Ideally, these should have been generated during the design and installation process and subjected to the process of DQ, IQ, and OQ as previously discussed.

- There must be a multidisciplinary approach to change control. Changes must be assessed for their impact from a wide perspective. This should include at least

  - Engineering

  - Quality control/assurance

  - Regulatory affairs

- System definition for a freeze dryer should include relevant utilities, including the steam supply. Any changes should be evaluated for their impact on the freeze dryer concerned. For example,

  - Changes to the steam supply system

  - Addition (or deletion) of other equipment to the steam supply

  - Changes in water quality or treatment regime

The replacement of valves or fittings on the freeze dryer must always be critically evaluated. A common issue is whether a genuine "like for like" transition is occurring. Where there is a question, specialist advice is essential.

Modern freeze dryers are typically computer controlled and changes to the hardware, or more particularly the software, are likely to have a significant effect on equipment operation and must be carefully controlled. Whilst this may be relatively simple to achieve for computer control hardware, it can be extremely difficult for software.

As with any successful change control process it should start with an adequate system definition. It is desirable for this to include the source code listing as an absolute reference. Proposed changes must be carefully evaluated for potential effects on the system operation and the need for revalidation.

Revalidation

The change control programme will identify the requirements for revalidation when changes have occurred. In addition, it is accepted practice to perform periodic revalidation of critical systems and processes to ensure that undetected or unknown changes or faults in the system have not occurred, and that it is functioning in essentially the same manner as when the original (commissioning) validation was performed. For freeze drying, periodic revalidation is normally limited to the equipment sterilisation process.

Annual revalidation has been widely accepted by the regulatory authorities. Since reproducibility has already been demonstrated (and any revalidation work will add to this body of information), a single validation exercise is normally all that is required.

- *Steam sterilisation:* temperature distribution throughout the equipment, particularly covering any "cold spots" previously identified.

- *Gas sterilisation:* distribution of appropriate BIs in the chamber, condenser and associated pipework, filters, and so on.

- *Surface sanitisation:* as noted earlier, it is not considered desirable to challenge such sanitisation programmes by deliberately contaminating surfaces with resistant organisms. However, since this process is less rigorous than both steam and gas sterilisation and also less amenable to true validation (since variation in, for instance, the natural flora that may challenge the process cannot be rigorously controlled), it is desirable to monitor the microbial cleanliness of the equipment on a frequent basis. How frequently such monitoring is performed (typically by the use of swabs or surface contact plates) will depend on the nature of the materials to be processed, throughput, conditions of equipment, and other factors. A weekly or monthly programme would probably be regarded as typical, but other intervals between testing may be appropriate in certain circumstances.

REFERENCE

Parenteral Society. 1993. *The use of process simulation tests in the evaluation of processes for the manufacture of sterile products.* Technical Monograph No. 4. Swindon, UK: Parenteral Society.

10

CYCLE OPTIMISATION AND PROCESS TRANSFER

Kevin Kinnarney

Bio Products Laboratory
Herts, United Kingdom

It is usual for most freeze drying processes to be developed as part of the protocol for the manufacture of a new product. In the past, many products have been generated up to the final dosage presentation before a decision was made as to how the product will be marketed. As freeze drying must rank as one of the most expensive ways to prepare a product for sale, all other presentations may well have been tried and discounted for a variety of reasons. There will always be pressure on any R&D unit to transfer products to production so that returns on investment may be obtained as soon as possible. This pressure, added to any delay in turning to freeze drying for final product presentation, may result in little time being allowed for either the development or the optimisation of the process. This may then result in the freeze drying cycle not being the best possible.

A well-planned process will take account of the needs of freeze drying and reduce the ingredients to those salts, sugars, or buffers that may be easily dried. This may also mean the addition of some of these types of components to assist the drying process. The ideal optimised cycle will be as short as possible. The cost of operating a freeze dryer for a few hours longer than necessary is not cheap; in addition a second batch cannot be processed until the first batch has been completed and removed from the equipment. Added up over a year, a few hours unnecessary freeze drying may mean the loss of a number of potential batches filled. The return on capital, and freeze dryers represent substantial investment, is reduced and could make the product uneconomical.

When a new product is formulated in R&D, only small-scale batches are usually made. This may be due to the high cost of the raw material and the reluctance to waste valuable assets, or the material itself may be difficult to obtain. If the freeze drying cycle is to be investigated fully, some wastage will inevitably take place. The quantity of material for processing may also be limited by the size of equipment available for manufacture. Much R&D freeze drying may be undertaken with a bench-top unit only holding a handful of containers. This is perfectly acceptable for early benchwork, but process development ought to be carried out on equipment that mimics the ability of production units.

The development of the actual freeze drying cycle may be carried out by people with a thorough knowledge of the requirements of the final production facility. Alternatively, less emphasis may be placed on this part of the process and freeze drying viewed as a necessary "evil" like packaging. Obviously, there are many shades between these two examples, but freeze drying must be considered as part of the production process.

In the past, many freeze drying cycles have "appeared from the mists of time" and were based on the customs and practice of a few of the development staff. This could mean that the product was frozen down to –50°C because that just happened to be the temperature of the laboratory chest freezer. Equally, overnight freezing was convenient as it allowed staff to put the product into the freezer at the end of the working day and then continue with the process the next morning. Using the above as an example, we would have a freezing cycle for the product of –50°C for 15 hours! A fully investigated, scientific approach may result in a freezing cycle far shorter in time, perhaps 3–4 hours, at only –40°C. with the subsequent savings in time and energy. Hopefully, this type of practice is diminishing and more attention is paid to optimisation. Other organisation priorities may play their part in curtailing the effort needed to produce a fully optimised cycle.

If a product has been successfully freeze dried and the freeze drying cycle proved to be repeatable to the point of being subject to validation, then the tendency to start aging trials exists. Once these stability trials are underway or completed, the pressure to introduce the product into full-scale production increases. Further cycle optimisation then relies on another set of stability trials taking place, with the added cost in material and manpower.

CYCLE OPTIMISATION

Successful optimisation actually starts with formulation, as previously mentioned, but can only be refined when it has been proved that the product can be freeze dried successfully. At this stage, we must assume that there can be no further changes in formulation, final dose size, or presentation. Carrying out this exercise successfully requires a solid commitment to the process before commencing any work. The aim is to supply a freeze drying cycle that requires the minimum operation time with the best operating parameters. There is always the possibility that the first freeze drying cycle attempted is close to the ideal, and further work will not be of much benefit. Optimisation studies will prove the case and support any later investigation into possible problems. There may be an acceptable compromise in time, for instance, if the end of the cycle is during the middle of the night, then it may be acceptable to allow the cycle extra time to finish for the start of the working day. It is not worth attempting to only save real time if this is meaningless to the work pattern.

The first parameter to optimise, therefore, is time. Operational time is always at a cost in, at the very least, power to allow the motors and so on to function. A short time equals low operating costs; lower plant utilisation allows other products to be processed, if required.

The second function to address is the control temperatures of, usually, the product shelves. The critical temperature of the product can be related to the shelf temperature and later, during freeze drying, the pressure. The speed at which the product can be frozen, or at least changed into a glass, and the effect of this stage on the drying regime should be explored. There is no hard and fast rule of what is the best method of freezing-this must be left in the hands of the development expert. Some products require rapid freezing, whilst others slow cooling. Some may have a cooling cycle followed by warming to just below the eutectic point to "temper" the material. If possible, we only need to achieve a temperature below the eutectic point of the product, if a measurable one can be identified, to allow freezing to occur. If the product is frozen, cooling further will have no effect, other than cooling!

To measure the temperature in the product under test, a thermocouple or some other type of sensor is used. These devices will, when connected to an indicator, display the temperature at the sensor, the tip in the case of a thermocouple, wherever it is positioned in the product mass. During any stage of the process, we should be concerned about the total volume of the product. Using a point sensor could be slightly misleading when trying to determine if complete freezing has taken place, as only the temperature at this point is indicated. If the probe shows us that the freezing temperature has been reached, we must be sure that the total mass has reached this temperature.

It is usual to have a hold time at this temperature to ensure "evenness" throughout the frozen plug. Whatever information can be obtained from the probes is helpful, however, by their presence in the container, they will have created an artificial environment. Results that have been obtained by these probes should be viewed carefully, and it is not unusual to have some extra time added to the freezing stage to ensure that the mass within containers without probes, are frozen.

The length of time needed to ensure complete freezing of the product should be kept as short as possible, as the refrigeration system fitted to the freeze dryer will be running unnecessarily if overlong freezing times are used. An increase in wear and tear of compressors results when they are operated at low pressures during cooling at a low temperature for a long period of time.

The freezing cycle may have various changes in temperature level within it and could also include rewarming to encourage crystallisation. Because every product has such different features, it is almost impossible to recommend any particular type of cycle. The component parts will indicate the likely trends of the freezing, but mixtures do not necessarily behave as expected. It is not unknown for a product to be considered totally unsuitable for freeze drying even if it has been successfully produced in this manner for many years.

The primary drying stage of the cycle follows freezing. During this stage, the solvent should be removed as quickly as possible, without any detriment to the active ingredients. Again, a cycle must be developed to ensure minimum effect on the contained product. It may be accepted that there is some activity loss in the active ingredient during this stage of the process. Care should be taken to ensure that this loss is not added to by stressing the system by over optimistic expectations.

The primary drying cycle must remove the solvent as quickly as possible, without risk to the product. High shelf temperatures at the initial stage of drying, with a decrease at a later stage, may be required to dry a product in the shortest period of time. However, too complicated a shelf temperature profile may not prove possible on production plant. High shelf temperatures also expose the product to the risk of melting if a short failure in processing occurs.

Pressure may also be controlled to arrive at the quickest sublimation rate. The speed at which the vapour can be removed relates to back pressure within the system caused by the pressure level and the rate of heat transfer to the product drying interface. Control of both these parameters is critical to the drying speed and the safety of the product. When using a production plant, it is preferable to have a relatively small differential between the shelf and product temperatures, as this allows recovery to be more easily achieved when there is some form of plant failure. It is fairly standard to have crash cooling of the shelves in the event of a vacuum failure, and it is obviously quicker to cool shelves from, say, 0°C to -40°C than from 30°C. Measurement of the completion of this part of the cycle must be addressed and this may be determined by traditional methods such as pressure rise tests. Weight measurement of the containers during this part of the process may indicate when stability has been achieved and no sublimation is occurring. When satisfied that this stage is complete, secondary drying can commence.

Secondary drying is usually carried out at a higher temperature and ensures that the final moisture content of the product is between set limits. Relationship between temperature during this stage and final moisture content can be found by experiment. Extended secondary drying can be used to ensure equilibrium of moisture to temperature figures are reproducible. When this has been achieved, then work must be done to determine the period required for the secondary drying cycle. This should be as short as possible to achieve this equilibrium, as extended drying is only a waste of process time. Final moisture can be determined while secondary drying is continuing by using a "thief" apparatus to withdraw samples from the freeze dryer and subjecting them to testing. As soon as the water content stabilises, then secondary drying is complete and the time for this stage set.

All stages of optimisation should have the needs of the process as the driving force, with the constraints of production processing not overlooked. Once this stage of development has been completed, it is more difficult to "revisit" as the savings generated by reexamining the process may be difficult to quantify.

TECHNOLOGY TRANSFER

Process

When the process has been finally developed in R&D, there remains the task of translating this work to the final production environment. This often entails a massive scale-up, and, consequently, a detailed programme of work should be undertaken. The original process should be as fully documented as possible, and all the steps necessary to ensure success taken and evaluated. At this stage, the only changes taking place should be location and quantity—this is not the time to experiment with changes in the formulation! It is usual to operate all the equipment and final process using a placebo that could be the product components minus the active ingredient. Whatever is used should be as close to the final product as possible.

As far as freeze drying is concerned, we should assume that the product will arrive at this stage resembling the method of preparation as defined during development. The vials, or containers, that will be regularly used must be of the same type as was used for the development of the freeze drying cycle. Similar vials from another manufacturer may not necessarily show the same results as the original vial, and results on the first real product batches could show some unexpected abnormalities. It is more prudent to remain with the same container that was part of the transfer information. Any changes should be carried out in a controlled manner at a later time. The preparation of the containers should also form part of the controlled process.

The above comments also hold true for the stoppers. The preparation of these, especially the pretreatment with silicon to assist the closure, should be paid close attention. It is also important to copy the poststerilisation regime of any drying or storage prior to use. The primary container system must, therefore, mirror the R&D process if changes in either component affecting the product are to be eliminated.

Although the load produced in the production environment will, inevitably, be much larger than had been seen up to this point, the packing density of the vials on the chamber shelves should be the same. This will render the cooling or heating capacity of the load to a similar level and not allow too much variation in the drying regime. Transfer of heat through the shelves is plant related and varies from plant to plant.

It is also advisable to run through some cycle simulation on the empty freeze dryer before any placebo trials to ensure there are no problems with any of the selected parameters. It is not always the case that a large production freeze dryer can meet the parameters that were achieved on a R&D plant or can react as quickly to changes in state. It may also be necessary at this stage to use some form of media fill to confirm the suitability of the process.

Loading Plant

The main concern at this stage centres around the time taken to load the plant; it is assumed that the loading temperature of the shelves is carefully controlled with the method of loading defined. Filling is often being carried out at the same time as loading the freeze dryer. As this can take several hours to complete, account must be made of this regarding any possible activity loss. Some products cannot remain at ambient temperature for long periods without subsequent loss of activity. It is relatively easy to control the temperature of the product before filling, for instance, in a jacketed vessel with controlled heating or cooling. Likewise, the shelf temperature is easily controlled, but the period of filling and loading may be more difficult to manage. If the product has been developed to be loaded at around 20°C and will remain stable at this temperature for a number of hours, then no problem exists; however, this is not always possible. Loading time and environmental impact on this part of the process should be considered.

Freezing

The shelf cooling rate must be matched to the cooling cycle developed, and it should be possible to replicate any slope of cooling or hold period relatively easily. There may prove to be differences in the heat transfer properties of the shelves themselves, which may then introduce some variation in the actual cooling of the product. There may be a need to modify the cycle slightly to take account of this phenomenon, if observed. The actual product temperature should also be monitored, as at this stage the readings obtained are useful in indicating the rate of heat transfer across the shelf/glass/product matrix.

The freezing time may just be observed, or the profile amended and matched to that expected. It may be that the freezing time is affected by the difficulty in heat transfer; although the temperature of the shelf and product eventually stabilise, this stabilisation time may be extended beyond the expected time. If there are difficulties in this stage due to heat transfer problems, the expected final product temperature in relation to the shelf may not be reached and a lower shelf temperature may be required.

Experience shows that the effect on supercooling of the product by the change in environment offered by the new process acts as a good indicator as to successful transfer of the freezing stage. Many products show supercooling during freezing; if this is carefully monitored, measured, and compared, a good indication of replication of the process is indicated if the same figure is found. Changes in the level of supercooling may not just be affected by different plants but can equally be affected by upstream processes. These things that may have changed the degree of supercooling may also affect both the freezing and drying of the product.

Primary Drying

During the stage of primary drying, the shelf temperature must be controlled and monitored. Assuming the eutectic temperature of the product is known, then this can indicate the maximum temperature allowable before total disaster. It is, obviously, usual to remain at least a few degrees below this temperature to ensure successful drying. When the primary drying cycle commences, care must be taken to ensure the correct conditions are achieved. Setting the shelf temperature and system pressure to levels that have previously been used may result in a different product temperature than that expected. It may then become necessary to adjust one of the above to maintain the correct product temperature for efficient drying. Small changes in pressure can show a more marked effect on product temperature than large changes in shelf temperature, due to the heat transfer effect of the gases present. If it is necessary to make these small adjustments to "tune" the system, it is recommended to try altering the pressure first. The reasons for this are twofold: (1) The reaction to pressure change is very rapid, and the results of any change are soon observed; changes in shelf temperature are relatively slow to become effective. (2) If the shelf temperature has been raised too much, the differential between the shelf and product temperatures becomes very large, with a greater heat gradient across the product. Whatever method is chosen, care must be exercised to ensure melting does not take place; remember the probe position is measuring one point in the product only.

Having achieved a product temperature close to the desirable level, the length of the process may be measured. This may relate to the time that the product probes take before rising in temperature to meet the shelf temperature. Again, care must be taken as the containers with the product probes do not mirror those without. If the probe is not positioned where the last vestiges of ice will be sublimed, then the indication as to completion is inaccurate. This temperature must be taken as an indicator only; provided the R&D work was carried out using the same method, a comparison may be made using this data. Experience gained during preliminary work may show, for instance, that allowing the drying to continue for a further number of hours will ensure that this stage is complete.

It is also possible to detect the end of primary drying by using a pressure rise test. This test consists of isolating the chamber containing the product from the condenser with the main valve and observing the rise in pressure on the pressure control instrumentation. If the pressure rises quickly, then there is still substantial sublimation taking place, and the drying must be allowed to continue by reopening the main valve. If this test is carried out too early in the cycle, then there is the risk of the product melting, as the resultant pressure rise is very rapid.

If the test is carried out after all drying has ceased, then the only pressure rise will be from the leaks that exist in the system. Testing during the final stages of drying should, therefore, give a good indication of how far this stage has progressed. Care must be taken with these observations, as the speed of pressure rise will also be related to the quantity of containers and volume of product available. The accuracy of pressure measurements is also related to the accuracy of the measuring system. By looking at pressure rise tests over a period of time, a subjective indication of dryness can be seen.

Both probe temperature and pressure rise measurements are not a particularly accurate method of determining the end of primary drying, but they act as a good guide as to the likely state of the process. If these observations are related to the same observations during pilot studies, and the two are similar, then some confidence may be gained. It would be hoped that the length of this part of the process is the same as on the pilot plant. This time should be added to the necessary parameters for checking.

The condenser temperature may not be particularly important to achieve the expected drying profile. This only becomes a problem if there are significant differences in the temperatures achieved on the two types of plants. When very low temperatures are achieved in the condensers, the difference in sublimation rates possible are negligible. It is worth noting the temperature and, certainly, any collapse in temperature that may occur during the main part of sublimation. It may not be possible to control this, but it may have an effect on the product that will call for modification later (e.g., slower sublimation by lowering the product temperature).

The chamber pressure must be controlled to allow the sublimation rate required to maintain the product temperature. This may have been adjusted to allow the shelf temperature level to be in an acceptable range, but now must be kept in control. If Pirani type gauges were used for initial trials, then the same type should be used for production. Although there are arguments about which type is more suitable for freeze drying and which is more accurate, the type used for process development should be used at this stage, regardless of these arguments. As we are looking for repeatability, a different type of gauge will cloud the issue.

The method of pressure control must be considered. There are many ways of controlling, including calibrated leak, vacuum valve control, and throttling the main valve. Whatever method is used, or combination of methods adopted, the method(s) should mirror that used for cycle determination. A further important point is to use the same gas for injection through the calibrated leak, if this was the chosen method of pressure regulation. There are many theories about the use of dry nitrogen compared to atmospheric air as a better aid to freeze drying, but this is not the time to experiment with these differences. If dry nitrogen was originally used as a control gas, then it should be used in production.

Finally, the recorder trace should be compared to the expected profile. If the monitoring system is sufficiently good to record all the usual parameters, this record will act as a template for future batches, and a comparison to the R&D data supplied (also in the form of a recorder graph, if possible).

Secondary Drying

Many of the same aspects of the cycle must be monitored as for primary drying. These will include shelf temperature, product temperature, duration, chamber pressure, and control. As for primary drying, these should mirror fairly closely the expected attributes of the cycle. Determining the end of the cycle is more difficult, as the rate of sublimation is minimal and the product and shelf temperature should be the same value. Often, the secondary drying is related to a time value only that must be matched.

Having finished the drying cycle, the product must be sealed and removed from the plant. Any backfilling pressure and the type of gas used should be as originally established, with final stoppering carried out in the plant. The product may then be removed, oversealed, and sent for testing.

Testing

Testing should not bring any surprises and should qualify the effort put into the transfer of the process. The first test that can be carried out quite rapidly is visual inspection. This is an area that should not be underestimated, as many faults can easily be detected with the human eye and subjective observations made. A sample of the R&D product to use for comparison purposes is a good guide to appearance, and allowing the product "champion" to view and check some of the batch is helpful. Unsatisfactory drying or failures resulting in partial or full melting can be observed, and the need for subsequent longterm testing reviewed. Reconstitution of the dried product is a further test that can soon be carried out. Longer than expected reconstitution times or undissolved "bits" in the solution can highlight shortcomings in the process. Assuming the appearance is as expected, then the full range of tests can be undertaken. These may include moisture determination and measurement of loss or denaturation of the active ingredient(s). Finally, stability trials must be undertaken to prove, at least, the relative success of freeze drying the product.

Summary

There are some aspects of transfer that can act as beneficial to the whole operation. The location of all interested parties on the same site allows easy passage of documentation and visual information. Physical distance is usually a hindrance to obtaining commonalty of approach and review of progress.

Full documentation at the conception and development of the cycle are necessary to the successful transfer and follow up of the process. Without the fallback of being able to see how the cycle was developed, then out-of-control processes or parameters cannot be fully investigated, understood, or corrected. Once the cycle has been successful, then a final process program may be incorporated into the operating procedures. This may form part of the standard operating procedures or be a computer program for completely automatic control. When this has been completed, the first product batch using these parameters will form part of the performance qualification of the process.

11

CFC REPLACEMENT

Kevin Murgatroyd

Biopharma Process Systems Ltd.
Winchester, United Kingdom

As the efficiency of refrigeration systems increased, and powerful refrigerants were introduced that were capable of generating temperatures as low as -90°C within the freeze dryer, the freeze drying community enjoyed a period where the performance of the freeze dryer was taken for granted. It is unfortunate that many cycles are developed with a freezing step that is dictated, not by the solidification temperature of the product, but by the ultimate shelf minimum temperature of the development freeze dryer. Once a cycle is described in a product licence it becomes difficult to change, even though equivalent results could be obtained at higher temperatures with a smaller energy consumption.

This state of affairs came to a sudden halt in the beginning of 1994, within Europe, when it became illegal to manufacture bulk quantities of the refrigerant R13b1; the design of equipment to utilise this chemical was also banned. At the time, R13b1 was the most popular refrigerant used in a freeze dryer. The alternative, R502, was to be banned a year later on 31 December 1994. The result was that it became extremely difficult to produce a refrigeration system, other than an expensive cascade system, that could match the performance that the market was demanding. The rest of the world, with a few excepted countries, followed Europe exactly 12 months later.

The full implications of this ban were not fully appreciated by the freeze drying community prior to 1991 and there was little that could be done. Refrigerant manufacturers had concentrated, since 1987, when the Montreal Protocol was signed, on alternatives for refrigerants R11 and R12 that accounted for the bulk of refrigeration applications. Little priority was placed on refrigerants with the performance required by a freeze dryer.

The challenge was eventually overcome by the development of hydrofluorocarbons (HFCs), although a full replacement for R13b1 has not yet been developed. Freeze dryer manufacturers made their plants more efficient, and the problem is now virtually solved. The freeze drying community was lucky; the refrigerant manufacturers failed to develop suitable replacements for R13b1 and R502, even though they had 6 years warning. Freeze dryer manufacturers did not recognise the problem until 1991 when it was almost too late, but there was little that they could do as they had to wait for alternative refrigerants. Users totally ignored the problem but still insisted on the temperatures that they had enjoyed in the past.

What follows is the background and the history. Fortunately, this time, the story has a happy ending, but should give a warning. Whilst ozone depletion has been addressed, the problem of global warming has not. New refrigerants still exhibit global warming properties and may be the subject of future scrutiny. Now is the time to formulate and optimise new freeze-dried products, without compromising efficacy, so that cycles are performed at higher temperatures and the impact of any future refrigeration bans are reduced to the minimum.

THE REFRIGERANTS

Chemistry

Refrigerants are composed, in the main, of one or more SP$_3$ hybridised carbon atoms, heavily substituted with halogens. The most common halogens are chlorine and fluorine, but a small number of refrigerants, notably R13b1, contain bromine. Few refrigerants contain more than two carbon atoms, and the majority have a molecular weight of less than 200.

These common chemicals have been known since the late 1800s, but their properties in terms of refrigeration were first investigated by Dr. Thomas Midgely of the Frigidaire division of General Motors in 1928. He predominantly worked with dichloro-difluoromethane, which later became known as R12.

Many refrigerants are a single chemical moiety, but some of the more powerful are blends of two or more refrigerants. Prior to the Montreal protocol, the refrigerants were blended as azeotropes. An azeotropic mixture has the same composition in either the vapour or liquid phase. As refrigeration involves two phase changes in the cycle it is important that this is so. Post-Montreal, the difficulty has been in producing blends that have the correct thermodynamic properties but are azeotropes; in general, this has not been achieved.

Properties

Refrigerants were initially selected as useful for refrigeration duty on the basis of their thermodynamic properties, but they were later shown to have other valuable properties as commodity chemicals. These properties are as follows:

- Very low toxicity
- Nonflammable
- Chemically stable
- Miscible with oils
- Relatively low priced
- Easy to manufacture
- Noncorrosive

These refrigerants rapidly replaced the chemicals that had been previously used. The only refrigerant that survived the advent of halogenated hydrocarbons was ammonia.

Classification

Halogenated hydrocarbon refrigerants can be placed in four classes:

1. *Halons.* The most notable member of this group is R13b1, bromotrifluoromethane, $CBrF_3$.

2. *CFCs, chlorofluorocarbons.* As the name suggests, these compounds contain chlorine and fluorine; they are characterised by the lack of hydrogen. The main CFCs are R11, R12, R13, R113, and R115. The azeotropes R500, R501, R502, and R503 contain CFCs as one or more of the components.

3. *HCFCs, hydrochlorofluorocarbons.* These refrigerants are similar to CFCs but contain at least one hydrogen atom. The most common HCFC is R22.

4. *HFCs. hydrofluorocarbons.* These refrigerants contain fluorine and hydrogen but no chlorine. They are seen as long-term replacements for the CFCs.

The R numbering system was developed by Du Pont shortly after they acquired Frigidaire in 1930. These chemicals have other uses, including foam blowing, aerosol propellants, carrier gases, and degreasers. The R prefix designates the chemical as a refrigerant, CFC12 and R12 are chemically identical.

The designated numbers are known as the ASRE numbers and the structure of the refrigerant can be elucidated from the number. ASRE (or ASHRAE) is a shortened acronym for the American Society of Heating, Refrigeration, and Air Conditioning Engineers who developed the system in 1957. The first number, reading from right to left is the number of fluorine atoms in the molecule, the second number is the number of hydrogen atoms plus one, and the third number is the number of carbon atoms minus one. The third number is omitted if it is zero (i.e., one carbon atom). Therefore, trichlorofluoromethane (CCl_3F) is R11.

Asymmetric molecules are suffixed by an "a". Azeotropes do not fit into this system, and their numbering is relatively arbitrary. Bromine atoms are added to the right by a "b", followed by the number of atoms. Bromotrifluoromethane (CF_3Br) is R13b1.

THE ENVIRONMENTAL IMPACT

History

The refrigeration industry thrived on the seemingly solid foundation of CFCs and HCFCs. However, the level of ozone in the atmosphere had been monitored since the 1950s, and when a thinning of the ozone layer was noticed above the Antarctic in 1982, the so-called "hole in the ozone layer", the ozone depletion theories forwarded by Rowland and Molina in 1974 began to be accepted.

The hole in the ozone layer is seasonal and varies in size; but in 1987, it covered an area the size of the United States. The ozone layer exists in the stratosphere at a height of 15–50 km. It is tenuous and at sea level would account for a layer about 3 mm thick.

The one hope is that the increase in the accuracy of instrumentation used to determine atmospheric ozone may be clouding the historical trend. There is an alternative theory that states that all we are observing is a fluctuation in a long-term cycle. The weight of evidence shows that these are probably forlorn hopes.

The Ozone Layer

Oxygen can exist in two stable forms: ozone, which contains three molecules of oxygen, and dioxygen, usually referred to as oxygen, which contains two. CFCs are accused of depleting the ozone layer by the following mechanism:

Ozone is split by ultraviolet (UV) light into oxygen and an oxygen radical. The oxygen radical reacts with another oxygen molecule to re-form ozone. The nett effect is the adsorption of UV and the dispersal of its energy as heat.

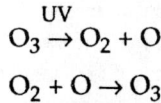

$$O_3 \xrightarrow{UV} O_2 + O$$

$$O_2 + O \rightarrow O_3$$

If a chlorine radical is formed by the breakdown of a CFC, again by UV light, then this radical will break down ozone, but will only combine with another radical, as the intermediate state is stable. The available radicals are oxygen and chlorine, but oxygen far outnumbers chlorine. If the chlorine intermediate combines with an oxygen radical, then oxygen is produced, and the chlorine radical is free to attack another ozone molecule. The nett result is that an ozone molecule and an oxygen atom combine to form two molecules of oxygen.

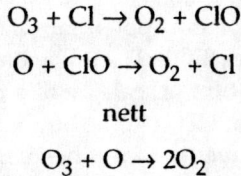

$$O_3 + Cl \rightarrow O_2 + ClO$$

$$O + ClO \rightarrow O_2 + Cl$$

nett

$$O_3 + O \rightarrow 2O_2$$

It is this chain reaction that causes the problem (each free chlorine radical will cause the splitting of many ozone molecules). The free chlorine in the atmosphere has risen from 2 to 3 parts per billion in the last two decades, and scientists are of the opinion that this rise is attributable to CFC releases.

The ozone layer adsorbs UV light that is harmful to life, and has even been used as a sterilant. If UV levels increase by 1 percent it has been calculated that there will be a 5 percent increase in nonmalignant skin cancers, coupled with a drastic increase in eye cataracts. The afflictions that would be caused in humans are the trivial part of the consequences of increased UV levels. Plants, especially some of the hybrid, high-yield food plants, would be devastated and famine could result. Also at risk would be phytoplankton, the first link in the food chain for the world's marine life.

The Greenhouse Effect

CFCs (and HCFCs and HFCs) are called greenhouse gases and contribute to the increase in global warming, which is often called the greenhouse effect. In actuality, the mechanisms of the greenhouse effect and a greenhouse are quite different. The greenhouse effect works by greenhouse gases adsorbing infrared radiation reflected from the earth. This infrared is then reradiated back to the earth, and the balance of heat striking the earth is increased, thereby increasing its temperature. A greenhouse works by reducing the cooling factor of wind and by not allowing air, which has been warmed by the sun, to rise and escape.

Global warming is a natural process and increases the average temperature of the earth by 3°C to a value of 18°C. What is the issue is the addition to this process that has been caused by the activities of man, "anthropogenic global warming"

The implications of global warming are well discussed. The rise in temperature will cause climatic shifts that will devastate forest and agriculture alike; sea levels will rise due to the melting polar ice caps and destroy useful land. The world will have difficulty supporting its population.

The Impact of Refrigerants

There can be no doubt that, with the exception of R13b1, CFCs have the greatest ozone depletion potential (ODP). The relative ODPs are shown on the chart (see Table 11.1). The baseline value is that R11 has an ODP of 1. R13b1 is off the scale, with a relative ODP of 12.

The long lifetime of CFCs in the atmosphere exacerbates the problems—R11 and R12 have lifetimes in excess of 50 years. By comparison, HCFCs have shorter lifetimes. R22 has a lifetime of 15 years, as it is degraded by reactions with hydroxyl radicals in the troposphere. HFCs do not contain chlorine and have virtually zero ODP; their atmospheric lifetime is largely irrelevant in terms of ozone depletion, but is important in terms of global warming.

All refrigerants contribute to anthropogenic global warming, although CFCs have the greatest effect. Refrigerants account for a very small percentage of the greenhouse gases within the atmosphere, but their effect is out of proportion to their presence. Estimates as to the total effect of refrigerants, or the same chemicals that have been released in other activities, varies from 10 percent to 25 percent of the total anthropogenic global warming.

Again, the global warming potential (GWP) is based on a value of R11 = 1, in order to compare refrigerants. If the alternative scale of carbon dioxide = 1 is used, then R11 has a value of 3,300 and R12 has a value of 10,000.

A little realised fact is that much of the global warming that is attributable to refrigeration actually comes from the burning of fossil fuels to power refrigeration compressors. Refrigerants have no effect on global warming, or ozone depletion, when they are within the refrigeration circuit.

Table 11.1. Commonly Used Refrigerants and Their Environmental Impact

Refrigerant	Components	Chemical Structure	ODP R11 = 1	GWP R11 = 1	To Replace
Bromofluorocarbons (BFC)					
R13b1	Monobromotrifluoromethane	$CBrF_3$	12.00		
Chlorofluorocarbons (CFC)					
R11	Trichloromonofluoromethane	CCl_3F	1.00	1.00	
R12	Dichlorodifluoromethane	CCl_2F_2	1.00	3.10	
R113	Trichlorotrifluoroethane	$CCl_2F_2CClF_2$	0.80	1.30	
R114	Dichlorotetrafluoroethane	$CClF_2CClF_2$	0.70	4.20	
R115	Monochloropentafluorethane	CF_3CClF_2	0.40	9.80	
Azeotropic chlorofluorocarbons					
R500	R12/R152a		0.75	2.20	
R501	R12/R22		0.70	3.40	
R502	R115/R22		0.33	5.10	
Hydrochlorofluorocarbons (HCFC)					
R123	Dichlorotrifluoroethane	CF_3CHCl_2	0.02	0.02	R11
R124	Monochlorotetrafluoroethane	CF_3CHClF	0.02	0.10	R114
R141b	Dichlorofluoroethane	CH_3CCl_2F	0.11	0.09	
R142b	Monochlorodifluoromethane	CH_3CClF_2	0.06	0.37	R12
R22	Monochlorodifluoromethane	$CHClF_2$	0.05	0.37	
Zeotropic hydrochlorofluorocarbons					
R69	R22/R218/R290		0.04		R502
R402	R22/R125/R290		0.03	0.62	R502
Hydrofluorocarbons (HFC)					
R125	Pentafluoroethane	CHF_2CF_3	0.00	0.61	R13b1
R134a	Tetrafluoroethane	CF_3CH_2F	0.00	0.29	R12
R143a	Trifluoroethane	CH_3CF_3	0.00	0.77	
R152a	Difluoroethane	CH_3CHF_2	0.00	0.03	
R218	Octofluoropropane	$CF_3CF_2CF_3$	0.00		
R23	Trifluormethane	CHF_3	0.00		
R32	Difluoromethane	CH_2F_2	0.00	0.14	
Azeotropic Hydrofluorocarbons					
R410a	R125/R32		0.00	0.47	R22
R507	R125/R143a		0.00	1.00	R502
Zeotropic Hydrofluorocarbons					
R404a	R125/R134a/R143a		0.00	0.94	R502
R407	3R125/R134a/R32		0.00	0.29	R22
Others					
R290	Propane	$CH_3CH_2CH_3$	0.00		

R22 was mooted as a R502 replacement before more efficient gases became commercially available. R22 was 30 percent less efficient than R502, so either a larger compressor or a longer running time was required with this gas. R22 may be less harmful in the atmosphere, but it resulted in the burning of 30 percent more fossil fuels, and the release of an extra 30 percent of carbon dioxide than would have otherwise been released.

THE LEGISLATION

History

The United Nationals Environment Programme negotiated to limit the use of CFCs once it was accepted that they were depleting the ozone layer. This resulted in an agreement that was signed by 27 nations in September 1987. The meeting was held in Montreal and the agreement became known as the Montreal Protocol. Initially, the Montreal Protocol called for a phased reduction of CFC manufacture, which would lead to a 50 percent reduction by 2000.

A subsequent meeting, held in London in June 1990, called for a complete ban on manufacture by 2000. An additional action of this meeting was to call for a reduction in the manufacture of what were termed "transitional substances". The original Montreal Protocol had not addressed these chemicals. Briefly, transitional substances were gases that could be used to assist the phasing out of CFCs and would substitute for CFCs in most applications until novel, environmentally friendly, alternatives could be developed. The most important of these transitional substances was chlorodifluoromethane, R22. R22 is an HCFC. Whilst HCFCs will deplete the ozone layer their lifetime is relatively short and their potential for depletion is approximately 5 percent of R11.

The November 1992 meeting, which was held in Copenhagen, called for a full CFC phaseout by 31 December 1995. Additionally, the phasing out of transitional substances underwent further agreement. Production of HCFCs was capped at 1989 levels, plus the equivalent of 3.1 percent of the ODP of CFCs in 1989. This allowed HCFCs to be available as substitutes or for blending. A phaseout schedule was agreed to,which called for the eventual ban of production by 2030.

Meanwhile, Europe was agreeing to a more rapid phaseout. Under European regulation number ER594/91, it was agreed that, amongst others, R13b1 production would cease on 31 December 1993 and CFC production by 31 December 1994. Two years later, in 1993, the regulation was further amended to introduce a reduction in HCFCs. At the time of writing, the phaseout of HCFC production is still under negotiation, but could occur this century.

Within the United Kingdom the Environmental Protection Act (1992) makes it illegal to deliberately allow the release of refrigerants into the atmosphere. Other countries have similar legislation.

The Montreal Protocol and ER594/91 only bind the countries that are signatory to these legislations. Some Third-World countries can still manufacture these banned substances, but their import into countries bound by the two agreements is illegal.

Implications

In order to gain a perspective, it is a fact that of all the CFCs manufactured in 1986, prior to Montreal only 15 percent were used in refrigeration. Many of the other uses were in applications where they were easily substituted (e.g., degreasers, foam blowers, aerosol propellants, and carrier gases). However, the proposed phaseout meant that there would not be a sufficient quantity available for refrigeration.

The initial long-term phaseout was probably agreed to because the total phaseout was sufficiently far into the future and not politically sensitive, whilst it showed a suitable attitude to the environment, which was politically expedient. Unfortunately, this long timescale did not give a sufficient impetus to the development of long-term, environmentally acceptable, alternatives.

At the time of writing, R13b1 and CFCs are no longer produced. The implication of the agreements was in terms of de novo manufacture and the design and manufacture of equipment to use these refrigerants. If a refrigeration system was in existence, then the requisite gas could be bought and stockpiled for future use. There are reports of companies buying large quantities of refrigerant and aerosol propellants, but this was a short-term measure, as the stored gas would eventually be used up.

It is not illegal to use a refrigeration system running on, for example, R502. If the system is leaktight, the R502 is not harming the environment. Indeed, until lately, it was a sensible strategy to keep the plant running on its original charge of R502, as the only alternatives were HCFC blends that would themselves have a limited availability because total HCFC phaseout was soon to come.

Users of refrigeration equipment that utilise phased out substances should now be contemplating changing to an environmentally acceptable gas, but only as an environmental concern. Refrigerant manufacturers will accept phased out gases, but, unfortunately, will reclaim it and resell it, thereby gaining profit on both disposal and resale. This is a necessary service, as there are some systems that cannot accept alternative refrigerants; obviously, the most acceptable environmental solution would be to dispose of these gases in a safe manner.

It is worth noting that global warming was not an issue in either the Montreal Protocol or ER594/91, which concentrated on the ODP of the gases. HFCs, which are seen as the gases of the present, and the future, are greenhouse gases. They have been discussed at international conferences, and the possibility does exist that at some stage international legislation will be introduced to phase out these greenhouse gases.

THE FREEZE DRYER

Implications

The implications to the new freeze dryer were that the temperatures previously accepted as usual were now extremely difficult to achieve. Existing freeze dryers had a potential problem in that if they lost their refrigerant, burned out a compressor, or the refrigerant became acidic then the replacement of the refrigerant would be difficult, if not impossible.

Alternative Refrigerants

In the few years prior to R13b1 and CFC phaseout, it was difficult to choose from all the refrigerant blends that were suddenly "available". Most of these gases were only available in test quantities, and it was not possible to obtain a sufficient quantity to charge a freeze dryer's refrigeration system. The issue of future availability was also of concern, and many of the blends have now disappeared. Compressor manufacturers could not test all of the available blends, and their long-term reliability and seal compatibility was not known.

Unsurprisingly, the first strategy developed by freeze dryer manufacturers was conservative and R22, a transition HCFC, was the recommended refrigerant for new freeze dryers. The use of R22 would mean the loss of 3–5°C on the shelves and up to 15°C on the condenser, when compared to an equivalent R13b1 system. The time taken to achieve these temperatures was also considerably extended. R22 was 30 percent less efficient, by the official performance yardstick, than R502. This implied that larger compressors had to be fitted, or the same compressors had to run under load for longer times. Running costs and power usage were, therefore, increased, and the environmental cost in terms of released greenhouse gases derived from the burning of fossil fuels increased by 30 percent.

Several blends came into prominence, notably R69, which was a nonazeotropic blend of R22, R218, and R290 (chlorodifluoromethane, octafluoropropane, and propane). This was claimed to be a drop in replacement for R502, and to a large extent it was, but it still contained a transition gas and, therefore, had a limited lifetime. However, R69 was tested, seal compatibility was not an issue, and the same oils and expansion valves could be used. R69 allowed a refrigerant change on an existing system to be a viable proposition.

Another issue regarding blends was that most of the new blends were not azeotropes. Previously, almost all refrigerants were either single chemical moieties or azeotropes. The introduction of nonazeotropes had four implications:

1. *Glide.* Glide is where the refrigerant will boil over a temperature range rather than at a single temperature. Slight changes in composition of the gas phase and the changing boiling point make the tuning of the refrigeration system more difficult.

2. *Leaks.* A gas leak would alter the composition of the remaining liquid, as one of the components would be enriched in the gas phase. After the leak had been repaired, the question had to be asked as to whether the whole charge had to be replaced or was the composition of the remaining liquid close enough to the specification to allow a top up.

3. *Flammability.* When a flammable component, is present there is the possibility that this component will become sufficiently enriched, in the presence of a leak, that an explosive mixture could be formed. This concept has largely been discounted on theoretical and experimental grounds.

4. *Filling.* Because the gas phase has a different composition to the liquid phase, it was necessary to charge the refrigeration system with the liquid phase. This is more cumbersome.

Refrigerant manufacturers reduced glide to a minimum and pronounced their blends usable. They were correct, but much debate and uncertainty followed these issues. Blends were never really used in freeze dryers, because HFCs were developed and became commercially available.

Refrigerant R125 (pentafluoroethane) was becoming noticed, and was available. This gas eventually led to the evolution of HFC blends that are seen as the present replacement. Those used in freeze dryers can give a performance equivalent to R502. R125 has been suggested as an R13b1 replacement. The most common usage to date has been that of R404a, which is a nonazeotropic blend of R125, R143a (trifluoroethane), and R134a (tetrafluoroethane). R404a has many trade names —404a, HP62 and FX-70. A similar refrigerant, R507, is composed of an azeotropic mix of R125 and R143a, and goes under the trade name of AZ-50.

R404a and R507 are seen as refrigerant gases that should, at present, be used in the freeze dryer's refrigeration system. Their performance is similar to that which was given by R502.

Oils

In order for an oil to be effective within a refrigeration system, it must exhibit a miscibility with the refrigerant. CFCs were compatible with conventional mineral oils, but if a HCFC was utilised, or used as a replacement, it was recommended that the oil have an alkylbenzene content of at least 50 percent. HFCs are not compatible with mineral or alkylbenzene oils, and polyol ester lubricants should be used.

Polyol ester lubricants are extremely hygroscopic, and care should be taken that any exposure to the atmosphere is minimal, in order to minimise the possibility of the lubricant picking up water vapour. A partly used can of a polyol ester lubricant cannot be stored (except possibly under a dried gas or a vacuum) and should be discarded. Several small containers are usually more economic in the long term than a single large container.

A new freeze dryer, with a refrigeration system that has been filled with R404a and a polyol ester lubricant presents no problem. Compressors that are built to operate with HFCs are marketed with an indication within the serial number that signifies that it has been assembled using compatible elastomers, and filled with a compatible lubricant.

The conversion of an existing system from a CFC to a HFC is a far more complicated process. Initially, refrigerant manufacturers had specified a 1 percent mineral oil content in the polyol ester lubricant. This figure was revised upward, to 5 percent, when it became obvious that 1 percent was extremely difficult to achieve; field experience has shown little adverse effect at this concentration of mineral oil.

Changing the lubricant in a compressor cannot be equated to changing the oil in a motor vehicle. Apart from the mechanical differences that occur because air must not enter the refrigeration system and the refrigerant must not escape, there is the other issue of where the lubricant is residing. Because the lubricant is miscible with the refrigerant, it is carried around the refrigeration circuit. Most of the lubricant is separated out by the oil separator and returned to the compressor crankcase, but some will travel all the way round the refrigeration circuit and eventually return to the compressor through the suction line. The lubricant in the circuit is not recovered by a compressor oil change.

In order to remove this entrapped lubricant, it is necessary to perform several flushes with the replacement oil to reduce the final content of the replaced oil. Typically three or four flushes with several days running in the interim between flushes would be necessary. During this time, the system would be running on the CFC refrigerant, the CFC would be reclaimed, and the HFC charged only after the last oil change. Many of the oil companies market test kits to indicate the proportion of mineral oil in the compressor lubricant.

The system filter dryer, phial, and expansion valve will have been changed at some time during the exchange of refrigerants; the refrigeration system can then be tuned and is then ready for use. If a performance test had been undertaken prior to the refrigerant change, then an indication of the change in performance is easily seen.

A planned refrigerant and lubricant change is a tedious business; an unplanned one is difficult in the extreme. A traumatic leak, burnout, or refrigerant acidification would result in a refrigeration circuit filled with the wrong type of oil and, once the system had been repaired, no refrigerant with which to charge it in order to enable the system to run to flush out the old oil. The choice is between charging with a HFC and polyol ester oil, and performing the first oil change after a very short interval, or charging with a HCFC, cleaning up the system, and then performing a refrigerant change.

Seals

The compatibility of elastomer seals is different for the different classes of refrigerant and there are many contradictions in the literature. In general, seals made from polytetrafluoroethane (PTFE), ethylene-propylene terpolymer (EPDM), neoprene, and probably Buna-N™ are acceptable. Concerns regarding elastomer compatibility should be referred to the compressor manufacturer or, if a list of elastomers is available, to the refrigerant distributor. Compressed fibre and compressed fibre/metal laminates used for flanged joints are compatible with all refrigerants.

The components of the electrical motor in a semihermetic compressor are in direct contact with the refrigerant and are cooled by it. Extensive testing has shown that there is no degradation of motor components during long-term exposure to HFCs.

Filter Dryers

Filter dryers should be changed to a grade suitable for the replacement refrigerant. This would be a usual activity during maintenance and is essential during a refrigerant change.

Leak Detection

It is worth noting that HFCs do not react to conventional halide leak detectors, even though fluorine is a halogen. Coated diode-type leak detectors are available for the leak detection of HFCs.

Liquid Nitrogen

If a new plant is being considered, then the ultimate, alternative refrigerant is liquid nitrogen. It is nonpolluting, has no effect on the ozone layer, is chemically compatible with almost everything, is non-poisonous, nonflammable, and will give a superb performance.

Unfortunately, it does not operate in a closed loop system, is bulky, and must be constantly replenished. The economics must be carefully investigated.

A freeze dryer utilising liquid nitrogen will usually control the condenser temperature by regulating the flow of liquid nitrogen through it. Liquid nitrogen boils at a temperature of -196°C; however, a condenser does not need to be colder than -75°C, and so the flow is regulated to give this temperature. This flow can be increased to adsorb heat at the peak demand at the beginning of primary drying. Shelf temperature control is by a secondary fluid circulation system, with liquid nitrogen cooling the circulating fluid in a heat exchanger. The circulating fluid in a liquid nitrogen–driven freeze dryer is still a silicone oil, and the lowest temperature of this oil is limited to approximately -70°C because of viscosity considerations.

Transfer from the holding tank is usually by vacuum insulated pipe to reduce heat ingress and gas formation. The tendency of liquid nitrogen to form an insulating layer of gas on all surfaces with which it is in contact results in the necessity to have turbulence promoters in the condenser coils and heat exchangers. The engineering issues involved in the use of a low temperature fluid have been solved many decades ago, and cryogenic valves are freely available. The efficiency of a liquid nitrogen system is such that the temperature of the outgoing nitrogen gas is only a few degrees below that of the shelves.

Liquid nitrogen consumption will be between 10 and 20 litres of liquid nitrogen per litre of wet product, but this is obviously cycle dependant. The requirement to store large quantities of liquid nitrogen has to be taken into account when the economics of the process are calculated.

The advantages of liquid nitrogen may be summarised as follows:

- Nonpolluting and environmentally friendly

- High cooling capacity

- Low temperature use

- Ideal for nonaqueous freeze drying

- Elimination of compressors and their maintenance

- Small installation footprint

- No cooling water requirement

- Reduced electrical power requirement

- Reduced noise

Of course, the pollution and electrical power consumption took place when the liquid nitrogen was manufactured and was increased as it was transported. However, if the economics are right, liquid nitrogen is a good alternative. The ideal freeze dryer user for a liquid nitrogen application is one who needs a large freeze dryer, already uses liquid nitrogen on-site and could possibly use the outgoing gas for another purpose. The outgoing gas is at low pressure and is not constantly flowing; its use is, therefore, limited. The usage in small applications is usually not viable, except in certain cases where low temperatures are essential. Liquid nitrogen retrofits are extensive, and expensive, projects and all alternative options should be investigated before this course is chosen.

Freeze Dryer Modifications

When it became apparent that alternatives to R13b1 and R502 would not be immediately available, freeze dryer manufacturers embarked on the exercise of making the freeze dryer more efficient to offset the lowered efficiency of the refrigerant. Now that refrigerants are approaching the efficiency of CFCs, the bonus has been that freeze dryers are more efficient.

The increase in efficiency was made in several ways:

- Shell-and-tube heat exchangers were replaced by plate-and-frame heat exchangers. Plate-and-frame heat exchangers have the double advantage of being more efficient in heat transfer and have a smaller volume. The smaller volume results in less silicone oil being required and a smaller thermal mass to be changed in temperature. Plate-and-frame heat exchangers could be foam insulated more efficiently than the shell-and-tube heat exchangers.

- Whenever possible, weight was reduced in the components that underwent the temperature cycle.

- Low heat input circulating pumps were utilised.

- Insulation was improved from the already high standard.

Formulation

Whilst efficacy, drug delivery, and safety are the greatest concerns for a drug formulation, it may be possible to optimise the formulation for freeze drying. If very low temperatures are not required for solidification, then the cycle can be performed at higher temperatures, which will be quicker and at a reduced cost. The vulnerability to a second crisis that will occur if global warming caused by refrigerants is ever addressed can now be largely overcome by serious formulation, with respect to freeze drying.

REPLACEMENT STRATEGY (FIGURE 11.1)

A new plant will be specified with either a viable refrigerant or a liquid nitrogen system and, unless global warming is addressed, will need no modification for its foreseeable lifetime. It is the plants that are currently operating with a CFC, or even a HCFC, that have problems that must be addressed.

On a basic level, the "do nothing" strategy appears to be attractive. It is not illegal to operate a plant on a CFC. The refrigerant is not damaging the environment whilst it is in the refrigeration circuit; performance is what was specified, and there are no lubricant, seal, or filter dryer compatibility problems.

Unfortunately, all semihermetic, and open, compressors will leak to some extent, and the refrigerant charge will slowly escape, although it may take decades before this is noticeable. The more important consideration is what will happen if the system develops a traumatic leak, the refrigerant becomes acidic or the compressor burns out. Production demands will make it difficult to take the plant out of commission for two weeks to flush the mineral oil out of the system fully and replace it with a polyol ester so that an HFC can be used to charge the system.

Figure 11.1. HFC replacement strategy.

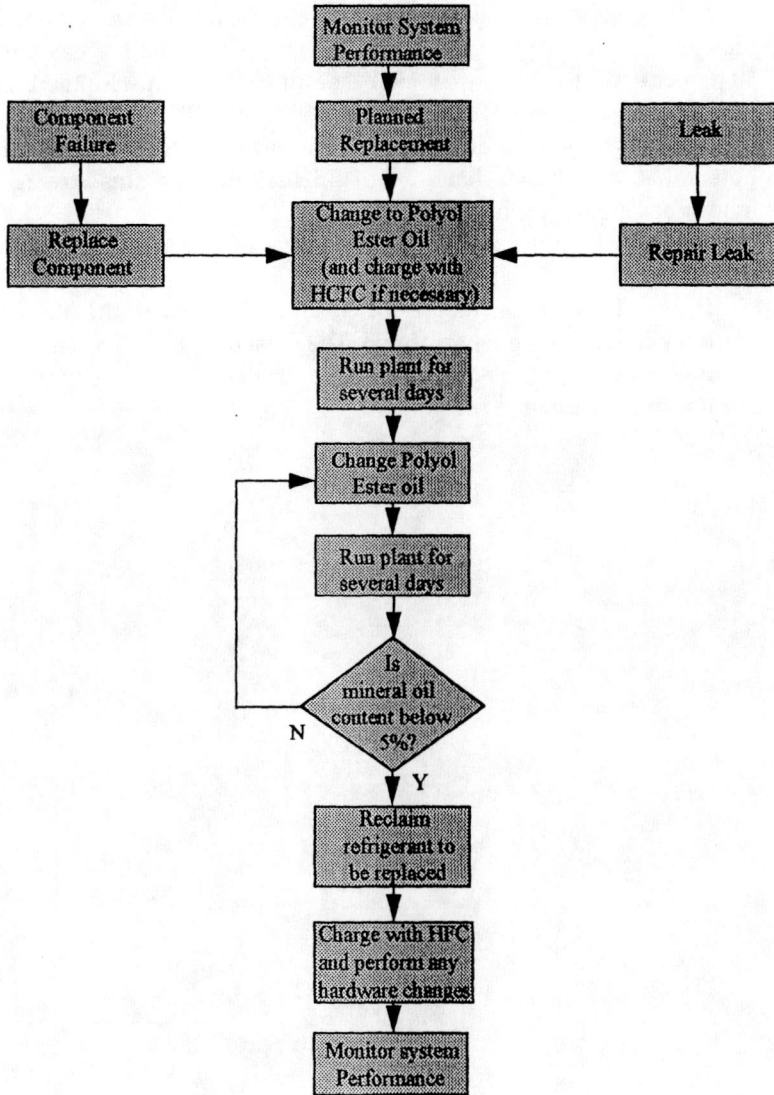

The second strategy would be to gradually replace the mineral oil in the refrigeration circuit over a period of time, whilst retaining the CFC, so that in the case of a traumatic incident, the changeover to an

HFC is relatively easy. This methodology depends on the compatibility of the polyol ester with the CFC in the system, and advice should be taken before commencing this strategy.

A third strategy would be to change to an alkylbenzene oil using one oil change to guarantee an alkylbenzene content greater than 50 percent and then using an HCFC or an HCFC blend. R22 will give poor performance when compared to R502 and will be well below that of R13b1. R69 will give an equivalent performance to R502. It must be noted that the HCFCs have a limited lifetime, and this strategy is merely saving the problem for a later date.

The fourth strategy is to set aside time to fully change over to a HFC.

If the refrigerant is changed, then several aspects of the plant validation will have to be reperformed. The most sensible option is, therefore, to plan for this and to have a controlled changeover with the minimum of risk.

RECOMMENDED READING

Avallone, H. L., and A. E. Wold. 1986. Regulatory Aspects of Lyophilization. *Journal of Parenteral Science and Technology* 40:81–82.

Cammack, K. A., and G. D. J. Adams. 1985. Formulation and Storage. In *Animal Cell Biotechnology*, Vol 2. London: Academic Press, Inc.

Carleton, F. J., and J. P. Agalloco. 1986. *Validation of Aseptic Pharmaceutical Processes*. New York: Marcel Dekker, Inc.

Edwards' Freeze Drying Handbook. 1978. Crawley, UK: Edwards High Vacuum.

FDA. 1993. *Guide to Inspections of Lyophilization of Parenterals*. Rockville, MD: Food and Drug Administration.

FDA. 1989. *Guideline on Sterile Drug Products Produced by Aseptic Processing*. Rockville, MD: Food and Drug Administration.

F-D-C Reports—"The Pink Sheet". F-D-C Reports, Inc. Chevy Chase, MD 20815-7278.

GMP Trends. GMP Trends, Inc. Boulder, CO 80306.

Jennings, T. A. 1986. Effect of Pressure on the Sublimation Rate of Ice. *Journal of Parenteral Science and Technology* 4:95.

Lee, J. Y. 1988. GMP Compliance for the Lyophilization of Parenterals: Part I. *Pharmaceutical Technology* (October): 54–60.

Lee, J. Y. 1988. GMP Compliance for the Lyophilization of Parenterals: Part II. *Pharmaceutical Technology* (November): 38–42.

Masterson, P. M. 1989. Applying Automated Process Control to Lyophilization. *Pharmaceutical Technology* (January): 48–54.

Parenteral Society Freeze Dryer Technical Group. 1994. *Sterilisation of Freeze Dryers*. Technical Monograph No. 5. Swindon, UK: Parenteral Society.

Parenteral Society Freeze Dryer Technical Group. 1995. *Leak Testing of Freeze Dryers*. Technical Monograph No. 7. Swindon, UK: Parenteral Society.

Parenteral Society Freeze Dryer Technical Group. 1995. *Integrity Testing of Freeze Dryer Inlet Filters*. Technical Monograph No. 8. Swindon, UK: Parenteral Society.

Patel, S. D., B. Gupta, and S. H. Yalkowsky. 1989. Acceleration of Heat Transfer in Vial Freeze Drying of Pharmaceuticals I: Corrugated Aluminum Quilt. *Journal of Parenteral Science and Technology* 43 (1): 8–14.

Quality Control Reports—"The Gold Sheet". F-D-C Reports, Inc. Chevy Chase, MD 20815-7278.

Snowman, J. W. 1991. Freeze Drying of Sterile Products. In *Sterile Pharmaceutical Manufacturing*, Vol. 1, edited by M. J. Groves, W. P. Olson, and M. H. Anisfeld. Buffalo Grove, IL: Interpharm Press.

Trappler, E. H. 1989. Validation of Lyophilization. *Pharmaceutical Technology* (January): 56–60.

Index